KAPLAN & SADOCK'S

Concise

Textbook of Child and Adolescent Psychiatry

Consulting Editor

Caroly S. Pataki, M.D.

Clinical Professor of Psychiatry and Behavioral Sciences, and Division Chief, Child and Adolescent Psychiatry, Keck School of Medicine at the University of Southern California, Los Angeles, California.

Contributing Editor

Samoon Ahmad, M.D.

Clinical Associate Professor of Psychiatry and Co-director of Continuing Medical Education, Department of Psychiatry, NYU School of Medicine, NYU Langone Medical Center, Attending Psychiatrist, Tisch Hospital, Bellevue Hospital, New York, New York.

KAPLAN & SADOCK'S

Concise
Textbook of
Child and Adolescent Psychiatry

Benjamin James Sadock, M.D.

Menas S. Gregory Professor of Psychiatry and Vice Chairman
Department of Psychiatry, New York University School of Medicine, NYU Langone Medical Center;
Attending Psychiatrist, Tisch Hospital;
Attending Psychiatrist, Bellevue Hospital Center;
Consulting Psychiatrist, Lenox Hill Hospital,
New York, New York

Virginia Alcott Sadock, M.D.

Professor of Psychiatry, Department of Psychiatry,
New York University School of Medicine, NYU Langone Medical Center;
Attending Psychiatrist, Tisch Hospital;
Attending Psychiatrist, Bellevue Hospital Center,
New York, New York

Wolters Kluwer Health | Lippincott Williams & Wilkins

New Delhi • Philadelphia • Baltimore • New York • London
Buenos Aires • Hong Kong • Sydney • Tokyo

530 Walnut Street
Philadelphia, PA 19106 USA
LWW.com

Care has been taken to confirm the accuracy of the information presented and to describe generally accepted practices. However, the authors, editors, and publishers are not responsible for errors or omissions or for any consequences from application of the information in this book and make no warranty, expressed or implied, with respect to the currency, completeness, or accuracy of the contents of the publication. Application of this information in a particular situation remains the professional responsibility of the practitioner.

The authors, editors, and publisher have exerted every effort to ensure that drug selection and dosage set forth in this text are in accordance with current recommendations and practice at the time publication. However, in view of ongoing research, changes in government regulations, and the constant flow of information relating to drug therapy and drug reactions, the reader is urged to check the package insert for each drug for any change in indications and dosage and for added warnings and precautions. This is particularly important when the recommended agent is a new or infrequently employed drug.

Some drugs and medical devices presented in this publication have Food and Drug Administration (FDA) clearance for limited use in restricted research settings. It is the responsibility of the health care provider to ascertain the FDA status of each drug or device planned for use in their clinical practice.

First Indian Reprint, 2009
Second Indian Reprint, 2009
Third Indian Reprint, 2011
Fourth Indian Reprint, 2013
Fifth Indian Reprint, 2014
Sixth Indian Reprint, 2016

Indian Reprint ISBN-13: 978-81-8473-204-7
Original ISBN-13: 978-0-7817-9387-2

Published by Wolters Kluwer (India) Pvt. Ltd., New Delhi.

Printed and bound at Gopsons Papers Ltd.

To
Emily and Celia

Preface

This book, *Concise Textbook of Child and Adolescent Psychiatry*, covers the diagnosis and treatment of mental disorders in children and adolescents. The reader will find detailed information about the diagnosis and treatment of every childhood and adolescent mental disorder listed in the latest fourth revised edition of the American Psychiatric Association's *Diagnostic and Statistical Manual of Mental Disorders* (DSM-IV-TR). This book evolved from our experience editing a larger volume, *Kaplan and Sadock's Synopsis of Psychiatry*, tenth edition, which covers the behavioral sciences and all clinical psychiatric disorders in children and adults. The elimination of the sections on the behavioral sciences and adult psychiatry accounts for this book's smaller and more manageable size. It is designed to meet the needs of the reader who requires a compact but thorough coverage of the field of child and adolescent psychiatry.

TEACHING SYSTEM

This textbook forms one part of a comprehensive system we have developed to facilitate the teaching of psychiatry and the behavioral sciences. At the head of the system is the *Comprehensive Textbook of Psychiatry*, which is global in depth and scope. It is designed for and used by psychiatrists, behavioral scientists, and all workers in the mental health field. *Synopsis of Psychiatry* is a relatively compact, highly modified, original, and current text useful for medical students, psychiatric residents, practicing psychiatrists, and mental health professionals. Another part of the system is *Study Guide and Self-Examination Review of Psychiatry*, which consists of multiple-choice questions and answers. It is designed for students of psychiatry who are preparing for a variety of examinations. Other parts of the system are the pocket handbooks: *Pocket Handbook of Clinical Psychiatry*, *Pocket Handbook of Psychiatric Drug Treatment*, and *Pocket Handbook of Emergency Psychiatric Medicine*. Those books cover the diagnosis and the treatment of psychiatric disorders, psychopharmacology, and psychiatric emergencies, respectively, and are compactly designed and concisely written to be carried in the pocket by clinical clerks and practicing physicians, whatever their specialty, to provide a quick reference. Another book, *Concise Textbook of Clinical Psychiatry* covers all clinical disorders in children and adults to provide a compact overview of all known mental disorders. Finally, the *Comprehensive Glossary of Psychiatry and Psychology* provides simply written definitions of all terms used in psychiatry including a complete glossary of signs and symptoms. Taken together, those seven books create a multipronged approach to the teaching, study, and learning of psychiatry. This text is a new addition to our teaching system.

NEW AND REVISED AREAS

Every section on clinical psychiatry has been updated to include the latest information about diagnosing and treating mental illness in children and adolescents. New advances since the publication of *Synopsis of Psychiatry* in 2007 have been added, particularly in the ever-changing area of child psychopharmacology. The reader will find completely updated material on medication such as dosages, methods of use, warnings and side-effects, including information about all drugs approved since the last edition was published. Data about posttraumatic stress disorders in children includes the latest information about the psychological effects on children exposed to terrorist activities and natural disasters. The section on Anxiety Disorders in Children and Adolescents was completely reorganized.

FORMAT

Case Histories

Case histories are an integral part of this book and are included to make the clinical disorders more interesting and vital for the student. All cases in this edition are new, derived from various sources: *ICD-10 Casebook*, *DSM-IV-TR Casebook*, *DSM-IV-TR Case Studies*, from contributors to the *Comprehensive Textbook of Psychiatry,* and from the authors' clinical experience at New York's Bellevue Hospital Center. We especially wish to thank the American Psychiatric Press and the World Health Organization for permission to use many of their cases. Cases appear in tinted type to help the reader find them easily.

References

To conserve space, references were not included at the end of each section. The interested reader can find a complete bibliography for each section by referring to either *Synopsis of Psychiatry* or the *Comprehensive Textbook of Psychiatry*. Those texts will also provide an in-depth, thorough, and detailed discussion of all the topics in this book. We also are mindful of the fact that modern-day readers consult internet sources, such as PsychInfo and Medline, to stay abreast of the most current literature and encourage that trend.

B.J.S.
V.A.S.

Acknowledgments

We deeply appreciate the work of our distinguished collaborator, Caroly Pataki, M.D., who was responsible for organizing, updating and revising the section on childhood and adolescent disorders in many of our books including the current ninth edition of the *Comprehensive Textbook of Psychiatry* and the tenth edition of *Synopsis of Psychiatry* for which she is consulting and contributing editor. She is Professor of Psychiatry and Division Chief of Child and Adolescent Psychiatry at Keck School of Medicine at the University of Southern California in Los Angeles, California, and an extraordinary talented educator and clinician. We thank her for her tremendous help in this area.

Samoon Ahmad, M.D. deserves special thanks for his role as Consulting Editor in the field of biological psychiatry and pharmacology.

Nitza Jones played a key and invaluable role as Project Editor, as she has for many of our other books. Her vast knowledge of every aspect of book publishing was indispensable, and she contributed heavily to editing the text. We also want to thank Sara Brown who was extraordinarily helpful. They worked with enthusiasm, alacrity, and intelligence. We thank Dorice Viera, Associate Curator of the Frederick L. Ehrman Medical Library at the New York University School of Medicine, for her assistance.

We also wish to acknowledge the contributions of James Sadock, M.D., and Victoria Gregg, M.D., for their help in their areas of expertise: emergency adult and emergency pediatric medicine, respectively. We also thank Alan and Marilyn Zublatt for their generous support and their friendship.

We want to take this opportunity to acknowledge those who have translated this and other *Kaplan & Sadock* books into foreign languages, including Chinese, Croatian, French, German, Greek, Indonesian, Italian, Japanese, Polish, Portuguese, Romanian, Russian, Spanish, and Turkish, in addition to a special Asian and international student edition.

Additionally, we wish to acknowledge our great and obvious debt to the more than 2,000 psychiatrists and behavioral scientists who contributed to the various editions of the *Comprehensive Textbook of Psychiatry*, especially to those in the field of child and adolescent mental health who allowed us to synopsize their work for this book. At the same time, we must accept responsibility for the modifications and changes in the new work.

The staff at Lippincott Williams & Wilkins was most efficient. We wish to thank Sirkka Howes at LWW. Chris Miller at Aptara also deserves our thanks. Joyce Murphy, Associate Director of Development, and Charley Mitchell, Publisher, have been loyal friends over the years and their encouragement and enthusiasm have been most welcome.

B.J.S.
V.A.S.

Contents

KAPLAN & SADOCK TEXTBOOKS

Published by Lippincott Williams & Wilkins

Comprehensive Textbook of Psychiatry
1st Edition, 1967 (with A.M. Freedman)
2nd Edition, 1975 (with A.M. Freedman)
3rd Edition, 1980 (with A.M. Freedman)
4th Edition, 1985
5th Edition, 1989
6th Edition, 1995
7th Edition, 1998 (with V.A. Sadock)
8th Edition, 2005 (with V.A. Sadock)

Synopsis of Psychiatry
1st Edition, 1972 (with A.M. Freedman)
2nd Edition, 1976 (with A.M. Freedman)
3rd Edition, 1981
4th Edition, 1985
5th Edition, 1988
6th Edition, 1991
7th Edition, 1994 (with J. Grebb)
8th Edition, 1998
9th Edition, 2003 (with V.A. Sadock)
10th Edition, 2007 (with V.A. Sadock)

Study Guide and Self-Examination Review of Psychiatry
1st Edition, 1983
2nd Edition, 1985
3rd Edition, 1989
4th Edition, 1991
5th Edition, 1994
6th Edition, 1999 (with V.A. Sadock)
7th Edition, 2003 (with V.A. Sadock and R.M. Jones)
8th Edition, 2007 (with V.A. Sadock and Z. Levin)

Comprehensive Group Psychotherapy
1st Edition, 1971
2nd Edition, 1983
3rd Edition, 1993

The Sexual Experience
1976 (with A.M. Freedman)

Concise Textbook of Clinical Psychiatry
1st Edition, 1996 (with V.A. Sadock)
2nd Edition, 2004 (with V.A. Sadock)
3rd Edition, 2008 (with V.A. Sadock)

Pocket Handbook of Clinical Psychiatry
1st Edition 1990
2nd Edition, 1996
3rd Edition, 2001 (with V.A. Sadock)
4th Edition, 2005 (with V.A. Sadock)

Comprehensive Glossary of Psychiatry and Psychology
1991

Pocket Handbook of Psychiatric Drug Treatment
1st Edition, 1993
2nd Edition, 1996
3rd Edition, 2001 (with V.A. Sadock)
4th Edition, 2006 (with V.A. Sadock and N. Sussman)

Pocket Handbook of Emergency Psychiatric Medicine
1993

Pocket Handbook of Primary Care Psychiatry
1996

Various editions of the above books have been translated and published in Bulgarian, Croatian, French, German, Greek, Indonesian, Italian, Japanese, Polish, Portuguese, Russian, Spanish, and Turkish. In addition, an International Asian edition has been published in English.

BY OTHER PUBLISHERS

Studies in Human Behavior, 1–5
1972 (with A.M. Freedman)
Athenaeum

1. Diagnosing Mental Illness: Evaluation in Psychiatry and Psychology
2. Interpreting Personality: A Survey of Twentieth-Century Views
3. Human Behavior: Biological, Psychological, and Sociological
4. Treating Mental Illness: Aspects of Modern Therapy
5. The Child: His Psychological and Cultural Development

Volume 1: Normal Development and Psychological Assessment
Volume 2: The Major Psychological Disorders and their Treatment

Modern Group Books I–VI
1972
E.P. Dutton

I. Origins of Group Analysis
II. Evolution of Group Therapy
III. Groups and Drugs
IV. Sensitivity through Encounter and Motivation
V. New Models for Group Therapy
VI. Group Treatment of Mental Illness

The Human Animal
1974 (with A.M. Freedman)
K.F.S. Publications
Volume 1: Man and His Mind
Volume 2: The Disordered Personality

KAPLAN & SADOCK'S

Concise

Textbook of
Child and Adolescent Psychiatry

1 Assessment, Examination, and Psychologic Testing

Psychiatric assessment of a child or adolescent includes identifying the reasons for referral; assessing the nature and extent of the child's psychologic and behavioral difficulties; and determining family, school, social, and developmental factors that may be influencing the child's emotional well-being.

A comprehensive evaluation of a child is composed of interviews with the parents, the child, and other family members; gathering information regarding the child's current school functioning; and, often, a standardized assessment of the child's intellectual level and academic achievement. In some cases, standardized measures of developmental level and neuropsychologic assessments are useful.

Psychiatric evaluations of children are rarely initiated by the child, so clinicians must obtain information from the family and the school to understand the reasons for the evaluation. In some cases, the court or a child protective service agency may initiate a psychiatric evaluation. Children can be excellent informants about symptoms related to mood and inner experiences, such as psychotic phenomena, sadness, fears, and anxiety, but they often have difficulty with the chronology of symptoms and are sometimes reticent about reporting behaviors that have gotten them into trouble. Very young children often cannot articulate their experiences verbally and do better showing their feelings and preoccupations in a play situation.

The first step in the comprehensive evaluation of a child or adolescent is to obtain a full description of the current concerns and a history of the child's previous psychiatric and medical problems. This part of the evaluation is often done with the parents for school-age children, whereas adolescents may be seen alone first, to get their perception of the situation. Direct interview and observation of the child is usually next, followed by psychologic testing, when indicated.

Clinical interviews offer the most flexibility in understanding the evolution of problems and in establishing the role of environmental factors and life events, but they may not systematically cover all psychiatric diagnostic categories. To increase the breadth of information generated, the clinician may use semistructured interviews, such as the *Kiddie Schedule for Affective Disorders and Schizophrenia for School-Age Children* (K-SADS); structured interviews, such as the *National Institute for Mental Health Diagnostic Interview Schedule for Children Version IV* (NIMH DISC-IV); and rating scales, such as the *Child Behavior Checklist* and *Connors Parent or Teacher Rating Scale for ADHD*.

It is not uncommon for interviews from different sources, such as parents, teachers, and school counselors, to reflect different or even contradictory information about a given child. When faced with conflicting information, the clinician must determine whether apparent contradictions actually reflect an accurate picture of the child in different settings. After a complete history is obtained from the parents, the child is examined, the child's current functioning at home and at school is assessed, and psychologic testing is completed, the clinician can use all the available information to make a best-estimate diagnosis and can then make recommendations.

After clinical information is obtained about a child or adolescent, it is the clinician's task to determine whether criteria are met for one or more psychiatric disorders according to the text revision of the 4th edition of the *Diagnostic and Statistic Manual of Mental Disorders* (DSM-IV-TR). This most current version is a categoric classification reflecting the consensus on constellations of symptoms believed to comprise discrete and valid psychiatric disorders. A psychiatric disorder is defined by the DSM-IV-TR as a clinically significant set of symptoms that is associated with impairment in one or more areas of functioning. Although clinical situations requiring intervention do not always fall within the context of a given psychiatric disorder, it is important to identify psychiatric disorders when they arise to facilitate meaningful investigation of childhood psychopathology.

CLINICAL INTERVIEWS

To conduct a useful interview with a child of any age, clinicians must be familiar with normal development to place the child's responses in the proper perspective. For example, a young child's discomfort on separation from a parent and a school-age child's lack of clarity about the purpose of the interview are both normal and should not be misconstrued as psychiatric symptoms. Furthermore, behavior that is normal in a child at one age, such as temper tantrums in a 2-year-old, takes on a different meaning, for example, in a 17-year-old.

The interviewer's first task is to engage the child and develop a rapport so that the child is comfortable. The interviewer should inquire about the child's concept of the purpose of the interview and should ask what the parents have told the child. If the child seems confused about the reason for the interview, the examiner may opt to summarize the parents' concerns in a developmentally appropriate and supportive manner. During the interview with the child, the clinician seeks to learn about the child's relationships with family members and peers, academic achievement and peer relationships in school, and the child's pleasurable activities. An estimate of the child's cognitive functioning is a part of the mental status examination.

The extent of confidentiality in child assessment is correlated with the age of the child. In most cases, almost all specific information can appropriately be shared with the parents of a very young child, whereas privacy and permission of an older child or adolescent are mandated before sharing information with parents. School-age and older children are informed that if the clinician becomes concerned that the child is dangerous to himself or herself or to others, this information must be shared with parents and, sometimes, additional adults. As part of a psychiatric assessment of a child of any age, the clinician must determine whether that child is safe in his or her environment and must develop an index of suspicion about whether the child is a victim of abuse or neglect. Whenever there is a suspicion of child maltreatment, the local child protective service agency must be notified.

Toward the end of the interview, the child may be asked in an open-ended manner whether he or she would like to bring up anything else. Each child should be complimented for his or her cooperation and thanked for participating in the interview, and the interview should end on a positive note.

Infants and Young Children

Assessments of infants usually begin with the parents present because very young children may be frightened by the interview situation; the interview with the parents present also allows the clinician to assess the parent–infant interaction. Infants may be referred for a variety of reasons, including high levels of irritability, difficulty being consoled, eating disturbances, poor weight gain, sleep disturbances, withdrawn behavior, lack of engagement in play, and developmental delay. The clinician assesses areas of functioning that include motor development, activity level, verbal communication, ability to engage in play, problem-solving skills, adaptation to daily routines, relationships, and social responsiveness.

The child's developmental level of functioning is determined by combining observations made during the interview with standardized developmental measures. Observations of play reveal a child's developmental level and reflect the child's emotional state and preoccupations. The examiner can interact with an infant 18 months or younger in a playful manner by using games such as peek-a-boo. Children 18 months to 3 years old can be observed in a playroom. Children 2 years or older may exhibit symbolic play with toys, revealing more in this mode than through conversation. The use of puppets and dolls with children younger than 6 years is often an effective way to elicit information, especially if questions are directed to the dolls, rather than to the child.

School-Age Children

Some school-age children are at ease when conversing with an adult; others are hampered by fear, anxiety, poor verbal skills, or oppositional behavior. School-age children can usually tolerate a 45-minute session. The room should be sufficiently spacious for the child to move around, but not so large as to reduce intimate contact between the examiner and the child. Part of the interview can be reserved for unstructured play, and various toys can be made available to capture the child's interest and to elicit themes and feelings. Children in lower grades may be more interested in the toys in the room, whereas by the sixth grade, children may be more comfortable with the interview process and less likely to exhibit spontaneous play.

The initial part of the interview explores the child's understanding of the reasons for the meeting. The clinician should confirm that the interview was not set up because the child is "in trouble" or as a punishment for "bad" behavior. Techniques that can facilitate disclosure of feelings include asking the child to draw peers, family members, a house, or anything else that comes to mind. The child can then be questioned about the drawings. Children may be asked to reveal three wishes, to describe the best and worst events of their lives, and to name a favorite person to be stranded with on a desert island. Games, such as Donald W. Winnicott's "squiggle" in which the examiner draws a curved line and then the child and the examiner take turns continuing the drawing, may facilitate conversation.

Questions that are partially open-ended with some multiple choices may elicit the most complete answers from school-age children. Simple, closed (yes or no) questions may not elicit sufficient information, and completely open-ended questions can overwhelm a school-age child who cannot construct a chronologic narrative. These techniques often result in a shoulder shrug from the child. The use of indirect commentary—such as, "I once knew a child who felt very sad when he moved away from all his friends"—is helpful, although the clinician must be careful not to lead the child into confirming what the child thinks the clinician wants to hear. School-age children respond well to clinicians who help them compare moods or feelings by asking them to rate feelings on a scale of 1 to 10.

Adolescents

Adolescents usually have distinct ideas about why the evaluation was initiated and can usually give a chronologic account of the recent events leading to the evaluation, although some may disagree with the need for the evaluation. The clinician should clearly communicate the value of hearing the story from the adolescent's point of view and must be careful to reserve judgment and not assign blame. Adolescents may be concerned about confidentiality, and clinicians can assure them that permission will be requested from them before any specific information is shared with parents except in situations involving danger to the adolescent or others, in which case confidentiality must be sacrificed. Adolescents can be approached in an open-ended manner; however, when silences occur during the interview, the clinician should attempt to reengage the patient. Clinicians can explore what the adolescent believes the outcome of the evaluation will be (e.g., change of school, hospitalization, removal from home, removal of privileges).

Some adolescents approach the interview with apprehension or hostility, but open up when it becomes evident that the clinician is neither punitive nor judgmental. Clinicians must be aware of their own responses to adolescents' behavior (countertransference) and stay focused on the therapeutic process even in the face of defiant, angry, or difficult teenagers. Clinicians should set appropriate limits and should postpone or discontinue an interview if they feel threatened, or if patients become destructive to property or engage in self-injurious behavior. Every interview should include an exploration of suicidal thoughts, assaultive behavior, psychotic symptoms, substance use, and knowledge of safe sexual practices along with a sexual history. When rapport has been established, many adolescents appreciate the opportunity to tell their side of the story and may reveal things that they have not disclosed to anyone else.

Family Interview

An interview with parents and the patient may take place first or may occur later in the evaluation. Sometimes, an interview with the entire family, including siblings, can be enlightening. The purpose is to observe the attitudes and behavior of the parents toward the patient and the responses of the children to their parents. The clinician's job is to maintain a nonthreatening atmosphere in which each member of the family can speak freely without feeling that the clinician is taking sides with any particular member. Although child psychiatrists generally function as advocates for the child, the clinician must validate each family member's feelings in this setting because lack of communication often contributes to the patient's problems.

Parents

The interview with the patient's parents or caretakers is necessary to get a chronologic picture of the child's growth and development. A thorough developmental history and details of any stressors or important events that have influenced the child's development must be elicited. The parents' view of the family dynamics, their marital history, and their own emotional adjustment are also elicited. The family's psychiatric history and the upbringing of the parents are pertinent. Parents are usually the best informants about the child's early development and previous psychiatric and medical illnesses. They may be better able to provide an accurate chronology of past evaluations and treatment. In some cases, especially with older children and adolescents, the parents may be unaware of significant current symptoms or social difficulties of the child. Clinicians elicit the parents' formulation of the causes and nature of their child's problems and ask about expectations about the current assessment.

DIAGNOSTIC INSTRUMENTS

The two main types of diagnostic instruments used by clinicians and researchers are diagnostic interviews and questionnaires. Diagnostic interviews are administered to either children or their parents and are often designed to elicit sufficient information on numerous aspects of functioning to determine whether criteria from the DSM-IV-TR are met.

Semistructured interviews, or "interviewer-based" interviews, such as the *Child and Adolescent Psychiatric Assessment* (CAPA), serve as guides for the clinician. They help the clinician clarify answers to questions about symptoms. Structured interviews, or "respondent-based" interviews, such as the *Children's Interview for Psychiatric Syndromes* (ChIPS), and the *Diagnostic Interview for Children and Adolescents* (DICA), basically provide a script for the interviewer without interpretation of the subject's responses. Two other diagnostic instruments use pictures, the *Dominic-R* and the *Pictorial Instrument for Children and Adolescents* (PICA-III-R). These instruments use pictures as cues, along with an accompanying question to elicit information about symptoms, especially for young children but also for adolescents.

Diagnostic instruments aid the collection of information in a systematic way. Diagnostic instruments, even the most comprehensive, however, cannot replace clinical interviews because clinical interviews are superior in understanding the chronology of symptoms, the interplay between environmental stressors and emotional responses, and developmental issues. Clinicians often find it helpful to combine the data from diagnostic instruments with clinical material gathered in a comprehensive evaluation.

Questionnaires can cover a broad range of symptom areas, such as the *Achenbach Child Behavior Checklist*, or they can be focused on particular types of symptoms. Questionnaires focused on symptoms are often called rating scales, such as the *Connors Parent Rating Scale for ADHD*.

Semistructured Diagnostic Interviews

Kiddie Schedule for Affective Disorders and Schizophrenia for School-Age Children. The K-SADS can be used for children 6 to 18 years of age. It presents multiple items with some space for further clarification of symptoms. It elicits information on current diagnosis and on symptoms present in the previous year. Another version can also ascertain lifetime diagnoses. It assesses diagnoses according to DSM-IV-TR. This instrument has been used extensively, especially in evaluation of mood disorders, and includes measures of impairment caused by symptoms. The schedule comes in a form for parents to give information about their child and in a version for use directly with the child. The schedule takes about 1 to 1.5 hours to administer. The interviewer should have some training in child psychiatry, but need not be a psychiatrist.

Child and Adolescent Psychiatric Assessment. The CAPA is an "interviewer-based" instrument that can be used for children 9 to 17 years old. It comes in modular form so that certain diagnostic entities can be administered without having to give the entire interview. It covers disruptive behavior disorders, mood disorders, anxiety disorders, eating disorders, sleep disorders, elimination disorders, substance use disorders, tic disorders, schizophrenia, posttraumatic stress disorder, and somatization symptoms. It focuses on the 3 months before the interview, called the "primary period." It generally takes about 1 hour to administer. It has a glossary to aid in decision making regarding symptoms and provides separate ratings of presence and severity of symptoms. It can be used to determine diagnoses according to DSM-IV, DSM-III-R, or the tenth revision of *International Statistical Classification of Diseases and Related Health Problems* (ICD-10). Training is necessary to administer this interview, and the interviewer must be prepared to use some clinical judgment in interpreting elicited symptoms.

Structured Diagnostic Interviews

National Institute of Mental Health Interview Schedule for Children Version IV. The NIMH DISC-IV is a highly structured interview designed to assess more than 30 DSM-IV diagnostic entities administered by trained "laypersons." It is available in parallel child and parent forms. The parent form can be used for children 6 to 17 years of age, and the direct child form of the instrument was designed for children 9 to 17 years old. It is applicable for a multitude of diagnoses keyed to DSM-IV-TR. A computer scoring algorithm is available. This instrument assesses the presence of diagnoses that have been present within the last 4 weeks and within the last year. Because it is a fully structured interview, the instructions serve as a complete guide for the questions, and the examiner need not have any knowledge of child psychiatry to administer the interview correctly.

Children's Interview for Psychiatric Syndromes. The ChIPS is a highly structured interview designed for use by trained interviewers with children 6 to 18 years of age. It is composed of 15 sections, and it elicits information on psychiatric symptoms and psychosocial stressors targeting 20 psychiatric disorders, according to DSM-IV criteria. There are parent and child forms. It takes approximately 40 minutes to administer the ChIPS. Diagnoses covered include depression, mania, attention-deficit/hyperactivity disorder (ADHD), separation disorder, obsessive-compulsive disorder (OCD), conduct disorder, substance use disorder, anorexia, and bulimia. The ChIPS was designed for use as a screening instrument for clinicians and a diagnostic instrument for clinical and epidemiologic research.

Diagnostic Interview for Children and Adolescents. The current version of the DICA was developed in 1997 to assess information resulting in diagnoses according to either DSM-IV or DSM-III-R. Although it was originally designed to be a highly structured interview, it can now be used in a semistructured format. This means that although interviewers are allowed to use additional questions and probes to clarify elicited information, the method of probing is standardized so that all interviewers follow a specific pattern. When using the interview with younger children, more flexibility is built in, allowing interviewers to deviate from written questions to ensure that the child understands the question. Parent and child interviews are expected to be used. It covers children 6 to 17 years old and generally takes 1 to 2 hours to administer. It covers externalizing behavior disorders, anxiety disorders, depressive disorders, and substance abuse disorders, among others.

Pictorial Diagnostic Instruments

Dominic-R. The Dominic-R is a pictorial, fully structured interview designed to elicit psychiatric symptoms from children 6 to 11 years of age. The pictures illustrate abstract emotional and behavioral content of diagnostic entities according to DSM-III-R. The instrument uses a picture of a child called "Dominic" who is experiencing the symptom in question. Some symptoms have more than one picture, with a brief story that is read to the child. Along with each picture is a sentence asking about the situation being shown and asking the child if he or she has experiences similar to the one that Dominic is having. Diagnostic entities covered by the Dominic-R include separation anxiety, generalized anxiety, depression and dysthymia, ADHD, oppositional defiant disorder, conduct disorder, and specific phobia. Although symptoms of the aforementioned diagnoses can be fully elicited from the Dominic-R, no specific provision within the instrument inquires about frequency of the symptom, duration, or age of onset. The paper version of this interview takes about 20 minutes, and the computerized version of this instrument takes about 15 minutes. Trained lay-interviewers can administer this interview. Computerized versions of this interview are available with pictures of a child who is white, black, Latino, or Asian.

Pictorial Instrument for Children and Adolescents. PICA-III-R is composed of 137 pictures organized in modules and designed to cover five diagnostic categories, including disorders of anxiety, mood, psychosis, disruptive disorders, and substance use disorder. It is designed to be administered by clinicians and can be used for children and adolescents ranging from 6 to 16 years of age. It provides a categoric (diagnosis present or absent) and a dimensional (range of severity) assessment. This instrument presents pictures of a child experiencing emotional, behavioral, and cognitive symptoms. The child is asked, "How much are you like him/her?" and a 5-point rating scale with pictures of a person with open arms in increasing degrees is shown to the child to help him or her identify the severity of the symptoms. It takes about 40 minutes to 1 hour to administer the interview. This instrument is currently keyed to DSM-III-R. It can be used to aid in clinical interviews and in research diagnostic protocols.

QUESTIONNAIRES AND RATING SCALES

Achenbach Child Behavior Checklist

The parent and teacher versions of the *Achenbach Child Behavior Checklist* were developed to cover a broad range of symptoms and several positive attributes related to academic and social competence. The checklist presents items related to mood, frustration tolerance, hyperactivity, oppositional behavior, anxiety, and various other behaviors. The parent version consists of 118 items to be rated 0 (not true), 1 (sometimes true), or 2 (very true). The teacher version is similar, but without the items that apply only to home life. Profiles were developed based on normal children of three different age groups (4 to 5 years, 6 to 11 years, and 12 to 16 years).

This checklist identifies specific problem areas that might otherwise be overlooked, and it may point out areas in which the child's behavior deviates from that of normal children of the same age group. The checklist is not used specifically to make diagnoses.

Revised Achenbach Behavior Problem Checklist

Consisting of 150 items that cover a variety of childhood behavioral and emotional symptoms, the *Revised Achenbach Behavior Problem Checklist* discriminates between clinic-referred and nonreferred children. Separate subscales have been found to correlate in the appropriate direction with other measures of intelligence, academic achievement, clinical observations, and peer popularity. As with the other broad rating scales, this instrument can help elicit a comprehensive view of a multitude of behavioral areas, but it is not designed to make psychiatric diagnoses.

Connors Abbreviated Parent-Teacher Rating Scale for ADHD

In its original form, the *Connors Abbreviated Parent-Teacher Rating Scale for ADHD* consisted of 93 items rated on a 0 to 3 scale and was subgrouped into 25 clusters, including problems with restlessness, temper, school, stealing, eating, and sleeping. Over the years, multiple versions of this scale were developed and used to aid in systematic identification of children with ADHD. A highly abbreviated form of this rating scale, the *Connors Abbreviated Parent-Teacher Questionnaire,* was developed for use with parents and teachers by Keith Connors in 1973. It consists of ten items that assess hyperactivity and inattention.

Brief Impairment Scale

A newly validated, 23-item instrument suitable to obtain information on children ranging from 4 to 17 years, the *Brief Impairment Scale* (BIS) evaluates three domains of functioning: interpersonal relations, school/work functioning, and care/self-fulfillment. This scale is administered to an adult informant about his or her child, does not take long to administer, and provides a global measure of impairment along the above-mentioned three dimensions. This scale cannot be used to make clinical decisions about individual patients, but it can provide information on the degree of impairment that a child is experiencing in a certain area.

COMPONENTS OF THE CHILD PSYCHIATRIC EVALUATION

Psychiatric evaluation of a child includes a description of the reason for the referral, the child's past and present functioning, and any test results. An outline of the evaluation is given in Table 1–1.

Table 1–1
Child Psychiatric Evaluation

- Identifying data
  - Identified patient and family members
  - Source of referral
  - Informants
- History
  - Chief complaint
  - History of present illness
  - Developmental history and milestones
  - Psychiatric history
  - Medical history, including immunizations
  - Family social history and parents' marital status
  - Educational history and current school functioning
  - Peer relationship history
  - Current family functioning
  - Family psychiatric and medical histories
  - Current physical examination
- Mental status examination
- Neuropsychiatric examination (when applicable)
- Developmental, psychologic, and educational testing
- Formulation and summary
- DSM-IV-TR diagnosis
- Recommendations and treatment plan

From American Psychiatric Association. *Diagnostic and Statistical Manual of Mental Disorders.* 4th ed. Text rev. Washington, DC: American Psychiatric Association; 2000, with permission.

Identifying Data

To understand the clinical problems to be evaluated, the clinician must first identify the patient and keep in mind the family constellation surrounding the child. The clinician must also pay attention to the source of the referral—that is, whether it is the child's family, school, or another agency—because this influences the family's attitude toward the evaluation. Finally, many informants contribute to the child's evaluation, and each must be identified to gain insight into the child's functioning in different settings.

History

A comprehensive history contains information about the child's current and past functioning, from the child's report, from clinical and structured interviews with the parents, and from information from teachers and previous treating clinicians. The chief complaint and the history of the present illness are generally obtained from both the child and the parents. Naturally, the child articulates the situation according to his or her developmental level. The developmental history is more accurately obtained from the parents. Psychiatric and medical histories, current physical examination findings, and immunization histories can be augmented with reports from psychiatrists and pediatricians who have treated the child in the past.

The child's report is critical in understanding the current situation regarding peer relationships and adjustment to school. Adolescents are the best informants regarding knowledge of safe sexual practices, drug or alcohol use, and suicidal ideation. The family's psychiatric and social histories and family function are best obtained from the parents.

Mental Status Examination

A detailed description of the child's current mental functioning can be obtained through observation and specific questioning. An outline of the mental status examination is presented in Table 1–2. Table 1–3 lists components of a comprehensive neuropsychiatry mental status.

Table 1–2
Mental Status Examination for Children

1. Physical appearance
2. Parent–child interaction
3. Separation and reunion
4. Orientation to time, place, and person
5. Speech and language
6. Mood
7. Affect
8. Thought process and content
9. Social relatedness
10. Motor behavior
11. Cognition
12. Memory
13. Judgment and insight

Table 1–3
Neuropsychiatric Mental Status Examination*

A. General Description
   1. General appearance and dress
   2. Level of consciousness and arousal
   3. Attention to environment
   4. Posture (standing and seated)
   5. Gait
   6. Movements of limbs, trunk, and face (spontaneous, resting, and after instruction)
   7. General demeanor (including evidence of responses to internal stimuli)
   8. Response to examiner (eye contact, cooperation, ability to focus on interview process)
   9. Native or primary language
B. Language and Speech
   1. Comprehension (words, sentences, simple and complex commands, and concepts)
   2. Output (spontaneity, rate, fluency, melody or prosody, volume, coherence, vocabulary, paraphasic errors, complexity of usage)
   3. Repetition
   4. Other aspects
      a. Object naming
      b. Color naming
      c. Body part identification
      d. Ideomotor praxis to command
C. Thought
   1. Form (coherence and connectedness)
   2. Content
      a. Ideational (preoccupations, overvalued ideas, delusions)
      b. Perceptual (hallucinations)
D. Mood and Affect
   1. Internal mood state (spontaneous and elicited; sense of humor)
   2. Future outlook
   3. Suicidal ideas and plans
   4. Demonstrated emotional status (congruence with mood)
E. Insight and Judgment
   1. Insight
      a. Self-appraisal and self-esteem
      b. Understanding of current circumstances
      c. Ability to describe personal psychologic and physical status
   2. Judgment
      a. Appraisal of major social relationships
      b. Understanding of personal roles and responsibilities
F. Cognition
   1. Memory
      a. Spontaneous (as evidenced during interview)
      b. Tested (incidental, immediate repetition, delayed recall, cued recall, recognition; verbal, nonverbal; explicit, implicit)
   2. Visuospatial skills
   3. Constructional ability
   4. Mathematics
   5. Reading
   6. Writing
   7. Fine sensory function (stereognosis, graphesthesia, two-point discrimination)
   8. Finger gnosis
   9. Right-left orientation
   10. "Executive functions"
   11. Abstraction

*Questions should be adapted to the age of the child.
Courtesy of Eric D. Caine, M.D., and Jeffrey M. Lyness, M.D.

Physical Appearances. The examiner should document the child's size, grooming, nutritional state, bruising, head circumference, physical signs of anxiety, facial expressions, and mannerisms.

Parent–Child Interaction. The examiner can observe the interactions between parents and child in the waiting area before the interview and in the family session. The manner in which parents and child converse and the emotional overtones are pertinent.

Separation and Reunion. The examiner should note the manner in which the child responds to the separation from a parent for an individual interview and the reunion behavior. Either lack of affect at separation and reunion or severe distress on separation or reunion can indicate problems in the parent–child relationship or other psychiatric disturbances.

Orientation to Time, Place, and Persons. Impairments in orientation can reflect organic damage, low intelligence, or a thought disorder. The age of the child must be kept in mind, however, because very young children are not expected to know the date, other chronologic information, or the name of the interview site.

Speech and Language. The examiner should evaluate the child's speech and language acquisition. Is it appropriate for the child's age? A disparity between expressive language usage and receptive language is notable. The examiner should also note the child's rate of speech, rhythm, latency to answer, spontaneity of speech, intonation, articulation of words, and prosody. Echolalia, repetitive stereotypical phrases, and unusual syntax are important psychiatric findings. Children who do not use words by age 18 months or who do not use phrases by age 2.5 to 3 years, but who have a history of normal babbling and responding appropriately to nonverbal cues, are probably developing normally. The examiner should consider the possibility that a hearing loss is contributing to a speech and language deficit.

Mood. A child's sad expression, lack of appropriate smiling, tearfulness, anxiety, euphoria, and anger are valid indicators of mood, as are verbal admissions of feelings. Persistent themes in play and fantasy also reflect the child's mood.

Affect. The examiner should note the child's range of emotional expressivity, appropriateness of affect to thought content, ability to move smoothly from one affect to another, and sudden labile emotional shifts.

Thought Process and Content. In evaluating a thought disorder in a child, the clinician must always consider what is developmentally expected for the child's age and what is deviant for any age group. The evaluation of thought form considers loosening of associations, excessive magical thinking, perseveration, echolalia, the ability to distinguish fantasy from reality, sentence coherence, and the ability to reason logically. The evaluation of thought content considers delusions, obsessions, themes, fears, wishes, preoccupations, and interests.

Suicidal ideation is always a part of the mental status examination for children who are sufficiently verbal to understand the questions and old enough to understand the concept. Children of average intelligence older than 4 years usually have some understanding of what is real and what is make-believe and may be asked about suicidal ideation, although a firm concept of the permanence of death may not be present until several years later.

Aggressive thoughts and homicidal ideation are assessed here. Perceptual disturbances, such as hallucinations, are also assessed. Very young children are expected to have short attention spans and may change the topic and conversation abruptly without exhibiting a symptomatic flight of ideas. Transient visual and auditory hallucinations in very young children do not necessarily represent major psychotic illnesses, but they do warrant further investigation.

Social Relatedness. The examiner assesses the appropriateness of the child's response to the interviewer, general level of social skills, eye contact, and degree of familiarity or withdrawal in the interview process. Overly friendly or familiar behavior may be as troublesome as extremely retiring and withdrawn responses. The examiner assesses the child's self-esteem, general and specific areas of confidence, and success with family and peer relationships.

Motor Behavior. The motor behavior part of the mental status examination includes observations of the child's coordination and activity level and ability to pay attention and carry out developmentally appropriate tasks. It also involves involuntary movements, tremors, motor hyperactivity, and any unusual focal asymmetries of muscle movement.

Cognition. The examiner assesses the child's intellectual functioning and problem-solving abilities. An approximate level of intelligence can be estimated by the child's general information, vocabulary, and comprehension. For a specific assessment of the child's cognitive abilities, the examiner can use a standardized test.

Memory. School-age children should be able to remember three objects after 5 minutes and to repeat five digits forward and three digits backward. Anxiety can interfere with the child's performance, but an obvious inability to repeat digits or to add simple numbers may reflect brain damage, mental retardation, or learning disabilities.

Judgment and Insight. The child's view of the problems, reactions to them, and suggested solutions may give the clinician a good idea of the child's judgment and insight. In addition, the child's understanding of what he or she can realistically do to help and what the clinician can do adds to the assessment of the child's judgment.

Neuropsychiatric Assessment

A neuropsychiatric assessment is appropriate for children who are suspected to have a neurologic disorder, a psychiatric impairment that coexists with neurologic signs, or psychiatric symptoms that may be caused by neuropathology. The neuropsychiatric evaluation combines information from neurologic, physical, and mental status examinations. The neurologic examination can identify asymmetric abnormal signs (hard signs) that may indicate lesions in the brain. A physical examination can evaluate the presence of physical stigmata of particular syndromes in which neuropsychiatric symptoms or developmental aberrations play a role (e.g., fetal alcohol syndrome, Down syndrome).

An important part of the neuropsychiatric examination is the assessment of neurologic soft signs and minor physical anomalies. The term *neurological soft signs* was first noted by Loretta Bender in the 1940s in reference to nondiagnostic abnormalities in the neurologic examinations of children with schizophrenia. Soft signs do not indicate focal neurologic disorders, but they are associated with a wide variety of developmental disabilities and occur frequently in children with low intelligence, learning disabilities, and behavioral disturbances. Soft signs may refer to behavioral symptoms (which are sometimes associated with brain damage, such as severe impulsivity and hyperactivity), physical findings (including contralateral overflow movements), and a variety of nonfocal signs (e.g., mild choreiform movements, poor balance, mild incoordination, asymmetry of gait, nystagmus, and the persistence of infantile reflexes).

Soft signs can be divided into those that are normal in a young child, but become abnormal when they persist in an older child, and those that are abnormal at any age. The *Physical and Neurological Examination for Soft Signs* (PANESS) is an instrument used with children 15 years or younger. It consists of 15 questions about general physical status and medical history and 43 physical tasks (e.g., touch your finger to your nose, hop on one foot to the end of the line, tap quickly with your finger). Neurologic soft signs are important to note, but they are not useful in making a specific psychiatric diagnosis.

Minor physical anomalies or dysmorphic features occur with a higher than usual frequency in children with developmental disabilities, learning disabilities, speech and language disorders, and hyperactivity. As with soft signs, the documentation of minor physical anomalies is part of the neuropsychiatric assessment, but it is rarely helpful in the diagnostic process and does not imply a good or bad prognosis. Minor physical anomalies include a high-arched palate, epicanthal folds, hypertelorism, low-set ears, transverse palmar creases, multiple hair whorls, a large head, a furrowed tongue, and partial syndactyly of several toes.

When a seizure disorder is being considered in the differential diagnosis or a structural abnormality in the brain is suspected, an electroencephalogram (EEG), computed tomography (CT) scan, or magnetic resonance imaging (MRI) study may be indicated.

Developmental, Psychologic, and Educational Testing

Psychologic tests are not always required to assess psychiatric symptoms, but they are valuable in determining a child's developmental level, intellectual functioning, and academic difficulties. A measure of adaptive functioning (including the child's competence in communication, daily living skills, socialization, and motor skills) is a prerequisite when a diagnosis of mental retardation is being considered. Table 1–4 outlines the general categories of psychologic tests.

Developmental Tests for Infants and Preschoolers. The *Gesell Infant Scale,* the *Cattell Infant Intelligence Scale,* the *Bayley Scales of Infant Development,* and the *Denver Developmental Screening Test* include developmental assessments of infants as young as 2 months of age. When used with very young infants, the tests focus on sensorimotor and social responses to a variety of objects and interactions. When these instruments are used with older infants and preschoolers, emphasis is placed on language acquisition. The *Gesell Infant Scale* measures development in four areas: motor, adaptive functioning, language, and social.

An infant's score on one of these developmental assessments is not a reliable way to predict a child's future intelligence quotient (IQ) in most cases. Infant assessments are valuable, however, in detecting developmental deviation and mental retardation and in raising suspicions of a developmental disorder. Although infant assessments rely heavily on sensorimotor functions, intelligence testing in older children and adolescents includes later-developing functions, including verbal, social, and abstract cognitive abilities.

Intelligence Tests for School-Age Children and Adolescents. The most widely used test of intelligence for school-age children and adolescents is the third edition of the *Wechsler Intelligence Scale for Children* (WISC-III-R). It can be given to children 6 to 17 years of age and yields a verbal IQ, a performance IQ, and a combined full-scale IQ. The verbal subtests consist of vocabulary, information, arithmetic, similarities, comprehension, and digit span (supplemental) categories. The performance subtests include block design, picture completion, picture arrangement, object assembly, coding, mazes (supplemental), and symbol search (supplemental). The scores of the supplemental subtests are not included in the computation of IQ.

Each subcategory is scored from 1 to 19, with 10 being the average score. An average full-scale IQ is 100; 70 to 80 represents borderline intellectual function; 80 to 90 is in the low average range; 90 to 109 is average; 110 to 119 is high average; and above 120 is in the superior or very superior range. The multiple breakdowns of the performance and verbal subscales allow great flexibility in identifying specific areas of deficit and scatter in

Table 1–4
Commonly Used Child and Adolescent Psychologic Assessment Instruments

Test	Age/Grades	Data Generated and Comments
Intellectual ability		
Wechsler Intelligence Scale for Children–Third Edition (WISC-III-R)	6–16	Standard scores: verbal, performance and full-scale IQ; scaled subtest scores permitting specific skill assessment
Wechsler Adult Intelligence Scale–Third Edition (WAIS-III)	16–adult	Same as WISC-III-R
Wechsler Preschool and Primary Scale of Intelligence–Revised (WPPSI-R)	3–7	Same as WISC-III-R
Kaufman Assessment Battery for Children (K-ABC)	2.6–12.6	Well grounded in theories of cognitive psychology and neuropsychology. Allows immediate comparison of intellectual capacity with acquired knowledge. Scores: Mental Processing Composite (IQ equivalent); sequential and simultaneous processing and achievement standard scores: scaled mental processing and achievement subtest scores; age equivalents; percentiles
Kaufman Adolescent and Adult Intelligence Test (KAIT)	11–>85	Composed of separate Crystallized and Fluid scales. Scores: Composite Intelligence Scale; Crystallized and Fluid IQ; scaled subtest scores; percentiles
Stanford-Binet, 4th Edition (SB:FE)	2–23	Scores: IQ; verbal, abstract/visual, and quantitative reasoning; short-term memory; standard age
Peabody Picture Vocabulary Test–III (PPVT-III)	4–adult	Measures receptive vocabulary acquisition; standard scores, percentiles, age equivalents
Achievement		
Woodcock-Johnson Psycho-Educational Battery–Revised (W-J)	K–12	Scores: reading and mathematics (mechanics and comprehension), written language, other academic achievement; grade and age scores, standard scores, percentiles
Wide Range Achievement Test–3, Levels 1 and 2 (WRAT-3)	Level 1: 1–5 Level 2: 12–75	Permits screening for deficits in reading, spelling, and arithmetic; grade levels, percentiles, stanines, standard scores
Kaufman Test of Educational Achievement, Brief and Comprehensive Forms (K-TEA)	1–12	Standard scores: reading, mathematics, and spelling; grade and age equivalents, percentiles, stanines. Brief Form is sufficient for most clinical applications; Comprehensive Form allows error analysis and more detailed curriculum planning
Wechsler Individual Achievement Test (WIAT)	K–12	Standard scores: basic reading, mathematics reasoning, spelling, reading comprehension, numeric operations, listening comprehension, oral expression, written expression. Conormal with WISC-III-R
Adaptive behavior		
Vineland Adaptive Behavior Scales	Normal: 0–19; Retarded: All ages	Standard scores: adaptive behavior composite and communication, daily living skills, socialization and motor domains; percentiles, age equivalents, developmental age scores. Separate standardization groups for normal, visually handicapped, hearing impaired, emotionally disturbed, and retarded
Scales of Independent Behavior–Revised	Newborn–adult	Standard scores: four adaptive (motor, social interaction/communication, personal living, community living) and three maladaptive (internalized, asocial, and externalized) areas; General Maladaptive Index and Broad Independence cluster
Attentional capacity		
Trail Making Test	8–adult	Standard scores, standard deviations, ranges; corrections for age and education
Wisconsin Card Sorting Test	6.6–adult	Standard scores, standard deviations, T-scores, percentiles, developmental norms for number of categories achieved, perseverative errors, and failures to maintain set; computer measures
Behavior Assessment System for Children (BASC)	4–18	Teacher and parent rating scales and child self-report of personality permitting multireporter assessment across a variety of domains in home, school, and community. Provides validity, clinical, and adaptive scales. ADHD component avails
Home Situations Questionnaire–Revised (HSQ-R)	6–12	Permits parents to rate child's specific problems with attention or concentration. Scores for number of problem settings, mean severity, and factor scores for compliance and leisure situations

(continued)

Table 1–4
(Continued)

Test	Age/Grades	Data Generated and Comments
ADHD Rating Scale	6–12	Score for number of symptoms keyed to DSM cutoff for diagnosis of ADHD; standard scores permit derivation of clinical significance for total score and two factors (Inattentive-Hyperactive and Impulsive-Hyperactive)
School Situations Questionnaire (SSQ-R)	6–12	Permits teachers to rate a child's specific problems with attention or concentration. Scores for number of problem settings and mean severity.
Child Attention Profile (CAP)	6–12	Brief measure allowing teachers' weekly ratings of presence and degree of child's inattention and overactivity. Normative scores for inattention, overactivity, and total score
Projective tests		
Rorschach Inkblots	3–adult	Special scoring systems. Most recently developed and increasingly universally accepted is John Exner's Comprehensive System (1974). Assesses perceptual accuracy, integration of affective and intellectual functioning, reality testing, and other psychologic processes
Thematic Apperception Test (TAT)	6–adult	Generates stories that are analyzed qualitatively. Assumed to provide especially rich data regarding interpersonal functioning
Machover Draw-A-Person Test (DAP)	3–adult	Qualitative analysis and hypothesis generation, especially regarding subject's feelings about self and significant others
Kinetic Family Drawing (KFD)	3–adult	Qualitative analysis and hypothesis generation regarding an individual's perception of family structure and sentient environment. Some objective scoring systems in existence
Rotter Incomplete Sentences Blank	Child, adolescent, and adult forms	Primarily qualitative analysis, although some objective scoring systems have been developed
Personality tests		
Minnesota Multiphasic Personality Inventory–Adolescent (MMPI-A)	14–18	1992 version of widely used personality measure, developed specifically for use with adolescents. Standard scores: 3 validity scales, 14 clinical scales, additional content and supplementary scales
Million Adolescent Personality Inventory (MAPI)	13–18	Standard scores for 20 scales grouped into three categories: personality styles, expressed concerns, behavioral correlates. Normed on adolescent population. Focuses on broad functional spectrum, not just problem areas. Measures 14 primary personality traits, including emotional stability, self-concept level, excitability, and self-assurance
Children's Personality Questionnaire	8–12	Generates combined broad trait patterns including extraversion and anxiety
Neuropsychologic screening tests and test batteries		
Developmental Test of Visual-Motor Integration (VMI)	2–16	Screening instrument for visual motor deficits. Standard scores, age equivalents, percentiles
Benton Visual Retention Test	6–adult	Assesses presence of deficits in visual-figure memory. Mean scores by age
Benton Visual Motor Gestalt Test	5–adult	Assesses visual-motor deficits and visual-figure retention. Age equivalents
Reitan-Indiana Neuropsychological Test Battery for Children	5–8	Cognitive and perceptual-motor tests for children with suspected brain damage
Halstead-Reitan Neuropsychological Test Battery for Older Children	9–14	Same as Reitan-Indiana
Luria-Nebraska Neuropsychological Battery: Children's Revision LNNB:C	8–12	Sensory-motor, perceptual, cognitive tests measuring 11 clinical and 2 additional domains of neuropsychologic functioning Provides standard scores
Developmental status		
Bayley Scales of Infant Development–Second Edition	16 days–42 mo	Mental, motor, and behavior scales measuring infant, development. Provides standard scores
Mullen Scales of Early Learning	Newborn–5 yr	Language and visual scales for receptive and expressive ability. Yields age scores and T-scores

Adapted from Racusin G, Moss N. Psychological assessment of children and adolescents. In: Lewis M, ed. *Child and Adolescent Psychiatry: A Comprehensive Textbook.* 3rd ed. Philadelphia: Lippincott Williams & Wilkins, 2002:558–559, with permission.)

intellectual abilities. Because a large part of intelligence testing measures abilities used in academic settings, the breakdown of the WISC-III-R can also be helpful in pointing out skills in which a child is weak and may benefit from remedial education.

The *Stanford-Binet Intelligence Scale* covers an age range from 2 to 24 years. It relies on pictures, drawings, and objects for very young children and on verbal performance for older children and adolescents. This intelligence scale, the earliest version of an intelligence test of its kind, leads to a mental age score as well as an intelligence quotient.

The *McCarthy Scales of Children's Abilities* and the *Kaufman Assessment Battery for Children* are two other intelligence tests that are available for preschool and school-age children. They do not cover the adolescent age group.

LONG-TERM STABILITY OF INTELLIGENCE. Although a child's intelligence is relatively stable throughout the school-age years and adolescence, some factors can influence intelligence and a child's score on an intelligence test. The intellectual functions of children with severe mental illnesses and of children from low socioeconomic levels may decrease over time, whereas the IQs of children whose environments have been enriched may increase over time. Factors that influence a child's score on a given test of intellectual functioning and affect the accuracy of the test are motivation, emotional state, anxiety, and cultural milieu.

Perceptual and Perceptual Motor Tests. The *Bender Visual Motor Gestalt Test* can be given to children 4 to 12 years old. The test consists of a set of spatially related figures that the child is asked to copy. The scores are based on the number of errors. Although not a diagnostic test, it is useful in identifying developmentally age-inappropriate perceptual performances.

Personality Tests. Personality tests are not of much use in making diagnoses, and they are less satisfactory than intelligence tests in regard to norms, reliability, and validity. They can be helpful, however, in eliciting themes and fantasies.

The Rorschach test is a projective technique in which ambiguous stimuli—a set of bilaterally symmetric inkblots—are shown to a child, who is asked to describe what he or she sees in each. The hypothesis is that the child's interpretation of the vague stimuli reflects basic characteristics of personality. The examiner notes the themes and patterns. Two sets of norms have been established for the Rorschach test, one for children 2 to 10 years old and one for adolescents 10 to 17 years old.

A more structured projective test is the *Children's Apperception Test* (CAT), which is an adaptation of the *Thematic Apperception Test* (TAT). The CAT consists of cards with pictures of animals in scenes that are somewhat ambiguous, but are related to parent–child and sibling issues, caretaking, and other relationships. The child is asked to describe what is happening and to tell a story about the scene. Animals are used because it was hypothesized that children might respond more readily to animal images than to human figures.

Drawings, toys, and play are also applications of projective techniques that can be used during the evaluation of children. Dollhouses, dolls, and puppets have been especially helpful in allowing a child a nonconversational mode in which to express a variety of attitudes and feelings. Play materials that reflect household situations are likely to elicit a child's fears, hopes, and conflicts about the family.

Projective techniques have not fared well as standardized instruments. Rather than being considered tests, projective techniques are best considered as additional clinical modalities.

Educational Tests. Achievement tests measure the attainment of knowledge and skills in a particular academic curriculum. The *Wide-Range Achievement Test–Revised* (WRAT-R) consists of tests of knowledge and skills and timed performances of reading, spelling, and mathematics. It is used with children from 5 years of age to adulthood. The test yields a score that is compared with the average expected score for the child's chronological age and grade level.

The *Peabody Individual Achievement Test* (PIAT) includes word identification, spelling, mathematics, and reading comprehension. The *Kaufman Test of Educational Achievement,* the *Gray Oral Reading Test–Revised* (GORT-R), and the *Sequential Tests of Educational Progress* (STEP) are achievement tests that determine whether a child has achieved the educational level expected for his or her grade level. Children with an average IQ whose achievement is significantly lower than expected for their grade level in one or more subjects are considered to be learning disabled. Achievement testing, combined with a measure of intellectual function, can identify specific learning disabilities for which remediation is recommended. Children who do not reach their grade level according to their chronologic age, but who function intellectually in the borderline range or lower, are not necessarily learning disabled, unless a disparity exists between their IQs and their levels of achievement.

Biopsychosocial Formulation. The clinician's task is to integrate all of the information obtained into a formulation that takes into account the biologic predisposition, psychodynamic factors, environmental stressors, and life events that have led to the child's current level of functioning. Psychiatric disorders and any specific physical, neuromotor, or developmental abnormalities must be considered in the formulation of etiologic factors for current impairment. The clinician's conclusions are an integration of clinical information along with data from standardized psychologic and developmental assessments. The psychiatric formulation includes an assessment of family function as well as the appropriateness of the child's educational setting. A determination of the child's overall safety in his or her current situation is made. Any suspected maltreatment must be reported to the local child protective service agency. The child's overall well-being regarding growth, development, and academic and play activities is considered.

Diagnosis

Current evidence suggests that the use of structured and semistructured (evidence-based) assessment tools enhance a clinician's ability to make the most accurate diagnoses. These instruments, described earlier, include the K-SADS, the CAPA, and the NIMH DISC-IV interviews. The advantages of including an evidence-based instrument in the diagnostic process include decreasing potential clinician bias to make a diagnosis without all of the necessary symptoms information, and serving as guides for the clinician to consider each symptom that could contribute to a given diagnosis. These data can enable the clinician to optimize his or her expertise to make challenging judgments regarding child and adolescent disorders that may possess overlapping symptoms.

The clinician's ultimate task includes making all appropriate diagnoses according to DSM-IV-TR. Some clinical situations do not fulfill criteria for DSM-IV-TR diagnoses, but cause impairment and require psychiatric attention and intervention. Clinicians who evaluate children are frequently in the position of determining the impact of behavior of family members on the child's well-being. In many cases, a child's level of impairment is related to factors extending beyond a psychiatric diagnosis, such as the child's adjustment to his or her family life, peer relationships, and educational placement.

RECOMMENDATIONS AND TREATMENT PLAN

The recommendations for treatment are derived by a clinician who integrates the data gathered during the evaluation into a coherent formulation of the factors that are contributing to the child's current problems, the consequences of the problems, and strategies that may ameliorate the difficulties. The recommendations can be broken down into their biologic, psychologic, and social components. That is, identification of a biologic predisposition to a particular psychiatric disorder may be clinically relevant to inform a psychopharmacologic recommendation. As part of the formulation, an understanding of the psychodynamic interactions between family members may lead a clinician to recommend treatment that includes a family component. Educational and academic problems are addressed in the formulation and may lead to a recommendation to seek a more effective academic placement. The overall social situation of the child or adolescent is taken into account when recommendations for treatment are developed. The physical and emotional safety of a child or adolescent is of the utmost importance and always at the top of the list of recommendations.

The child or adolescent's family, school life, peer interactions, and social activities often have a direct impact on the child's success in overcoming his or her difficulties. The psychologic education and cooperation of a child or adolescent's family are essential ingredients in successful application of treatment recommendations. Communications from clinicians to parents and family members that balance the observed positive qualities of the child and family with the weak areas are often perceived as more helpful than a focus only on the problem areas. Finally, the most successful treatment plans are plans developed cooperatively between the clinician, child, and family members during which each member of the team perceives that he or she has been given credit for positive contributions.

2 Mental Retardation

The conceptualization of mental retardation includes deficits in cognitive abilities and in behaviors required for social and personal sufficiency, known as *adaptive functioning.* Wide acceptance of this definition has led to the consensus that assessments of social adaptation and intelligence quotient (IQ) are necessary to determine the level of mental retardation. Measures of adaptive function assess competency in performance of everyday tasks, whereas measures of intellectual function focus on cognitive abilities. Evidence shows that all individuals with a given intellectual level do not have the same adaptive function, yet IQ likely contributes an upper limit or ceiling to adaptive accomplishments.

In the mid-1800s, many children with mental retardation were placed in residential educational facilities in conjunction with the belief that if these children received sufficient intensive training, they would be able to return to their families and function in society at a higher level. The original plan of educating the children so that they could overcome their disabilities was not realized. Gradually, these residential programs became larger, and eventually the focus began to shift from intensive education to custodial care. These residential institutional settings for children with mental retardation received their maximal use in the mid-1900s, until public awareness of the crowded, unsanitary, and, in some cases, abusive conditions sparked the movement toward "deinstitutionalization." An important force in the deinstitutionalization of children with mental retardation was the philosophy of "normalization" in living situations and "inclusion" in educational settings. Since the late 1960s, few children with mental retardation have been placed in institutional settings, and the concepts of "normalization" and inclusion became prominent issues among advocacy groups and most citizens.

The passage of Public Law 94-142 (Education for all Handicapped Children Act) in 1975 mandated the public school system to provide appropriate educational services to all children with disabilities. The Individuals with Disabilities Act in 1990 extended and modified the aforementioned legislation. Currently, provision of public education for all children, including children with disabilities, "within the least restrictive environment" is mandated by law.

In addition to the educational system, advocacy groups, including the Council for Exceptional Children (CEC) and the National Association for Retarded Citizens (NARC), are well-known parental lobbying organizations for children with mental retardation and were instrumental in advocating for Public Law 94-142. The most prominent advocacy organization in this field is the American Association on Mental Retardation (AAMR), which has been most influential in educating the public about mental retardation and in supporting research and legislation relating to mental retardation.

The AAMR promotes a view of mental retardation as a functional interaction between an individual and the environment, instead of a static description of a person'san 's limitations. Within this conceptual framework, a person is designated as needing intermittent, limited, extensive, or pervasive "environmental support" with respect to a specific set of adaptive function domains. These areas of function are communication, self-care, home living, social or interpersonal skills, use of community resources, self-direction, functional academic skills, work, leisure, health, and safety.

The AAMR promotes designating an IQ of 75, rather than 70, as the beginning level of the mild mental retardation range, enabling many more individuals to receive services as mentally retarded. The advantage of the AAMR view is that, instead of defining a person's degree of mental retardation by the level of cognitive and adaptive impairment, the degree of "support" necessary for functioning becomes the defining feature. The disadvantage of this nomenclature is that it is difficult to quantify the "supports," and it would be problematic to match new research with the existing body of research using an IQ cutoff of 70. The decision of the work group of the 4th edition of *Diagnostic and Statistical Manual of Mental Disorders* (DSM-IV) and its text revision (DSM-IV-TR) was that an IQ cutoff of 70 would be retained, and the adaptive function domains recommended by the AAMR would be included in the diagnostic criteria for mental retardation.

NOMENCLATURE

Accurately defining mental retardation has challenged clinicians over the centuries. In the 1800s, the notion that mental retardation was based primarily on a deficit in social or moral reasoning was promoted. Since then, the addition of intellectual deficit was added to the concept of inadequate social function. All current classification systems retain the understanding that mental retardation is based on more than intellectual deficits; that is, it also depends on a lower than expected level of adaptive function. According to DSM-IV-TR, a diagnosis of mental retardation can be made only when the IQ, as measured by a standardized test, is subaverage, and a measure of adaptive function reveals deficits in at least two of the areas of adaptive function. Mental retardation diagnoses are coded on Axis II in the DSM-IV-TR.

CLASSIFICATION

According to the DSM-IV-TR, mental retardation is defined as significantly subaverage general intellectual functioning resulting in, or associated with, concurrent impairment in adaptive behavior and manifested during the developmental period, before age 18 years. The diagnosis is made regardless of whether the individual has a coexisting physical disorder or other mental disorder. Table 2–1 presents an overview of developmental levels in communication, academic functioning, and vocational skills expected of persons with various degrees of mental retardation.

General intellectual functioning is determined by the use of standardized tests of intelligence, and the term *significantly subaverage* is defined as an IQ of approximately 70 or below or two standard deviations below the mean for the particular test. Adaptive functioning can be measured by using a standardized scale, such as the *Vineland Adaptive Behavior Scale*. This scale scores communications, daily living skills, socialization, and motor skills (up to 4 years, 11 months), and generates an adaptive behavior composite that is correlated with the expected skills at a given age.

Approximately 85 percent of persons who are mentally retarded fall within the mild mental retardation category (IQ between 50 and 70). The adaptive functions of mildly retarded persons are effective in several areas, such as communications, self-care, social skills, work, leisure, and safety. Mental retardation is influenced by genetic, environmental, and psychosocial factors; previously, the development of mild retardation was often attributed to severe psychosocial deprivation. More recently, however, researchers have increasingly recognized the likely contribution of a host of subtle biologic factors, including chromosomal abnormalities; subclinical lead intoxication; and prenatal exposure to drugs, alcohol, and other toxins.

Evidence is increasing that subgroups of persons who are mentally retarded, such as those with fragile X syndrome, Down syndrome, and Prader-Willi syndrome, have characteristic patterns of social, linguistic, and cognitive development and typical behavioral manifestations.

The DSM-IV-TR has included in its text on mental retardation additional information regarding the etiologic factors and their association with mental retardation syndromes (e.g., fragile X syndrome).

DEGREES OF SEVERITY OF MENTAL RETARDATION

The degrees, or levels, of mental retardation are expressed in various terms. DSM-IV-TR presents four levels of mental

Table 2–1
Developmental Characteristics of Mentally Retarded Persons

Degree of Mental Retardation	Preschool Age (0–5 yrs) Maturation and Development	School Age (6–20 yrs) Training and Education	Adult (≥21 yrs) Social and Vocational Adequacy
Profound	Gross retardation; minimal capacity for functioning in sensorimotor areas; needs nursing care; constant aid and supervision required	Some motor development present; may respond to minimal or limited training in self-help	Some motor and speech development; may achieve very limited self-care; needs nursing care
Severe	Poor motor development; speech minimal; generally unable to profit from training in self-help; little or no communication skills	Can talk or learn to communicate; can be trained in elemental health habits; profits from systematic habit training; unable to profit from vocational training	May contribute partially to self-maintenance under complete supervision; can develop self-protection skills to a minimal useful level in controlled environment
Moderate	Can talk or learn to communicate; poor social awareness; fair motor development; profits from training in self-help; can be managed with moderate supervision	Can profit from training in social and occupational skills; unlikely to progress beyond second-grade level in academic subjects; may learn to travel alone in familiar places	May achieve self-maintenance in unskilled or semiskilled work under sheltered conditions; needs supervision and guidance when under mild social or economic stress
Mild	Can develop social and communication skills; minimal retardation in sensorimotor areas; often not distinguished from normal until later age	Can learn academic skills up to approximately sixth-grade level by late teens; can be guided toward social conformity	Can usually achieve social and vocational skills adequate for minimal self-support, but may need guidance and assistance when under unusual social or economic stress

Adapted from *Mental Retarded Activities of the US Department of Health, Education and Welfare.* Washington, DC: US Government Printing Office; 1989:2. DSM-IV criteria are adapted essentially from this chart.

retardation: mild, moderate, severe, and profound. The category borderline mental retardation (between one and two standard deviations below the test mean) was eliminated in 1973. Borderline intellectual functioning, according to DSM-IV-TR, is not within the diagnostic boundary of mental retardation and refers to a full-scale IQ in the 71 to 84 range that is a focus of psychiatric attention.

Mild mental retardation (IQ range 50 to 70) accounts for approximately 85 percent of persons with mental retardation. In general, children with mild mental retardation are not identified until after first or second grade, when academic demands increase. By late adolescence, they often acquire academic skills at approximately a 6th-grade level. Specific causes of mental retardation are often unidentified in this group. Many adults with mild mental retardation can live independently with appropriate support and raise their own families.

Moderate mental retardation (IQ range 35 to 50) accounts for about 10 percent of persons with mental retardation. Most children with moderate mental retardation acquire language and can communicate adequately during early childhood. They are challenged academically and often are unable to achieve academically above a 2nd- to 3rd-grade level. During adolescence, socialization difficulties often set these individuals apart, and a great deal of social and vocational support is beneficial. As adults, persons with moderate mental retardation may be able to perform semiskilled work under appropriate supervision.

Severe mental retardation (IQ range 20–35) accounts for about 4 percent of individuals with mental retardation. These individuals may be able to develop communication skills in childhood and often can learn to count and recognize words that are critical to functioning. In this group, the cause of mental retardation is more likely to be identified than it is in milder forms of mental retardation. In adulthood, persons with severe mental retardation may adapt well to supervised living situations, such as group homes, and may be able to perform work-related tasks under supervision.

Profound mental retardation (IQ range <20) accounts for approximately 1 to 2 percent of persons with mental retardation. Most individuals with profound mental retardation have identifiable causes for their condition. Children with profound mental retardation may be taught some self-care skills and learn to communicate their needs given the appropriate training.

The DSM-IV-TR lists mental retardation, severity unspecified, as a type reserved for persons who are strongly suspected of having mental retardation, but who cannot be tested by standard intelligence tests or are too impaired or uncooperative to be tested. This type may be applicable to infants whose significantly subaverage intellectual functioning is clinically judged but for whom the available tests (e.g., *Bayley Scales of Infant Development* and *Cattell Infant Scale*) do not yield numeric IQ values. This type should not be used when the intellectual level is presumed to be >70.

EPIDEMIOLOGY

The prevalence of mental retardation at any one time is estimated to range from 1 percent to 3 percent of the population. The incidence of mental retardation is difficult to calculate because mild mental retardation sometimes goes unrecognized until middle childhood. In some cases, even when intellectual function is limited, good adaptive skills are not challenged until late childhood or early adolescence, and the diagnosis is not made until that time. The highest incidence is in school-age children, with the peak at age 10 to 14 years. Mental retardation is about 1.5 times more common among men than among women. In older persons, prevalence is lower; those with severe or profound mental retardation have high mortality rates because of the complications of associated physical disorders.

COMORBIDITY

Prevalence

Epidemiologic surveys indicate that two thirds of children and adults with mental retardation have comorbid mental disorders; this rate is several times higher than that in the community samples of those not mentally retarded. The prevalence of psychopathology seems to be correlated with the severity of mental retardation; the more severe the mental retardation, the higher the risk for other mental disorders. A more recent epidemiologic study found that 40.7 percent of intellectually disabled children between 4 and 18 years of age met criteria for at least one psychiatric disorder. The severity of retardation affected the type of psychiatric disorder. Disruptive and conduct-disorder behaviors occurred more commonly in the mildly retarded group; the more severely retarded group exhibited psychiatric problems more often associated with autistic disorder, such as self-stimulation and self-mutilation. In contrast to the epidemiology of psychopathology in children in general, age and sex did not affect the prevalence of psychiatric disorders in this study. Children with profound mental retardation were less likely to exhibit psychiatric symptoms.

The mental disorders that occur among persons who are mentally retarded seem to run the gamut of those seen in persons not mentally retarded, including mood disorders, schizophrenia, attention-deficit/hyperactivity disorder (ADHD), and conduct disorder. Individuals with severe mental retardation have a particularly high rate of autistic disorder and pervasive developmental disorders. About 2 to 3 percent of mentally retarded persons meet the criteria for schizophrenia; this percentage is several times higher than the rate for the general population. When instruments such as the *Kiddie Schedule for Affective Disorders and Schizophrenia*, the *Beck Depression Inventory*, and the *Children's Depression Inventory* were used in pilot studies, 50 percent of mentally retarded children and adults had a mood disorder, but because these instruments have not been standardized within the mentally retarded population, these findings must be considered preliminary.

Highly prevalent psychiatric symptoms that can occur in mentally retarded persons outside the context of a mental disorder include hyperactivity and short attention span, self-injurious behaviors (e.g., head-banging and self-biting), and repetitive stereotypical behaviors (hand-flapping and toe-walking). Personality styles and traits in mentally retarded persons are not unique to them, but negative self-image, low self-esteem, poor frustration tolerance, interpersonal dependence, and a rigid problem-solving style are overrepresented. Specific causal syndromes seen in mental retardation can also predispose affected persons to various types of psychopathologies.

Neurologic Disorders

Comorbid psychiatric disorders are increased in individuals with mental retardation who also have known neurologic conditions, such as seizure disorders. Rates of psychopathology increase with the severity of mental retardation; neurologic impairment increases as intellectual impairment increases. In a review of psychiatric disorders in children and adolescents with mental retardation and epilepsy, approximately one third also had autistic disorder or an autistic-like condition. The combination of mental retardation, active epilepsy, and autism or an autistic-like condition occurs at a rate of 0.07 percent in the general population.

Psychosocial Features

A negative self-image and poor self-esteem are common features of mildly and moderately mentally retarded persons, who are well aware of being different from others. They experience repeated failure and disappointment in not meeting their parents' and society's expectations and in falling progressively behind their peers and even their younger siblings. Communication difficulties further increase their vulnerability to feelings of ineptness and frustration. Inappropriate behaviors, such as withdrawal, are common. The perpetual sense of isolation and inadequacy has been linked to feelings of anxiety, anger, dysphoria, and depression.

ETIOLOGY

Etiologic factors in mental retardation can be primarily genetic, developmental, acquired, or a combination. Genetic causes include chromosomal and inherited conditions, developmental factors include prenatal exposure to infections and toxins, and acquired syndromes include perinatal trauma (e.g., prematurity) and sociocultural factors. The severity of the resulting mental retardation is related to the timing and duration of the trauma as well as to the degree of exposure to the central nervous system (CNS). The more severe the mental retardation, the more likely it is that the cause is evident. In about three fourths of persons with severe mental retardation, the cause is known, whereas the cause is apparent in only half of those with mild mental retardation. A study of 100 consecutive children with mental retardation admitted to a clinical genetics unit of a university pediatric hospital reported that in 41% of cases, a causative diagnosis was made. In general, etiologic classifications used included genetic, multifactorial, environmental, and unknown etiology.

No cause is known for three fourths of persons with borderline intellectual functioning. Overall, in up to two thirds of all mentally retarded persons, the probable cause can be identified. Among chromosomal and metabolic disorders, Down syndrome, fragile X syndrome, and phenylketonuria (PKU) are the most common disorders that usually produce at least moderate mental retardation. Individuals with mild mental retardation sometimes have a familial pattern apparent in parents and siblings. Deprivation of nutrition, nurturance, and social stimulation can contribute to the development of mental retardation. Current knowledge suggests that genetic, environmental, biologic, and psychosocial factors work additively in mental retardation.

Genetic Etiologic Factors in Mental Retardation

Abnormalities in autosomal chromosomes are frequently associated with mental retardation, whereas aberrations in sex chromosomes can result in characteristic physical syndromes that do not include mental retardation (e.g., Turner's syndrome with XO and Klinefelter's syndrome with XXY, XXXY, and XXYY variations). Some children with Turner's syndrome have normal to superior intelligence. Agreement exists on a few predisposing factors for chromosomal disorders, including advanced maternal age, increased age of the father, and X-ray radiation.

Genetic Mental Retardation Syndromes and Behavioral Phenotypes

Many researchers in the field of mental retardation have noted specific and predictable behaviors are associated with certain genetic mental retardation syndromes. These behavioral phenotypes are defined as a syndrome of observable behaviors that occur with a greater probability than expected among individuals with a specific genetic abnormality.

Examples of behavioral phenotypes occur in genetically determined syndromes, such as fragile X syndrome, Prader-Willi syndrome, and Down syndrome, in which specific behavioral manifestations can be expected. Persons with fragile X syndrome have extremely high rates (up to three fourths of those studied) of ADHD. High rates of aberrant interpersonal behavior and language function often meet the criteria for autistic disorder and avoidant personality disorder. Prader-Willi syndrome is almost always associated with compulsive eating disturbances, hyperphagia, and obesity. Children with the syndrome have been described as oppositional and defiant. Socialization is an area of weakness, especially in coping skills. Externalizing behavior problems—such as temper tantrums, irritability, and arguing—seem to be heightened in adolescence. Researchers and clinicians are working toward developing specific questionnaires to identify behavioral phenotypes of the aforementioned and other mental retardation syndromes.

Down Syndrome. The description of Down syndrome, first made by the English physician Langdon Down in 1866, was based on the physical characteristics associated with subnormal mental functioning. Since then, Down syndrome has been the most investigated, and most discussed, syndrome in mental retardation. Children with this syndrome were originally called *mongoloid* because of their physical characteristics of slanted eyes, epicanthal folds, and flat nose. Despite a plethora of theories and hypotheses advanced in the past 100 years, the cause of Down syndrome is still unknown.

The problem of cause is complicated even further by the recent recognition of three types of chromosomal aberrations in Down syndrome:

1. Patients with trisomy 21 (three chromosome 21, instead of the usual two) represent most cases of Down syndrome; they have 47 chromosomes, with an extra chromosome 21. The mothers' karyotypes are normal. A nondisjunction during meiosis, occurring for unknown reasons, is responsible for the disorder.
2. Nondisjunction occurring after fertilization in any cell division results in mosaicism, a condition in which normal and trisomic cells are found in various tissues.
3. In translocation, a fusion occurs of two chromosomes, usually 21 and 15, resulting in a total of 46 chromosomes, despite the presence of an extra chromosome 21. The disorder, in contrast to trisomy 21, is usually inherited, and the translocated chromosome may be found in unaffected parents and siblings. The asymptomatic carriers have only 45 chromosomes.

The incidence of Down syndrome in the United States is about 1 in every 700 births. In his original description, Down mentioned the frequency of 10 percent among all mentally retarded patients. For a middle-aged mother (>32 years old), the risk of having a child with Down syndrome with trisomy 21 is about 1 in 100 births, but when translocation is present, the risk is about 1 in 3. These facts assume special importance in genetic counseling.

Mental retardation is the overriding feature of Down syndrome. Most persons with the syndrome are moderately or severely retarded, with only a few having an IQ >50. Mental development seems to progress normally from birth to 6 months of age; IQ scores gradually decrease from near normal at 1 year of age to about 30 at older ages. The decline in intelligence may not be readily apparent. Infantile tests may not reveal the full extent of the defect, which may become manifest when sophisticated tests are used in early childhood. According to many sources, children with Down syndrome are placid, cheerful, and cooperative, and adapt easily at home. With adolescence, the picture changes: Youngsters may experience various emotional difficulties, behavior disorders, and (rarely) psychotic disorders.

In Down syndrome, language function is a relative weakness, whereas sociability and social skills, such as interpersonal cooperation and conformity with social conventions, are relative strengths. Most studies have noted muted affect in children with Down syndrome relative to children of the same mental age who are not retarded. Children with Down syndrome also manifest deficiencies in scanning the environment; they are likely to focus on a single stimulus and have difficulty noticing environmental changes. Various mental disorders occur in persons with Down syndrome, but the rates seem to be lower than those of other mental retardation syndromes, especially autistic disorder.

The diagnosis of Down syndrome is made with relative ease in an older child, but is often difficult in newborns. The most important signs in a newborn include general hypotonia; oblique palpebral fissures; abundant neck skin; a small, flattened skull; high cheekbones; and a protruding tongue. The hands are broad and thick, with a single palmar transversal crease, and the little fingers are short and curved inward. Moro reflex is weak or absent. More than 100 signs or stigmata are described in Down syndrome, but rarely are all found in one person. Life expectancy was once about 12 years; with the advent of antibiotics, few young patients die from Down syndrome, but many do not live beyond the age of 40. Life expectancy is increasing, however.

Persons with Down syndrome tend to exhibit marked deterioration in language, memory, self-care skills, and problem-solving in their 30s. Postmortem studies of patients with Down syndrome older than 40 have shown a high incidence of senile plaques and neurofibrillary tangles, as seen in Alzheimer's disease. Neurofibrillary tangles are known to occur in a variety of degenerative diseases, whereas senile plaques seem to be found most often in Alzheimer's disease and in Down syndrome. The two disorders may share some pathophysiology.

Fragile X Syndrome. Fragile X syndrome is the second most common single cause of mental retardation. The syndrome results from a mutation on the X chromosome at what is known as the fragile site (Xq27.3). The fragile site is expressed in only some cells, and it may be absent in asymptomatic males and female carriers. Much variability is present in genetic and phenotypic expression. Fragile X syndrome is believed to occur in about 1 of every 1,000 males and 1 of every 2,000 females. The typical phenotype includes a large, long head and ears; short stature; hyperextensible joints; and postpubertal macroorchidism. Mental retardation ranges from mild to severe.

The behavioral profile of persons with fragile X syndrome includes a high rate of ADHD, learning disorders, and pervasive developmental disorders, such as autism. Deficits in language function include rapid perseverative speech with abnormalities in combining words into phrases and sentences. Persons with fragile X syndrome seem to have relatively strong skills in communication and socialization; their intellectual functions seem to decline in the pubertal period. Female carriers are often less impaired than males with fragile X syndrome, but females also can manifest the typical physical characteristics and can be mildly retarded.

Prader-Willi Syndrome. Prader-Willi syndrome is postulated to result from a small deletion involving chromosome 15, usually occurring sporadically. Its prevalence is less than 1 of 10,000. Persons with the syndrome exhibit compulsive eating behavior and often obesity, mental retardation, hypogonadism, small stature, hypotonia, and small hands and feet. Children with the syndrome often have oppositional and defiant behavior.

Cat's Cry (Cri-du-Chat) Syndrome. Children with cat's cry syndrome lack part of chromosome 5. They are severely retarded and show many signs often associated with chromosomal aberrations, such as microcephaly, low-set ears, oblique palpebral fissures, hypertelorism, and micrognathia. The characteristic cat-like cry caused by laryngeal abnormalities that gave the syndrome its name gradually changes and disappears with increasing age.

Other Chromosomal Abnormalities. Other syndromes of autosomal aberrations associated with mental retardation are much less prevalent than Down syndrome.

Phenylketonuria. PKU was first described by Ivar Asbjörn Fölling in 1934 as the paradigmatic inborn error of metabolism. PKU is transmitted as a simple recessive autosomal mendelian trait and occurs in about 1 of every 10,000 to 15,000 live births; for parents who have already had a child with PKU, the chance of having another child with PKU is 1 of every 4 to 5 successive pregnancies. Although the disease is reported predominantly in persons of North European origin, a few cases have been described in blacks, Yemenite Jews, and Asians. The frequency among institutionalized retarded patients is about 1 percent. The basic metabolic defect in PKU is an inability to convert phenylalanine, an essential amino acid, to paratyrosine because of the absence or inactivity of the liver enzyme phenylalanine hydroxylase, which catalyzes the conversion. Two other types of hyperphenylalaninemia have recently been described. One is caused by a deficiency of the enzyme dihydropteridine reductase, and the other is caused by a deficiency of a cofactor, biopterin. The first defect can be detected in fibroblasts, and biopterin can be measured in body fluids. Both of these rare disorders carry a high risk of fatality.

Most patients with PKU are severely retarded, but some are reported to have borderline or normal intelligence. Eczema, vomiting, and convulsions occur in about a third of all patients. Although the clinical picture varies, typical children with PKU are hyperactive; they exhibit erratic, unpredictable behavior and are difficult to manage. They frequently have temper tantrums and often display bizarre movements of their bodies and upper extremities, including twisting hand mannerisms; their behavior sometimes resembles that of children with autism or schizophrenia. Verbal and nonverbal communication is usually severely impaired or nonexistent. The children's coordination is poor, and they have many perceptual difficulties.

The disease was previously diagnosed on the basis of a urine test: Phenylpyruvic acid in the urine reacts with ferric chloride solution to yield a vivid green color. The test, however, has its limitations; it may not detect the presence of phenylpyruvic acid in urine before an infant is 5 or 6 weeks of age, and it may give positive responses with other aminoacidurias. Currently, a more reliable screening test, the Guthrie inhibition assay, is more widely applied; it uses a bacteriologic procedure to detect phenylalanine in the blood.

In the United States, newborns are routinely screened for PKU. Early diagnosis is important because a low-phenylalanine diet, in use since 1955, significantly improves behavior and developmental progress. The best results seem to be obtained with early diagnosis and the start of dietary treatment before the child is 6 months old. Dietary treatment, however, is not without risk. Phenylalanine is an essential amino acid, and its omission from the diet can lead to severe complications such as anemia, hypoglycemia, edema, and even death. Dietary treatment of PKU should be continued indefinitely. Children who receive a diagnosis before age 3 months and are placed on an optimal dietary regimen may have normal intelligence. A low-phenylalanine diet does not influence the level of mental retardation in untreated older children and adolescents with PKU, but the diet does decrease irritability and abnormal electroencephalogram (EEG) changes, and does increase social responsiveness and attention span. The parents of children with PKU and some of the children's normal siblings are heterozygous carriers. The disease can be detected by a phenylalanine tolerance test, which may be important in genetic counseling of the family members.

Rett's Disorder. Rett's syndrome is caused by mutations in the MECP2 gene of the X chromosome. Retts syndrome affects 1 in every 10,000–15,000 live births. Boys suffering from the MECP2 mutations that cause Rett's syndrome in girls die shortly after birth, as they do not have a back up X chromosome to compensate for the deficit.

In 1966, Andreas Rett reported on 22 girls with a serious progressive neurologic disability. Deterioration in communications skills, motor behavior, and social functioning starts at about 1 year of age. Autistic-like symptoms are common, as are ataxia, facial grimacing, teeth-grinding, and loss of speech. Intermittent hyperventilation and a disorganized breathing pattern are characteristic while the child is awake. Stereotypical hand movements, including hand-wringing, are typical. Progressive gait disturbance, scoliosis, and seizures occur. Severe spasticity is usually present by middle childhood. Cerebral atrophy occurs with decreased pigmentation of the substantia nigra, which suggests abnormalities of the dopaminergic nigrostriatal system.

Neurofibromatosis. Also called *von Recklinghausen's disease,* neurofibromatosis is the most common of the neurocutaneous syndromes caused by a single dominant gene, which may be inherited or be a new mutation. The disorder occurs in about 1 of 5,000 births and is characterized by café au lait spots on the skin and by neurofibromas, including optic gliomas and acoustic neuromas, caused by abnormal cell migration. Mild mental retardation occurs in up to one third of those with the disease.

Tuberous Sclerosis. Tuberous sclerosis is the second most common neurocutaneous syndrome; a progressive mental retardation occurs in two thirds of all affected persons. It occurs in about 1 of 15,000 persons and is inherited by autosomal dominant transmission. Seizures are present in all those who are mentally retarded and in two thirds of those who are not. Infantile spasms may occur as early as 6 months of age. The phenotypic presentation includes adenoma sebaceum and ash-leaf spots that can be identified with a slit lamp.

Lesch-Nyhan Syndrome. Lesch-Nyhan syndrome is a rare disorder caused by a deficiency of an enzyme involved in purine metabolism. The disorder is X-linked; patients have mental retardation, microcephaly, seizures, choreoathetosis, and spasticity. The syndrome is also associated with severe compulsive self-mutilation by biting the mouth and fingers. Lesch-Nyhan syndrome is another example of a genetically determined syndrome with a specific, predictable behavioral pattern.

Adrenoleukodystrophy. The most common of several disorders of sudanophilic cerebral sclerosis, adrenoleukodystrophy is characterized by diffuse demyelination of the cerebral white matter resulting in visual and intellectual impairment, seizures, spasticity, and progression to death. The cerebral degeneration in adrenoleukodystrophy is accompanied by adrenocortic insufficiency. The disorder is transmitted by a sex-linked gene located on the distal end of the long arm of the X chromosome. The clinical onset is generally between 5 and 8 years of age, with early seizures, disturbances in gait, and mild intellectual impairment. Abnormal pigmentation reflecting adrenal insufficiency sometimes precedes the neurologic symptoms, and attacks of crying are common. Spastic contractures, ataxia, and swallowing disturbances are also frequent. Although the course is often rapidly progressive, some patients may have a relapsing and remitting course. The story of a child with the disorder was presented in the 1992 film *Lorenzo's Oil*.

Maple Syrup Urine Disease. The clinical symptoms of maple syrup urine disease appear during the first week of life. The infant deteriorates rapidly and has decerebrate rigidity, seizures, respiratory irregularity, and hypoglycemia. If untreated, most patients die in the first months of life, and the survivors are severely retarded. Some variants have been reported with transient ataxia and only mild retardation. Treatment follows the general principles established for PKU and consists of a diet very low in the three involved amino acids—leucine, isoleucine, and valine.

Other Enzyme Deficiency Disorders. Several enzyme deficiency disorders associated with mental retardation have been identified, and still more diseases are being added as new discoveries are made, including Hartnup disease, galactosemia, and glycogen-storage disease. Table 2–2 lists 30 important disorders with inborn errors of metabolism, hereditary transmission patterns, defective enzymes, clinical signs, and relation to mental retardation.

Acquired and Developmental Factors

Prenatal Period. Important prerequisites for the overall development of the fetus include the mother's physical, psychologic, and nutritional health during pregnancy. Maternal chronic illnesses and conditions affecting the normal development of the fetus's CNS include uncontrolled diabetes, anemia, emphysema, hypertension, and long-term use of alcohol and narcotic substances. Maternal infections during pregnancy, especially viral infections, have been known to cause fetal damage and mental retardation. The extent of fetal damage depends on such variables as the type of viral infection, the gestational age of the fetus, and the severity of the illness. Although numerous infectious diseases have been reported to affect the fetus's CNS, the following medical disorders have been definitely identified as high-risk conditions for mental retardation.

Rubella (German Measles). Rubella has replaced syphilis as the major cause of congenital malformations and mental retardation caused by maternal infection. Children of affected mothers may show several abnormalities, including congenital heart disease, mental retardation, cataracts, deafness, microcephaly, and microphthalmia. Timing is crucial because the extent and frequency of the complications are inversely related to the duration of the pregnancy at the time of maternal infection. When mothers are infected in the first trimester of pregnancy, 10 to 15 percent of children are affected, but the incidence increases to almost 50 percent when the infection occurs in the first month of pregnancy. The situation is often complicated by subclinical forms of maternal infection that frequently go undetected. Maternal rubella can be prevented by immunization.

Cytomegalic Inclusion Disease. In many cases, cytomegalic inclusion disease remains dormant in the mother. Some children are stillborn, and others have jaundice, microcephaly, hepatosplenomegaly, and radiographic findings of intracerebral calcification. Children with mental retardation from the disease frequently have cerebral calcification, microcephaly, or hydrocephalus. The diagnosis is confirmed by positive findings of the virus in throat and urine cultures and the recovery of inclusion-bearing cells in the urine.

Syphilis. Syphilis in pregnant women was once the main cause of various neuropathologic changes in their offspring, including mental retardation. Today, the incidence of syphilitic complications of pregnancy fluctuates with the incidence of syphilis in the general population. Some recent alarming

Table 2–2
Thirty Impairment Disorders with Inborn Errors of Metabolism

Disorder	Hereditary Transmission*	Enzyme Defect	Prenatal Diagnosis	Mental Retardation	Clinical Signs
I. LIPID METABOLISM					
Niemann-Pick disease					
Group A, infantile		Unknown			Hepatomegaly
Group B, adult	AR	Sphingomyelinase	+	±	Hepatosplenomegaly
Groups C and D, intermediate		Unknown	−	+	Pulmonary infiltration
Infantile Gaucher's disease	AR	β-Glucosidase	+	±	Hepatosplenomegaly, pseudobulbar palsy
Tay-Sachs disease	AR	Hexosaminidase A	+	+	Macular changes, seizures, spasticity
Generalized gangliosidosis	AR	β-Galactosidase	+	+	Hepatosplenomegaly, bone changes
Krabbe's disease	AR	Galactocerebroside β-Galactosidase	+	+	Stiffness, seizures
Metachromatic leukodystrophy	AR	Cerebroside sulfatase	+	+	Stiffness, developmental failure
Wolman's disease	AR	Acid lipase	+	−	Hepatosplenomegaly, adrenal calcification, vomiting, diarrhea
Farber's lipogranulomatosis	AR	Acid ceramidase	+	+	Hoarseness, arthropathy, subcutaneous nodules
Fabry's disease	XR	β-Galactosidase	+	−	Angiokeratomas, renal failure
II. MUCOPOLYSACCHARIDE METABOLISM					
Hurler's syndrome MPS I	AR	Iduronidase	+	+	?
Hurler's disease II	XR	Iduronate sulfatase	+	+	?
Sanfilippo's syndrome III	AR	Various sulfatases (types A–D)	+	+	Varying degrees of bone changes, hepatosplenomegaly, joint restriction
Morquio's disease IV	AR	N-Acetylgalactosamine-6-sulfate sulfatase	+	−	?
Maroteaux-Lamy syndrome VI	AR	Arylsulfatase B	+	±	?
III. OLIGOSACCHARIDE AND GLYCOPROTEIN METABOLISM					
I-cell disease	AR	Glycoprotein N-acetylglucosaminyl-phosphotransferase	+	+	Hepatomegaly, bone changes, swollen gingivae
Mannosidosis	AR	Mannosidase	+	+	Hepatomegaly, bone changes, facial coarsening
Fucosidosis	AR	Fucosidase	+	+	Same as above
IV. AMINO ACID METABOLISM					
Phenylketonuria	AR	Phenylalanine hydroxylase	−	+	Eczema, blonde hair, musty odor
Hemocystinuria	AR	Cystathionine β-synthetase	+	+	Ectopia lentis, Marfan-like phenotype, cardiovascular anomalies
Tyrosinosis	AR	Tyrosine amine transaminase	−	+	Hyperkeratotic skin lesions, conjunctivitis
Maple syrup urine disease	AR	Branched-chain ketoacid decarboxylase	+	+	Recurrent ketoacidosis
Methylmalonic acidemia	AR	Methylmalonyl-CoA mutase	+	+	Recurrent ketoacidosis, hepatomegaly, growth retardation
Propionic acidemia	AR	Propionyl-CoA carboxylase	+	+	Same as above
Nonketotic hyperglycinemia	AR	Glycine cleavage enzyme	+	+	Seizures
Urea cycle disorders	Mostly AR	Urea cycle enzymes	+	+	Recurrent acute encephalopathy, vomiting
Hartnup disease	AR	Renal transport disorder	−	−	None consistent
V. OTHERS					
Galactosemia	AR	Galactose-1-phosphate uridyltransferase	+	+	Hepatomegaly, cataracts, ovarian failure
Wilson's hepatolenticular degeneration	AR	Unknown factor in copper metabolism	−	±	Liver disease, Kayser-Fleischer ring, neurologic problems
Menkes' kinky-hair disease	XR	Same as above	+	−	Abnormal hair, cerebral degeneration
Lesch-Nyhan syndrome	XR	Hypoxanthine guanine phosphoribosyltrans-ferase	+	+	Behavioral abnormalities

*AR, autosomal recessive transmission; XR, X-linked recessive transmission.
Adapted from Leroy JC. Hereditary, development, and behavior. In: Levine MD, Carey WB, Crocker AC, eds. *Developmental-Behavioral Pediatrics.* Philadelphia: WB Saunders; 1983:315, with permission.

statistics from several major cities in the United States indicate that there is still no room for complacency.

Toxoplasmosis. Toxoplasmosis can be transmitted by the mother to the fetus. It causes mild or severe mental retardation and, in severe cases, hydrocephalus, seizures, microcephaly, and chorioretinitis.

Herpes Simplex. The herpes simplex virus can be transmitted transplacentally, although the most common mode of infection is during birth. Microcephaly, mental retardation, intracranial calcification, and ocular abnormalities may result.

Acquired Immunodeficiency Syndrome (AIDS). Many fetuses of mothers with AIDS never come to term because of stillbirth or spontaneous abortion. Of infants born infected with human immunodeficiency virus (HIV), half have progressive encephalopathy, mental retardation, and seizures within the first year of life. Children born with HIV infection often live only a few years; however, most infants born to HIV-infected mothers are not infected with the virus.

Fetal Alcohol Syndrome. Fetal alcohol syndrome results in mental retardation and a typical phenotypic picture of facial dysmorphism that includes hypertelorism; microcephaly; short palpebral fissures; inner epicanthal folds; and a short, turned-up nose. Often, affected children have learning disorders and ADHD. Cardiac defects are also frequent. The entire syndrome occurs in 15 percent of infants born to women who regularly ingest large amounts of alcohol. Infants born to women who consume alcohol regularly during pregnancy have a high incidence of ADHD, learning disorders, and mental retardation without the facial dysmorphism.

Prenatal Drug Exposure. Prenatal exposure to opioids, such as heroin, often results in infants who are small for gestational age, with a head circumference below the 10th percentile, and withdrawal symptoms that appear within the first 2 days of life. The withdrawal symptoms of infants include irritability, hypertonia, tremor, vomiting, a high-pitched cry, and an abnormal sleep pattern. Seizures are unusual, but the withdrawal syndrome can be life-threatening to infants if it is untreated. Diazepam (Valium), phenobarbital (Luminal), chlorpromazine (Thorazine), and paregoric have been used to treat neonatal opioid withdrawal.

The long-term sequelae of prenatal opioid exposure are not fully known; children's developmental milestones and intellectual functions may be within the normal range, but they have an increased risk for impulsivity and behavioral problems. Infants prenatally exposed to cocaine are at high risk for low birthweight and premature delivery. In the early neonatal period, they may have transient neurologic and behavioral abnormalities, including abnormal results on EEGs, tachycardia, poor feeding patterns, irritability, and excessive drowsiness. Rather than a withdrawal reaction, the physiologic and behavioral abnormalities are a response to the cocaine, which may be excreted for 1 week postnatally.

Complications of Pregnancy. Toxemia of pregnancy and uncontrolled maternal diabetes present hazards to the fetus and sometimes result in mental retardation. Maternal malnutrition during pregnancy often results in prematurity and other obstetric complications. Vaginal hemorrhage, placenta previa, premature separation of the placenta, and prolapse of the cord can damage the fetal brain by causing anoxia. The potential teratogenic effect of pharmacologic agents administered during pregnancy was widely publicized after the thalidomide tragedy (the drug produced a high percentage of deformed infants when given to pregnant women). So far, with the exception of metabolites used in cancer chemotherapy, no usual dosages of medications are known to damage the fetus's CNS, but caution and restraint in prescribing drugs to pregnant women are certainly indicated. The use of lithium during pregnancy was implicated more recently in some congenital malformations, especially of the cardiovascular system (e.g., Ebstein's anomaly).

Perinatal Period. Some evidence indicates that premature infants and infants with low birthweight are at high risk for neurologic and intellectual impairments that appear during their school years. Infants who sustain intracranial hemorrhages or show evidence of cerebral ischemia are especially vulnerable to cognitive abnormalities. The degree of neurodevelopmental impairment generally correlates with the severity of the intracranial hemorrhage. More recent studies have documented that, among children with very low birthweight (<1,000 g), 20% had significant disabilities, including cerebral palsy, mental retardation, autism, and low intelligence with severe learning problems. Very premature children and children who suffered intrauterine growth retardation were found to be at high risk for developing both social problems and academic difficulties. Socioeconomic deprivation can also affect the adaptive function of these vulnerable infants. Early intervention may improve cognitive, language, and perceptual abilities.

Acquired Childhood Disorders. Occasionally, a child's developmental status changes dramatically as a result of a specific disease or physical trauma. In retrospect, it is sometimes difficult to ascertain the full picture of the child's developmental progress before the insult, but the adverse effects on the child's development or skills are apparent afterward.

Infection. The most serious infections affecting cerebral integrity are encephalitis and meningitis. Measles encephalitis has been virtually eliminated by the universal use of measles vaccine, and the incidence of other bacterial infections of the CNS has been markedly reduced with antibacterial agents. Most episodes of encephalitis are caused by viruses. Sometimes a clinician must retrospectively consider a probable encephalitic component in a previous obscure illness with high fever.

Meningitis that was diagnosed late, even when followed by antibiotic treatment, can seriously affect a child's cognitive development. Thrombotic and purulent intracranial phenomena secondary to septicemia are rarely seen today except in small infants.

Head Trauma. The best-known causes of head injury in children that produces developmental handicaps, including seizures, are motor vehicle accidents, but more head injuries are caused by household accidents, such as falls from tables, from open windows, and on stairways. Child abuse also is a cause of head injury.

Other Issues. Brain damage from cardiac arrest during anesthesia is rare. One cause of complete or partial brain damage is asphyxia associated with near-drowning. Long-term exposure to lead is a well-established cause of compromised intelligence and learning skills. Intracranial tumors of various types and origins, surgery, and chemotherapy can also adversely affect brain function.

Environmental and Sociocultural Factors

Mild retardation can result from significant deprivation of nutrition and nurturance. Children who have endured these conditions are subject to long-lasting damage to their physical and emotional development. A prenatal environment compromised by poor medical care and poor maternal nutrition can be a contributing factor in the development of mild mental retardation. Teenage pregnancies are risk factors, and they are associated with obstetric complications, prematurity, and low birthweight. Poor postnatal medical care, malnutrition, exposure to toxic substances such as lead, and physical trauma are risk factors for mild mental retardation. Family instability, frequent moves, and multiple but inadequate caretakers may deprive an infant of necessary emotional relationships, leading to failure to thrive and potential risk to the developing brain.

An incapacitating mental disorder in a parent may interfere with appropriate child care and stimulation and cause developmental risk. Children of parents with mood disorders and schizophrenia are known to be at risk for these and related disorders. Some studies indicate a higher than expected prevalence of motor skills disorder and developmental disorders, but not mental retardation, among the children of parents with chronic mental disorders.

DIAGNOSIS

The diagnosis of mental retardation can be made after the history, a standardized intellectual assessment, and a measure of adaptive function indicate that a child's current behavior is significantly below the expected level (Table 2–3). The diagnosis itself does not specify either the cause or the prognosis. A history and psychiatric interview are useful in obtaining a longitudinal picture of the child's development and functioning, and examination of physical signs, neurologic abnormalities, and laboratory tests can be used to ascertain the cause and prognosis.

History

The history is most often obtained from the parents or the caretaker, with particular attention to the mother's pregnancy, labor, and delivery; the presence of a family history of mental retardation; consanguinity of the parents; and hereditary disorders. As part of the history, the clinician assesses the overall level of functioning and intellectual capacity of the parents and the emotional climate of the home.

Psychiatric Interview

Two factors are of paramount importance when interviewing the patient: the interviewer's attitude and manner of communicating. The interviewer should not be guided by the patient's mental age, which cannot fully characterize the person. A mildly retarded adult with a mental age of 10 is not a 10-year-old child.

Table 2–3
DSM-IV-TR Diagnostic Criteria for Mental Retardation

A. Significantly subaverage intellectual functioning: an IQ of approximately ≤70 on an individually administered IQ test (for infants, a clinical judgment of significantly subaverage intellectual functioning)
B. Concurrent deficits or impairments in present adaptive functioning (i.e., the person's effectiveness in meeting the standards expected for his or her age by his or her cultural group) in at least two of the following areas: communication, self-care, home living, social/interpersonal skills, use of community resources, self-direction, functional academic skills, work, leisure, health, and safety
C. The onset is before age 18 years

Code based on degree of severity reflecting level of intellectual impairment:

Mild mental retardation:	IQ level 50–55 to approximately 70
Moderate mental retardation:	IQ level 35–40 to 50–55
Severe mental retardation:	IQ level 20–25 to 35–40
Profound mental retardation:	IQ level <20 or 25
Mental retardation, severity unspecified:	When there is strong presumption of mental retardation but the person's intelligence is untestable by standard tests

From American Psychiatric Association. *Diagnostic and Statistical Manual of Mental Disorders.* 4th ed. Text rev. Washington, DC: American Psychiatric Association; 2000, with permission.

When addressed as if they were children, some retarded persons become justifiably insulted, angry, and uncooperative. Passive and dependent persons, alternatively, may assume the child's role that they think is expected of them. In neither case can valid diagnostic data be obtained.

The patient's verbal abilities, including receptive and expressive language, should be assessed as soon as possible by observing the communication between the caretakers and the patient and by taking the history. The clinician often finds it helpful to see the patient and the caretakers together. If the patient uses sign language, the caretaker may have to stay during the interview as an interpreter. Retarded persons often have the lifelong experience of failing in many areas, and they may be anxious about seeing an interviewer. The interviewer and the caretaker should attempt to give such patients a clear, supportive, concrete explanation of the diagnostic process, particularly patients with sufficiently receptive language. Patients should not be given the impression that their bad behavior is the cause of the referral. Support and praise should be offered in language appropriate to the patient's age and understanding. Leading questions should be avoided because retarded persons may be suggestible and wish to please others. Subtle direction, structure, and reinforcement may be necessary to keep them focused on the task or topic.

The patient's control over motility patterns should be ascertained, and clinical evidence of distractibility and distortions in perception and memory may be evaluated. The use of speech, reality testing, and the ability to generalize from experiences should be noted. The nature and maturity of the patient's defenses—particularly exaggerated or self-defeating uses of avoidance, repression, denial, introjection, and isolation—should be observed. Frustration, tolerance, and impulse control—especially over motor, aggressive, and sexual drives—should be assessed. Also important are self-image and its role in the development of self-confidence, and an assessment of tenacity, persistence, curiosity, and willingness to explore the unknown. Generally, the psychiatric examination of a retarded person should reveal how the patient has coped with the stages of development.

Physical Examination

Various parts of the body may have certain characteristics that have prenatal causes and are commonly found in persons who are mentally retarded. For example, the configuration and the size of the head offer clues to a variety of conditions, such as microcephaly, hydrocephalus, and Down syndrome. The patient's face may have some signs of mental retardation that greatly facilitate the diagnosis, such as hypertelorism, a flat nasal bridge, prominent eyebrows, epicanthal folds, corneal opacities, retinal changes, low-set and small or misshapen ears, a protruding tongue, and a disturbance in dentition. Facial expression, such as a dull appearance, can be misleading and should not be relied on without other supporting evidence. The color and texture of the skin and hair, a high-arched palate, the size of the thyroid gland, and the size of the child and his or her trunk and extremities should also be explored. The circumference of the head should be measured as part of the clinical investigation. Dermatoglyphics may offer another diagnostic tool because uncommon ridge patterns and flexion creases on the hand are often found in persons who are retarded. Abnormal dermatoglyphics occur in chromosomal disorders and in persons who were prenatally infected with rubella.

Table 2–4 lists the multiple handicaps associated with various mental retardation syndromes. The clinician should bear in mind during the examination that mentally retarded children, particularly children with associated behavioral problems, are at increased risk for child abuse.

Neurologic Examination

Sensory impairments occur frequently in persons who are mentally retarded; for example, 10 percent are hearing impaired, a rate that is four times that of the general population. Sensory disturbances include hearing difficulties, ranging from cortical deafness to mild hearing deficits, and visual disturbances, ranging from blindness to disturbances of spatial concepts, design recognition, and concepts of body image. Various other neurologic impairments also occur frequently in mentally retarded persons; seizure disorders occur in about 10 percent of all mentally retarded persons and in one third of those with severe retardation. When neurologic abnormalities are present, their incidence and severity generally increase in direct proportion to the degree of retardation. Many severely retarded children, however, have no neurologic abnormalities; conversely, about 25 percent of all children with cerebral palsy have normal intelligence. Disturbances in motor areas are manifested in abnormalities of muscle tone (spasticity or hypotonia), reflexes (hyperreflexia), and involuntary movements (choreoathetosis). Less disability is revealed in clumsiness and poor coordination.

Infants with the poorest prognoses are those who manifest a combination of inactivity, general hypotonia, and exaggerated response to stimuli. In older children, hyperactivity, short attention span, distractibility, and a low frustration tolerance are often signs of brain damage. In general, the younger the child at the time of investigation, the more caution is indicated in predicting future ability because the recovery potential of the infantile brain is very good. Observing the child's development at regular intervals is probably the most reliable approach.

Skull X-rays are usually taken routinely, but are illuminating in only a few conditions, such as craniosynostosis, hydrocephalus, and other disorders that result in intracranial calcifications (e.g., toxoplasmosis, tuberous sclerosis, cerebral angiomatosis, and hypoparathyroidism). Computed tomography (CT) scans and magnetic resonance imaging (MRI) have become important tools for uncovering CNS pathology associated with mental retardation. Occasionally, findings include internal hydrocephalus, cortical atrophy, or porencephaly in severely retarded, brain-damaged children.

Table 2–4
Representative Sample of Mental Retardation Syndromes and Behavioral Phenotypes

Disorder	Pathophysiology	Clinical Features and Behavioral Phenotype
Down syndrome	Trisomy 21, 95% nondisjunction, approximately 4% translocation; 1:1,000 live births: 1:2,500 in women <30 years old, 1:80 >40 years old, 1:32 at 45 years old; possible overproduction of β-amyloid due to defect at 21q21.1	Hypotonia, upward-slanted palpebral fissures, midface depression, flat wide nasal bridge, simian crease, short stature, increased incidence of thyroid abnormalities and congenital heart disease Passive, affable, hyperactivity in childhood, stubborn; verbal > auditory processing, increased risk of depression, and dementia of the Alzheimer type in adulthood
Fragile X syndrome	Inactivation of *FMR-1* gene at X q27.3 due to CGG base repeats, methylation; recessive; 1:1,000 male births, 1:3,000 female; accounts for 10–12% of mental retardation in males	Long face, large ears, midface hypoplasia, high arched palate, short stature, macroorchidism, mitral valve prolapse, joint laxity, strabismus Hyperactivity, inattention, anxiety, stereotypies, speech and language delays, IQ decline, gaze aversion, social avoidance, shyness, irritability, learning disorder in some females; mild mental retardation in affected females, moderate to severe in males; verbal IQ > performance IQ
Prader-Willi syndrome	Deletion in 15q12 (15q11–15q13) of paternal origin; some cases of maternal uniparental disomy; dominant 1:10,000 live births; 90% sporadic; candidate gene: small nuclear ribonucleoprotein polypeptide (SNRPN)	Hypotonia, failure to thrive in infancy, obesity, small hands and feet, microorchidism, cryptorchidism, short stature, almond-shaped eyes, fair hair and light skin, flat face, scoliosis, orthopedic problems, prominent forehead and bitemporal narrowing Compulsive behavior, hyperphagia, hoarding, impulsivity, borderline to moderate mental retardation, emotional lability, tantrums, excess daytime sleepiness, skin picking, anxiety, aggression
Angelman syndrome	Deletion in 15q12 (15q11–15q13) of maternal origin; dominant; frequent deletion of γ-aminobutyric acid (GABA) B-3 receptor subunit, prevalence unknown but rare, estimated 1:20,000–1:30,000	Fair hair and blue eyes (66%); dysmorphic faces including wide smiling mouth, thin upper lip, and pointed chin; epilepsy (90%) with characteristic EEG; ataxia; small head circumference, 25% microcephalic Happy disposition, paroxysmal laughter, hand flapping, clapping; profound mental retardation; sleep disturbance with nighttime waking; possible increased incidence of autistic features; anecdotal love of water and music
Cornelia de Lange syndrome	Lack of pregnancy associated plasma protein A (PAPPA) linked to chromosome 9q33; similar phenotype associated with trisomy 5p, ring chromosome 3; rare (1:40,000–1:100,000 live births); possible association with 3q26.3	Continuous eyebrows, thin downturning upper lip, microcephaly, short stature, small hands and feet, small upturned nose, anteverted nostrils, malformed upper limbs, failure to thrive Self-injury, limited speech in severe cases, language delays, avoidance of being held, stereotypic movements, twirling, severe to profound mental retardation
Williams syndrome	1:20,000 births; hemizygous deletion that includes elastin locus chromosome 7q11–23; autosomal dominant	Short stature, unusual facial features including broad forehead, depressed nasal bridge, stellate pattern of the iris, widely spaced teeth, and full lips; elfinlike facies; renal and cardiovascular abnormalities; thyroid abnormalities; hypercalcemia Anxiety, hyperactivity, fears, outgoing, sociable, verbal skills > visual spatial skills
Cri-du-chat syndrome	Partial deletion 5p; 1:50,000; region may be 5p15.2	Round face with hypertelorism, epicanthal folds, slanting palpebral fissures, broad flat nose, low-set ears, micrognathia; prenatal growth retardation; respiratory and ear infections; congenital heart disease; gastrointestinal abnormalities Severe mental retardation, infantile catlike cry, hyperactivity, stereotypies, self-injury
Smith-Magenis syndrome	Incidence unknown, estimated 1:25,000 live births; complete or partial deletion of 17p11.2	Broad face; flat midface; short, broad hands; small toes; hoarse, deep voice Severe mental retardation; hyperactivity; severe self-injury including hand biting, head banging, and pulling out fingernails and toenails; stereotyped self-hugging; attention seeking; aggression; sleep disturbance (decreased REM)

(*continued*)

Table 2–4 (Continued)

Disorder	Pathophysiology	Clinical Features and Behavioral Phenotype
Rubinstein-Taybi syndrome	1:250,000, approximately male = female; sporadic; likely autosomal dominant; documented microdeletions in some cases at 16p13.3	Short stature and microcephaly, broad thumb and big toes, prominent nose, broad nasal bridge, hypertelorism, ptosis, frequent fractures, feeding difficulties in infancy, congenital heart disease, EEG abnormalities, seizures Poor concentration, distractible, expressive language difficulties, performance IQ > verbal IQ; anecdotally happy, loving, sociable, responsive to music, self-stimulating behavior; older patients have mood lability and temper tantrums
Tuberous sclerosis complex 1 and 2	Benign tumors (hamartomas) and malformations (hamartias) of central nervous system (CNS), skin, kidney, heart; dominant; 1:10,000 births; 50% TSC 1, 9q34; 50% TSC 2, 16p13	Epilepsy, autism, hyperactivity, impulsivity, aggression; spectrum of mental retardation from none (30%) to profound; self-injurious behaviors, sleep disturbances
Neurofibromatosis type 1 (NF1)	1:2,500–1:4,000; male = female; autosomal dominant; 50% new mutations; >90% paternal NF1 allele mutated; *NF1* gene 17q11.2; gene product is neurofibromin thought to be tumor suppressor gene	Variable manifestations; café au lait spots, cutaneous neurofibromas, Lisch nodules; short stature and macrocephaly in 30–45% Half with speech and language difficulties; 10% with moderate to profound mental retardation; verbal IQ > performance IQ; distractible, impulsive, hyperactive, anxious; possibly associated with increased incidence of mood and anxiety disorders
Lesch-Nyhan syndrome	Defect in hypoxanthine guanine phosphoribosyltransferase with accumulation of uric acid; Xq26–27; recessive; rare (1:10,000–1:38,000)	Ataxia, chorea, kidney failure, gout Often severe self-biting behavior; aggression; anxiety; mild to moderate mental retardation
Galactosemia	Defect in galactose-1-phosphate uridyltransferase or galactokinase or empiramase; autosomal recessive; 1:62,000 births in the U.S.	Vomiting in early infancy, jaundice, hepatosplenomegaly; later cataracts, weight loss, food refusal, increased intracranial pressure and increased risk for sepsis, ovarian failure, failure to thrive, renal tubular damage Possible mental retardation even with treatment, visuospatial deficits, language disorders, reports of increased behavioral problems, anxiety, social withdrawal, and shyness
Phenylketonuria	Defect in phenylalanine hydroxylase (PAH) or cofactor (biopterin) with accumulation of phenylalanine; approximately 1:11,500 births; varies with geographic location; gene for PAH, 12q22–24.1; autosomal recessive	Symptoms absent neonatally, later development of seizures (25% generalized), fair skin, blue eyes, blond hair, rash Untreated: mild to profound mental retardation, language delay, destructiveness, self-injury, hyperactivity
Hurler's syndrome	1:100,000; deficiency in α-L-iduronidase activity; autosomal recessive	Early onset; short stature, hepatosplenomegaly; hirsutism, corneal clouding, death before age 10 years, dwarfism, coarse facial features, recurrent respiratory infections Moderate-to-severe mental retardation, anxious, fearful, rarely aggressive
Hunter's syndrome	1:100,000, X-linked recessive; iduronate sulfatase deficiency; X q28	Normal infancy; symptom onset at age 2–4 yrs; typical coarse faces with flat nasal bridge, flaring nostrils; hearing loss, ataxia, hernia common; enlarged liver and spleen, joint stiffness, recurrent infections, growth retardation, cardiovascular abnormality Hyperactivity, mental retardation by 2 yrs; speech delay; loss of speech at 8–10 yrs; restless, aggressive, inattentive, sleep abnormalities; apathetic, sedentary with disease progression
Fetal alcohol syndrome	Maternal alcohol consumption (trimester 3 > 2 > 1); 1:3,000 live births in Western countries; 1:300 with fetal alcohol effects	Microcephaly, short stature, midface hypoplasia, short palpebral fissure, thin upper lip, retrognathia in infancy, micrognathia in adolescence, hypoplastic long or smooth philtrum Mild to moderate mental retardation, irritability, inattention, memory impairment

Table courtesy of B. H. King, M.D., R. M. Hodapp, Ph.D., and E. M. Dykens, Ph.D.

An EEG is best interpreted with caution in cases of mental retardation. The exceptions are patients with hypsarrhythmia and grand mal seizures, in whom the EEG may help establish the diagnosis and suggest treatment. In most other conditions, a diffuse cerebral disorder produces nonspecific EEG changes, characterized by slow frequencies with bursts of spikes and sharp or blunt wave complexes. The confusion over the significance of the EEG in the diagnosis of mental retardation is best illustrated by the reports of frequent EEG abnormalities in Down syndrome, which are in the range of 25 percent in most patients examined.

CLINICAL FEATURES

Mild mental retardation may not be diagnosed until affected children enter school; their social skills and communication may be adequate in the preschool years. As they get older, however, cognitive deficits, such as poor ability to abstract and egocentric thinking, may distinguish them from others of their age. Although mildly retarded persons can function academically at the high elementary level, and their vocational skills suffice to support themselves in some cases, social assimilation can be difficult. Communication deficits, poor self-esteem, and dependence can contribute to their relative lack of social spontaneity. Some persons who are mildly retarded may fall into relationships with peers who exploit their shortcomings. In most cases, persons with mild mental retardation can achieve some social and vocational success in a supportive environment.

Moderate mental retardation is likely to be diagnosed at a younger age than mild mental retardation; communication skills develop more slowly in persons who are moderately retarded, and their social isolation may begin in the elementary school years. Although academic achievement is usually limited to the middle-elementary level, moderately retarded children benefit from individual attention focused on the development of self-help skills. Children with moderate mental retardation are aware of their deficits and often feel alienated from their peers and frustrated by their limitations. They continue to require a high level of supervision, but can become competent at occupational tasks in supportive settings.

Severe mental retardation is generally obvious in the preschool years; speech of affected children is minimal, and their motor development is poor. Some language development may occur in the school-age years. By adolescence, if language is poor, nonverbal forms of communication may have evolved; the inability to articulate needs fully may reinforce the physical means of communicating. Behavioral approaches can help promote some self-care, although individuals with severe mental retardation generally need extensive supervision.

Children with profound mental retardation require constant supervision and are severely limited in communication and motor skills. By adulthood, some speech development may be present, and simple self-help skills may be acquired. Even in adulthood, nursing care is needed.

Surveys have identified several clinical features that occur with greater frequency in persons who are mentally retarded than in the general population. These features, which can occur in isolation or as part of a mental disorder, include hyperactivity, low frustration tolerance, aggression, affective instability, repetitive and stereotypic motor behaviors, and various self-injurious behaviors. Self-injurious behaviors seem to be more frequent and more intense with increasingly severe mental retardation. It is often difficult to decide whether these clinical features are comorbid mental disorders or direct sequelae of the developmental limitations imposed by mental retardation.

Robert was a full-term infant, the last of three children born to his 38-year-old mother, a high school music teacher, and 40-year-old father, a high school science teacher. Pregnancy was unremarkable, and Robert's two older sisters were healthy and developing well. The family lived in a rural town in the Midwest.

Robert was an extremely fussy newborn and had extended periods of crying that the pediatrician labeled classic colic. At 2 months of age, the parents were told that Robert had a mild case of supravalvular aortic stenosis, one that warranted monitoring but no surgeries. Although Robert became slightly less fussy over time, he was a picky eater, refusing solid foods. Robert's parents also noted that he was more "high-strung" than his siblings, often quick to cry or cringe when his sisters played too loudly.

Milestones were slightly delayed, with Robert sitting unassisted at 10 months and walking at 18 months. Language was also delayed. Although his first words appeared at 20 months, Robert had always made his wants and needs known. Although his parents were concerned that he was delayed compared with his sisters, they were reassured by the pediatrician's sense that boys often had slight delays and that he was a lively, social boy who would quickly catch up.

When Robert was 3 years old, his parents insisted on a developmental evaluation, which showed modest delays in cognitive, linguistic, and motor functioning, with a developmental quotient (DQ) of 74. He was described as friendly and engaging, a real "charmer," with a cute face that endeared him to many. Robert was enrolled in a special kindergarten, and he remained in a combination of special education and mainstreamed classes throughout his academic career. Similar to his mother and sisters, Robert enjoyed listening to music and singing, and he took an active interest in tinkering on the piano.

When Robert was 7 years old, the school psychologist evaluated him and believed that he fit a "learning disability" profile. Robert had an overall IQ of 66, with close to average functioning in short-term memory and expressive language and pronounced deficits in long-term memory and expressive language and pronounced deficits in visual-spatial functioning. He struggled with writing tasks and arithmetic, but loved science and music and was amazingly conversant with anyone who would listen to him. Indeed, his parents feared he was "too friendly," as well as too active, and with transient, intense interests in unusual items, such as vacuum cleaners.

As he entered adolescence, Robert became increasingly anxious, so much so that he occasionally rubbed his hands or rocked, and he "fretted" about day-to-day issues and what would happen next. His long-term sensitivities to loud sounds seemed to wane slightly, but he developed fears of storm clouds and dogs and refused to ride on elevators. He became tearful and upset after one of his older sisters left for college and worried about her health and ability to watch the weather at college. Although Robert experienced nightmares and would occasionally pace with worry and complain of stomachaches, he attended school and had a small group of friends in the Special Olympics bowling league. He enjoyed singing with the high school chorus and was delighted to be routinely selected to play the piano at school concerts.

When Robert was 17 years old, his parents happened to watch a television documentary on Williams syndrome. They were overwhelmed by the similarities between Robert and the people described in the program. They later described the experience like a "jolt." They had always accepted Robert, quirks and all, and had stopped pushing their doctors for reasons "why" when Robert was a preschooler. Nevertheless, they immediately called the informational number offered in the show, and, within 2 months, they had the genetic tests done that confirmed their strong suspicion that Robert had Williams syndrome.

Although Robert's day-to-day life did not change dramatically since his diagnosis, his parents' report a big difference in Robert's outlook. He met new Williams syndrome friends at a conference, he applied to go to a summer music camp for young adults with Williams syndrome, and he states that he feels less alone. Robert's parents report a mixture of feelings at having such a late diagnosis—disappointment in their doctors, relief in finally knowing, and twinges of guilt. They are energized by having a new community of Williams syndrome families with whom to share their feelings and worries; similar to their son, they also feel less alone.

LABORATORY EXAMINATION

Laboratory tests used to elucidate the causes of mental retardation include chromosomal analysis, urine and blood testing for metabolic disorders, and neuroimaging. Chromosomal abnormalities are the most common cause of mental retardation found in individuals for whom a cause can be identified.

Chromosome Studies

The determination of the karyotype in a genetic laboratory is considered whenever a chromosomal disorder is suspected or when the cause of the mental retardation is unknown. Amniocentesis, in which a small amount of amniotic fluid is removed from the amniotic cavity transabdominally at about the 15th week of gestation, has been useful in diagnosing prenatal chromosomal abnormalities. Amniocentesis is often considered when an increased fetal risk exists, such as with increased maternal age. Amniotic fluid cells, mostly fetal in origin, are cultured for cytogenetic and biochemical studies. Many serious hereditary disorders can be predicted with amniocentesis, and it should be considered by pregnant women older than age 35.

Chorionic villi sampling (CVS) is a screening technique to determine fetal chromosomal abnormalities. It is done at 8 to 10 weeks of gestation, 6 weeks earlier than amniocentesis is done. The results are available in a short time (hours or days), and if the result is abnormal, the decision to terminate the pregnancy can be made within the first trimester. The procedure has a miscarriage risk between 2 and 5 percent; the risk in amniocentesis is lower (1 in 200).

Urine and Blood Analysis

Lesch-Nyhan syndrome, galactosemia, PKU, Hurler's syndrome, and Hunter's syndrome are examples of disorders that include mental retardation that can be identified through assays of the appropriate enzyme or organic or amino acids. Enzymatic abnormalities in chromosomal disorders, particularly Down syndrome, promise to become useful diagnostic tools. Unexplained growth abnormality, seizure disorder, poor muscle tone, ataxia, bone or skin abnormalities, and eye abnormalities are some indications for testing metabolic function.

Electroencephalography

Electroencephalography is indicated whenever a seizure disorder is suspected.

Neuroimaging

Neuroimaging studies are currently used to gather data that may uncover biologic mechanisms contributing to mental retardation syndromes. MRI, including structural MRI, functional MRI, and other forms of neuroimaging, is currently used by researchers seeking to identify specific etiologies of mental retardation syndromes. For example, current data suggest that individuals with fragile X syndrome who exhibit attentional deficits are also more likely to show aberrant frontal-striatal pathways seen on MRI. MRI can show abnormalities in the brain such as myelination patterns. MRI studies can also provide a baseline for comparison of a later, potentially degenerative process in the brain.

Hearing and Speech Evaluations

Hearing and speech should be evaluated routinely. Speech development may be the most reliable criterion in investigating mental retardation. Various hearing impairments often occur in persons who are mentally retarded, but in some instances impairments can simulate mental retardation. The commonly used methods of hearing and speech evaluation, however, require the patient's cooperation and, thus, are often unreliable in severely retarded persons.

Psychologic Assessment

Examining clinicians can use several screening instruments for infants and toddlers. As in many areas of mental retardation, the controversy over the predictive value of infant psychologic tests is heated. Some experts report the correlation of abnormalities during infancy with later abnormal functioning as very low, and others report it to be very high. The correlation increases in direct proportion to the age of the child at the time of the developmental examination; however, copying geometric figures, the *Goodenough Draw-a-Person Test,* the *Kohs Block Test,* and geometric puzzles all may be used as quick screening tests of visual-motor coordination.

Psychologic testing, performed by an experienced psychologist, is a standard part of an evaluation for mental retardation. The Gesell and Bayley scales and the *Cattell Infant Intelligence Scale* are most commonly used with infants. For children, the *Stanford-Binet Intelligence Scale* and the third edition of the *Wechsler Intelligence Scale for Children* (WISC-III) are the scales most widely used in the United States. Both tests have been criticized for penalizing culturally deprived children, for being culturally biased, for testing mainly the potential for academic achievement and not for adequate social functioning, and for their unreliability in children with IQs <50. Some clinicians have tried to overcome the language barrier of persons who are mentally retarded by devising picture vocabulary tests, of which the *Peabody Vocabulary Test* is the most widely used. The tests often found useful in detecting brain damage are the *Bender Gestalt Test* and the *Benton Visual Retention Test.* These tests are also useful for mildly retarded children. In addition, a psychologic evaluation should assess perceptual, motor, linguistic, and cognitive abilities. Information about motivational, emotional, and interpersonal factors is also important.

COURSE AND PROGNOSIS

In most cases of mental retardation, the underlying intellectual impairment does not improve, but the affected person's level of adaptation can be influenced positively by an enriched and supportive environment. In general, persons with mild and moderate mental retardation have the most flexibility in adapting to various environmental conditions. As in those who are not mentally retarded, the more comorbid mental disorders there are, the more guarded the overall prognosis. When clear-cut mental disorders are superimposed on mental retardation, standard treatments for the comorbid mental disorders are often beneficial. Yet, clarity about the classification of such aberrant behaviors as hyperactivity, emotional lability, and social dysfunction is still lacking.

DIFFERENTIAL DIAGNOSIS

By definition, mental retardation must begin before the age of 18. A mentally retarded child has to cope with so many difficult social and academic situations that maladaptive patterns often complicate the diagnostic process. Children whose family life provides inadequate stimulation may manifest motor and mental retardation that can be reversed if an enriched, stimulating environment is provided in early childhood. Several sensory disabilities, especially deafness and blindness, can be mistaken for mental retardation if no compensation is allowed during testing. Speech deficits and cerebral palsy often make a child seem retarded, even in the presence of borderline or normal intelligence. Chronic, debilitating diseases of any kind can depress a child's functioning in all areas. Convulsive disorders can give an impression of mental retardation, especially in the presence of uncontrolled seizures. Chronic brain syndromes can result in isolated handicaps—failure to read (alexia), failure to write (agraphia), failure to communicate (aphasia), and several others—that can exist in a person of normal and even superior intelligence. Children with learning disorders (which can coexist with mental retardation) experience a delay or failure of development in a specific area, such as reading or mathematics, but they develop normally in other areas. In contrast, children with mental retardation show general delays in most areas of development.

Mental retardation and pervasive developmental disorders often coexist; 70 to 75 percent of patients with pervasive developmental disorders have an IQ <70. A pervasive developmental disorder results in distortion of the timing, rate, and sequence of many basic psychologic functions necessary for social development. Because of their general level of functioning, children with pervasive developmental disorders have more problems with social relatedness and more deviant language than those with mental retardation. In mental retardation, generalized delays in development are present, and mentally retarded children behave in some ways as though they were passing through an earlier normal developmental stage, rather than one with completely aberrant behavior.

A difficult differential diagnostic problem concerns children with severe mental retardation, brain damage, autistic disorder, schizophrenia with childhood onset, or, according to some, Heller's disease. The confusion stems from details of the child's early history that are often unavailable or unreliable. In addition, when the children are evaluated, many with these conditions display similar bizarre and stereotyped behavior—mutism, echolalia, or functioning on a retarded level. By the time the children are usually seen, it does not matter from a practical point of view whether their retardation is secondary to a primary early infantile autistic disorder or schizophrenia, or whether the personality and behavioral distortions are secondary to brain damage or mental retardation. In a recent epidemiologic study, pervasive developmental disorders (such as autistic disorder) were found in 19.8% of children with mental retardation.

Children younger than 18 years who meet the diagnostic criteria for dementia and who have an IQ <70 are given the diagnoses of dementia and mental retardation. Individuals whose IQs become <70 after age 18 years and who have new onsets of cognitive disorders are not given the diagnosis of mental retardation but only the diagnosis of dementia.

TREATMENT

The treatment of individuals with mental retardation is based on an assessment of social, educational, psychiatric, and environmental need. Mental retardation is associated with a variety of comorbid psychiatric disorders that often require specific treatment, in addition to psychosocial support. When preventive measures are available, optimal treatment of conditions that could lead to mental retardation include primary, secondary, and tertiary prevention.

Primary Prevention

Primary prevention concerns actions taken to eliminate or reduce the conditions that lead to development of the disorders associated with mental retardation. Such measures include education to increase the general public's knowledge and awareness of mental retardation, continuing efforts of health professionals to ensure and upgrade public health policies, legislation to provide optimal maternal and child health care, and eradication of the known disorders associated with CNS damage. Family and genetic counseling helps reduce the incidence of mental retardation in a family with a history of a genetic disorder associated with mental retardation. For children and mothers of low socioeconomic status, proper prenatal and postnatal medical care and various supplementary enrichment programs and social service assistance may help minimize medical and psychosocial complications.

Secondary and Tertiary Prevention

When a disorder associated with mental retardation has been identified, the disorder should be treated to shorten the course of the illness (secondary prevention) and to minimize the sequelae or consequent disabilities (tertiary prevention). Hereditary metabolic and endocrine disorders, such as PKU and hypothyroidism, can be treated effectively in an early stage by dietary control or hormone replacement therapy. Mentally retarded children frequently have emotional and behavioral difficulties requiring psychiatric treatment. Their limited cognitive and social capabilities require modified psychiatric treatment modalities based on their level of intelligence.

Education for the Child. Educational settings for children who are mentally retarded should include a comprehensive program that addresses training in adaptive skills, social skills, and vocation. Particular attention should focus on communication and efforts to improve the quality of life. Group therapy has often been a successful format in which mentally retarded children can learn and practice hypothetical real-life situations and receive supportive feedback.

Behavioral, Cognitive, and Psychodynamic Therapies. The difficulties in adaptation among mentally retarded persons are widespread and so varied that several interventions alone or in combination may be beneficial. Behavioral therapy has been used for many years to shape and enhance social behaviors and to control and minimize aggressive and destructive behaviors. Positive reinforcement for desired behaviors and benign punishment (e.g., loss of privileges) for objectionable behaviors have been helpful. Cognitive therapy, such as dispelling false beliefs and relaxation exercises with self-instruction, has also been recommended for mentally retarded persons who can follow the instructions. Psychodynamic therapy has been used with patients and their families to decrease conflicts about expectations that result in persistent anxiety, rage, and depression.

Family Education. One of the most important areas that a clinician can address is educating the family of a mentally retarded patient about ways to enhance competence and self-esteem, while maintaining realistic expectations for the patient. The family often finds it difficult to balance the fostering of independence and the providing of a nurturing and supportive environment for a mentally retarded child, who is likely to experience some rejection and failure outside the family context. The parents may benefit from continuous counseling or family therapy and should be allowed opportunities to express their feelings of guilt, despair, anguish, recurring denial, and anger about their child's disorder and future. The psychiatrist should be prepared to give the parents all the basic and current medical information regarding causes, treatment, and other pertinent areas (e.g., special training and the correction of sensory defects). Table 2–5 lists some important needs of families of children with mental retardation and resources for them.

Social Intervention. One of the most prevalent problems among persons who are mentally retarded is a sense of social isolation and social skills deficits. Thus, improving the quantity and quality of social competence is a critical part of their care. Special Olympics International is the largest recreational sports program geared for this population. In addition to providing a forum to develop physical fitness, Special Olympics enhances social interactions, friendships, and (it is hoped) general self-esteem. A recent study confirmed positive effects of the Special Olympics on the social competence of the mentally retarded adults who participated.

Pharmacology. Pharmacologic approaches to the treatment of behavioral and psychologic symptoms in mentally retarded patients are much the same as for patients who are not mentally retarded. Increasing data support the use of a variety of medications for patients with mental disorders who are not mentally retarded, and some studies have focused on the use of medications for the following behavioral syndromes that are frequent among persons who are mentally retarded.

COMMON COMORBID PSYCHIATRIC DISORDERS

Attention-Deficit/Hyperactivity Disorder. Studies of methylphenidate (Ritalin) treatment in mildly retarded patients with ADHD have shown significant improvement in the ability to maintain

Table 2–5
Service Needs and Resources for Families of Disabled Children at Different Ages

	Needs	Resources
Age 0–3 yrs		
Child	Evaluation: physical, motor, cognitive, linguistic, social-emotional; early intervention services	Multidisciplinary evaluation, which results in an Individualized Family Service Plan (IFSP), with child and family receiving either center- or home-based early intervention services for a set number of hours per week
Mother	Emotional support, caregiving behaviors	Support groups by disability, region, and etiology; part of early intervention evaluation, intervention, and IFSP
Family	Support, financial assistance, information	Support groups; depending on problem, state of developmental disabilities or insurance payment for some services; hospitals, agencies, groups
Age 3–21 yrs		
Child	Evaluation, referral, and Individualized Educational Program (IEP)	School system: involves legal process of evaluation and placement (notification, hearings, appeals if necessary); information on transition to adult services as child nears age 21 (and school services end)
Family	Information, financial assistance, support	Local and national groups; state departments in some states; includes respite care, camps, art (Very Special Arts) or athletic activities (Special Olympics), scholarships for adolescents with some disabilities (deafness, blindness)
>21 yrs		
Offspring	Residential services, work	Both run by state developmental disability departments (parents and offspring have major say concerning whether residential or work placements are appropriate)
Family	Support, information, guardianship issues	Continuation of many of the services provided during the school years; particularly for individuals with severe disabilities, provisions for residential and work status after parents can no longer serve as legal guardians

Adapted from Hodapp RD. *Development and Disabilities.* New York: Cambridge University Press; 1998, with permission.

attention and to stay focused on tasks. Methylphenidate treatment studies have not shown evidence of long-term improvement in social skills or learning. In a treatment study of ADHD in a group of children and adolescents with moderate mental retardation, risperidone (Risperdal) was compared with methylphenidate with respect to reduction of impulsivity and short attention span. Risperidone was found to be highly beneficial in reducing symptoms of ADHD in this population. In another large open study, 500 children with disruptive behavior disorders and mental retardation treated with risperidone at a mean dose of 1.6 mg per day for 1 year showed improvement and tolerated the medication well. They concluded that adverse events at this dose of medication were mild, and the only clinically relevant laboratory test change was an increase in serum prolactin level. Although risperidone has been shown to be associated with significant symptom reduction of hyperactivity and disruptive behavior, and in general, adverse events during a year of treatment were mild, given its side-effect profile compared with methylphenidate, it is still prudent to begin with a trial of a stimulant medication before the use of antipsychotic preparations for the treatment of ADHD.

Aggression and Self-Injurious Behavior. There are few well-controlled clinical trials to guide optimal treatment of aggression and self-injurious behavior. Some evidence from controlled and uncontrolled studies indicates that lithium (Eskalith) has been useful in decreasing aggression and self-injurious behavior. Narcotic antagonists such as naltrexone have not been systematically shown to diminish aggression or self-injurious behaviors. Anticonvulsants, such as carbamazepine (Tegretol) and valproic acid (Depakene), have been used clinically for aggressive behavior in children and adolescents. Double-blind, placebo-controlled studies in mentally retarded adults and open clinical trials in mentally retarded children and adolescents have indicated that risperidone is efficacious in decreasing aggression and self-injurious behavior. Persons with mental retardation seem to be at higher risk for the development of tardive dyskinesia after use of a variety of antipsychotic medications. The atypical antipsychotics, including risperidone and clozapine (Clozaril), may provide some relief with a decreased risk of tardive dyskinesia.

Depressive Disorders. The diagnosis of depressive disorders among individuals with mental retardation may be overlooked when behavioral problems are prominent, and the need for antidepressant treatment for individuals with mental retardation may be underestimated. Some clinicians have reported disinhibition in response to serotonin reuptake inhibitors (e.g., fluoxetine [Prozac], paroxetine, sertraline [Zoloft]) in mentally retarded individuals who also have a diagnosis of pervasive developmental disorder. In general, given the relative safety of these medications, their use is indicated when a depressive disorder is diagnosed.

Table 2–6
Prominent Organizations in Mental Retardation*

The Association of Retarded Citizens of the United States
1010 Wayne Avenue
Suite 650
Silver Spring, MD 20910

American Association on Mental Retardation (AAMR)
1710 Kalorama Road, NW
Washington, DC 20009-2683
(800) 424-3688

Council for Exceptional Children (CEC)
1920 Association Drive
Reston, VA 22091-1589

American Association of University-Affiliated Programs for Persons with Developmental Disabilities
8630 Fenton Street, Suite 410
Silver Spring, MD 20910

TASH: The Association for People with Severe Handicaps
1025 Vermont Avenue
NW 7th floor
Washington, DC 2005
(202) 263-5600

CAPP National Parent Resource Center Federation for Children with Special Needs
95 Berkeley Street, Suite 104
Boston, MA 02116

National Information Center for Children and Youth with Disabilities
P.O. Box 1492
Washington, DC 20013
(800) 695-0285

National Organization for Rare Disorders (NORD)
100 Route 37
P.O. Box 8923
New Fairfield, CT 06812

Alliance of Genetic Support Groups
4301 Connecticut Avenue
NW Suite 404
Washington, DC 2008
(202) 966-5557

Sibling Information Network
1775 Ellington Road
South Windsor, CT 07074
(203) 648-1205

Resources for Children with Special Needs, Inc.
200 Park Avenue South, Suite 816
New York, NY 10003
(212) 677-4650

National Down Syndrome Society
666 Broadway
New York, NY 10012
(800) 221-4602

National Down Syndrome Congress
1800 Dempster Street
Park Ridge, IL 60068
(800) 232-6372

National Fragile X Syndrome Foundation
1441 York Street, Suite 215
Denver, CO 80206

The Prader-Willi Syndrome Association
8588 Potter Park Drive
Suite 500
Sarasota, FL 34238
(941) 312-0400

Williams Syndrome Association
P.O. Box 297
Clawson, MI 48017-0297
(248) 244-2229

*Accurate as of June 2008.

Stereotypical Motor Movements. Antipsychotic medications, such as haloperidol (Haldol) and chlorpromazine, decrease repetitive self-stimulatory behaviors in mentally retarded patients, but these medications have not increased adaptive behavior. Some mentally retarded children and adults (up to one third) face a high risk for tardive dyskinesia with the continued use of antipsychotic medications. Obsessive-compulsive symptoms often overlap with the repetitive stereotypical behaviors seen in mentally retarded children and adolescents and in those with mental retardation and a pervasive developmental disorder. Serotonin reuptake inhibitors, such as fluoxetine, fluvoxamine (Luvox), paroxetine, and sertraline, have been shown to have efficacy in treating obsessive-compulsive symptoms in children and adolescents and may have some efficacy for stereotyped motor movements.

Explosive Rage Behavior. β-adrenergic receptor antagonists (beta-blockers), such as propranolol (Inderal), reportedly result in fewer explosive rages in patients with mental retardation and autistic disorder. Antipsychotic medications have also been used in the treatment of explosive rage. Systematic controlled studies are indicated to confirm the efficacy of these drugs in the treatment of rage outbursts.

SERVICES AND SUPPORT FOR CHILDREN WITH MENTAL RETARDATION

Early Intervention

Early intervention programs serve individuals for the first 3 years of life. Such services are generally provided by the state and begin with a specialist visiting the home for several hours per week. Since the passage of Public Law 99-447, the Education of the Handicapped Amendments of 1986, early intervention services for the entire family are emphasized. Agencies are required to develop an Individualized Family Service Plan (IFSP) for each family identifying specific interventions to help the family and child best.

School

From age 3 years until 21 years, school is responsible by law to provide appropriate educational services to children with mental retardation. These mandates were created by the passage of Public Law 94-142, the Education for all Handicapped Children Act of 1975, and expanded with the addition of the Individuals with Disabilities Act (IDEA) of 1990. Through these two laws, public schools must develop and provide an individualized educational program for each student with mental retardation, determined at a meeting designated as the Individualized Education Plan (IEP) with school personnel and the family. The educational plan must be provided for the child in the "least restrictive environment" that would allow the child an education.

Supports

A wide variety of organized groups and services are available for children with mental retardation and their families. These include short-term respite care, allowing families a break, generally set up by state agencies. Other programs include the Special Olympics, which allows children with mental retardation to participate in team sports and in sports competitions. Many organizations (Table 2–6) also exist for families who wish to connect with others who have children with mental retardation syndromes.

Reference

Rett Syndrome fact sheet. National Institute of Neurological Disorders and Stroke. NIH Publication No. 04-4863.

3 Learning Disorders

Learning disorders in a child or adolescent are characterized by academic underachievement in reading, written expression, or mathematics in comparison with the overall intellectual ability of the child. Children with learning disorders often find it difficult to keep up with their peers in certain academic subjects, whereas they excel in others. Learning disorders affect at least 5 percent of school-age children. This represents approximately half of all public school children who receive special education services in the United States. In 1975, Public Law 94-142 (the Education for All Handicapped Children Act) mandated all states to provide free and appropriate educational services to all children. Since that time, the number of children identified with learning disorders has increased, and a variety of definitions of learning disabilities has arisen. The term *learning disorders,* formally referred to as *academic skills disorders,* was introduced by the fourth edition of the *Diagnostic and Statistical Manual of Mental Disorders* (DSM-IV). To meet the criteria for a diagnosis of learning disorder, a child's achievement in the particular learning area must be significantly lower than expected, and the learning problems interfere with academic achievement or activities of daily living.

The most recent revised version of the DSM-IV (DSM-IV-TR) includes four diagnostic categories of learning disorders: reading disorder, mathematics disorder, disorder of written expression, and learning disorder not otherwise specified. Children with a learning disorder, such as reading disorder, can be identified in two different ways: children who read poorly compared with most other children of the same age and children whose achievement in reading is significantly lower than their overall IQ would predict. DSM-IV-TR criteria for learning disorders require a substantial IQ–achievement discrepancy and significantly poor achievement in reading compared with that of most children of the same age. Research studies have led to questions regarding inclusion of an IQ–achievement discrepancy component in the definition of a learning disorder because current data suggest that most children with reading disorders, for example, have similar deficits in phonologic processing skills, regardless of their IQ. That is, most children with reading disorders have trouble with word recognition and "sounding out" words because they cannot understand and use phonemes, the smaller bits of words that are associated with particular sounds.

READING DISORDER

Reading disorders are present in approximately 75 percent of children and adolescents with learning disorders. Students who have learning problems in other academic areas most commonly experience difficulties with reading as well.

Reading disorder is defined as reading achievement below the expected level for a child's age, education, and intelligence, with the impairment interfering significantly with academic success or the daily activities that involve reading. According to DSM-IV-TR, if a neurologic condition or sensory disturbance is present, the reading disability exhibited exceeds that usually associated with the other condition.

Reading disorder is characterized by an impaired ability to recognize words, slow and inaccurate reading, and poor comprehension. In addition, children with attention-deficit/hyperactivity disorder (ADHD) are at high risk for reading disorder. Historically, many different labels have been used to describe reading disabilities, including word blindness, reading backward, learning disability, alexia, and developmental word blindness. The term *developmental alexia* was accepted and defined as a developmental deficit in the recognition of printed symbols. This term was simplified by adopting the term *dyslexia* in the 1960s. Dyslexia was used extensively for many years to describe a reading disability syndrome that often included speech and language deficits and right-left confusion.

Epidemiology

An estimated 4 percent of school-age children in the United States have reading disorder; prevalence studies find rates ranging between 2 and 8 percent. Three to four times as many boys as girls are reported to have reading disability in clinically referred samples. Careful epidemiologic studies have found closer to equal rates of reading disorder among boys and girls. Boys with reading disorder may be referred for evaluation more often than girls because of frequently associated behavior problems. No clear gender differential is seen among adults who report reading difficulties.

Comorbidity

Children with reading disorder are at higher than average risk for attentional problems, disruptive behavior disorders, and depressive disorders, particularly older children and adolescents. Data suggest that 25 percent of children with reading disorder also have ADHD. Conversely, it is estimated that between 15 and 30 percent of children diagnosed with ADHD have a learning disorder. Although these disorders frequently occur concurrently, they are distinct conditions and require separate interventions. Family studies indicate, however, that in some cases, ADHD and reading disorder may be genetically transmitted together. That is, some common genetic factors are producing both reading disorder and attentional syndromes. Some evidence also suggests that higher than random incidence of aggressive behavior is present in young children with reading disorders. In samples of children and adolescents with conduct disorders, reading disorder was more frequent than expected. Children with reading disorders experience higher levels of anxiety symptoms than children without learning disorders. Furthermore, children with reading disorders tend to be at increased risk for problematic peer relationships and have less skills responding to subtle social cues.

Etiology

Data from cognitive, neuroimaging, and genetic studies indicate that reading disorder is most accurately described as a neurobiologic disorder with a genetic origin. It is currently believed to reflect a deficiency in processing sounds of spoken language. That is, children who struggle with reading have a deficit in phonologic processing skills. These children cannot identify effectively the parts of words that denote specific sounds, which leads to grave difficulty in recognizing and sounding out words. Children with reading disorders are slower than average in naming letters and numbers, even when controlling for IQ. Thus, the core deficit for children with reading disorders lies within the domain of language use.

Given that reading disorder is essentially a language deficit, the left brain has been hypothesized to be the anatomic site of the dysfunction. Several research studies using magnetic resonance imaging (MRI) studies have suggested that the planum temporale in the left brain shows less asymmetry than the same site in the right brain in children with language and learning disorders. Positron emission tomographic (PET) studies have led some researchers to conclude that left temporal blood flow patterns during language tasks differ between children with and without learning disorders. Also, some cell analysis studies suggest that in reading-disordered persons, the visual magnocellular system (which normally contains large cells) contains more disorganized and smaller cell bodies than expected. None of the aforementioned studies provide conclusive evidence regarding brain differences between individuals with reading disorder and individuals without reading disorder.

Many studies support the hypothesis that genetic factors play a major role in the presence of reading disorders. Studies indicate that 35 to 40 percent of first-degree relatives of children with reading disorder also have some reading disability. Several more recent studies have suggested that phonologic awareness (i.e., the ability to decode sounds and sound out words) is linked to chromosome 6. Furthermore, the ability to identify single words has been linked to chromosome 15. Impairment in reading and spelling has now been linked to susceptibility loci on multiple chromosomes, including chromosomes 1, 2, 3, 6, 15, and 18. Although a recent research study identified a locus on chromosome 18 as a strong influence on single-word reading and phoneme awareness, generalist genes have also been implicated as responsible for learning disorders. Many genes associated with common learning disorders, such as reading disability, mathematics impairment, and language disorders, are believed to be generalists in the following ways. First, genes that affect common learning disorders may also influence normal variation in learning abilities. In addition, genes that affect one learning disorder are also more likely to affect other learning disorders.

Several historic hypotheses about the origin of reading disorders are now known to be untrue. The first myth is that reading disorders are primarily caused by visual-motor problems, or what has been termed *scotopic sensitivity syndrome*. No evidence indicates that children with reading disorders have visual problems or difficulties with their visual-motor system. The second theory with no supporting evidence is that allergies can cause, or contribute to, reading disabilities. Finally, unsubstantiated theories have implicated the cerebellar–vestibular system as the source of reading disorder.

Research in the fields of cognitive neuroscience and neuropsychology supports the hypothesis that encoding processes and working memory, rather than attention or long-term memory, are areas of weakness for children with reading disorder. Developmental factors have been hypothesized to play a role in reading disorders. Another recent study found an association between dyslexia and birth in the months of May, June, and July, which suggests that prenatal exposure to a maternal infectious illness, such as influenza, in the winter months may contribute to reading disorder. Studies in the 1930s attempted to explain reading disorder according to the cerebral hemispheric function model, which suggested positive correlations of reading disorder with left-handedness, left-eyedness, or mixed laterality. Subsequent epidemiologic studies did not find any consistent association between reading disorder and laterality of handedness or eyedness, but right-left confusion has been shown to be associated with reading difficulties.

Complications during pregnancy and prenatal and perinatal difficulties are common in the histories of children with reading disorder. Extremely low birthweight and severely premature children are at higher risk for reading disorder and other learning disorders than children who are born full term and have normal birthweight. A recent study reviewed the relationship between critical periods for brain growth and infants born significantly preterm. Children who are born very preterm who attend mainstream schools have been noted to be at increased risk of minor motor, behavioral, and learning disorders. These disorders appear to be associated with postnatal growth, particularly of the head. Although intrauterine growth retardation may play a role in compromised intellectual capacity, interventions that aim to improve motor ability and potentially learning disorders should focus on optimal nutrition and care postnatally.

A higher than average incidence of reading disorder occurs among children of normal intelligence who have cerebral palsy, and epileptic children exhibit a slightly increased incidence of reading disorder. Children with postnatal brain lesions in the left occipital lobe, which results in right visual-field blindness, may have secondary reading disorder, as may children with lesions in the splenium of the corpus callosum that blocks transmission of visual information from the intact right hemisphere to the language areas of the left hemisphere.

Data have documented an association of developmental delays and learning disabilities in fetal alcohol syndrome. Recent evidence suggests that certain peptides, such as those derived from activity-dependent neurotrophic factor-12, may mitigate alcohol-induced fetal death and developmental learning disabilities. This demonstrates that a single treatment with a peptide may be efficacious in preventing and mitigating alcohol-induced fetal damage. Other studies suggest an association between malnutrition and subsequent reading disorder. Children who were malnourished for long periods during early childhood are at increased risk of subaverage performance in many cognitive areas, including reading. Their cognitive performances appear to be lower than those of siblings who were not subjected to the same degree of malnutrition.

Diagnosis

Reading disorder is diagnosed when a child's reading achievement is significantly below that expected of a child of the same age and intellectual capacity (Table 3–1). Characteristic diagnostic features include difficulty recalling, evoking, and sequencing printed letters and words; processing sophisticated grammatical constructions; and making inferences. Clinically, a child may be first identified with a reading disorder after becoming demoralized or exhibiting symptoms of depression related to being unable to succeed in school. School failure and ensuing poor self-esteem can exacerbate the problems as the child becomes more consumed with a sense of failure and spends less time focusing on academic work. Students suspected of having reading disorders are entitled to an educational evaluation through the school district to determine eligibility for special education services. Special education classification, however, is not uniform across states or regions, and students with identical reading difficulties may be eligible for services in one region, but ineligible in another. In some cases, an evaluation is requested on the basis of disruptive behavioral problems that occur in conjunction with the reading disorder.

Table 3–1
DSM-IV-TR Diagnostic Criteria for Reading Disorder

A. Reading achievement, as measured by individually administered standardized tests of reading accuracy or comprehension, is substantially below that expected given the person's chronologic age, measured intelligence, and age-appropriate education.

B. The disturbance in Criterion A significantly interferes with academic achievement or activities of daily living that require reading skills.

C. If a sensory deficit is present, the reading difficulties are in excess of those usually associated with it.

Coding note: If a general medical (e.g., neurologic) condition or sensory deficit is present, code the condition on Axis III.

From American Psychiatric Association. *Diagnostic and Statistical Manual of Mental Disorders.* 4th ed. Text rev. Washington, DC: American Psychiatric Association; copyright 2000, with permission.

Clinical Features

Children who have reading disorder can usually be identified by the age of 7 years (second grade). Reading difficulty may be apparent among students in classrooms where reading skills are expected in the first grade. Children can sometimes compensate for reading disorder in the early elementary grades by the use of memory and inference, particularly when the disorder is associated with high intelligence. In such instances, the disorder may not be apparent until age 9 (fourth grade) or later. Children with reading disorder make many errors in their oral reading. The errors are characterized by omissions, additions, and distortions of words. Such children have difficulty in distinguishing between printed letter characters and sizes, especially those that differ only in spatial orientation and length of line. The problems in managing printed or written language can pertain to individual letters, sentences, and even a page. The child's reading speed is slow, often with minimal comprehension. Most children with reading disorder have an age-appropriate ability to copy from a written or printed text, but nearly all spell poorly.

Associated problems include language difficulties, exhibited often as impaired sound discrimination and difficulty in sequencing words properly. A child with disorders may start a word either in the middle or at the end of a printed or written sentence. At times, because of a poorly established left-right tracking sequence, such children transpose letters to be read. Failures in both memory recall and sustained elicitation result in poor recall of letter names and sounds.

Most children with reading disorder dislike and avoid reading and writing. Their anxiety is heightened when they are confronted with demands that involve printed language. Many children with the disorder who do not receive remedial education have a sense of shame and humiliation because of their continuing failure and subsequent frustration. These feelings grow more intense with time. Older children tend to be angry and depressed and exhibit poor self-esteem.

Jason, an 11-year-old boy, was referred for evaluation of increasing problems at school, including failing to complete in-class assignments and homework; failing tests in reading, spelling, and arithmetic; skipping classes; and some truancy. For the past 2 years (grades 5 and 6), he had been attending a special education class every morning in the local community school, based on placement recommendations from a prior assessment when he was in grade 2. At that time, he did not meet DSM-IV-TR criteria for any externalizing disorder, but was not doing well in school, and a specific learning disorder was queried. A subsequent psychoeducational assessment by a clinical psychologist confirmed reading problems, but he did not meet the school board's criteria for learning disorder, which was based on IQ–achievement discrepancy. Thus, he was not eligible for special education services. A change in the following year in the school board's policy regarding the need for a discrepancy-based definition of learning disorder meant that Jason was now eligible for special education, whereupon he started attending the half-day program. He was in a class with eight other students ranging from 6 to 12 years of age.

Clinical interview with his parents revealed a normal pregnancy, but a history of language delay. In preschool and kindergarten, he was reported to have had difficulty with rhyming games and showed a marked lack of interest in books and preferred to play with construction toys. In the primary grades, he had more difficulty learning to read than other boys in his class and continued to have problems pronouncing multisyllabic words (e.g., he said "aminals" for "animals" and "sblanation" for "explanation"). Family history was positive for reading disorder and ADHD. Specifically, Jason's father admitted a history of reading problems but commented that, although he still cannot read too well (and never for pleasure), he runs a successful business. The older brother, 15 years of age, had ADHD, which was responding fairly well to stimulant medication. The parents' main concern was that Jason seemed to "be getting just like his brother and not focusing on school work," and they queried whether he also had ADHD. In the clinical interview with Jason, it was noted that he rarely made eye contact with the clinician, mumbled a lot, and struggled to find the right word (e.g., manifested many false starts, hesitations, and nonspecific terms, such as "the thing that you draw . . . um . . . pencil—no . . . um . . . lines with"). He admitted to skipping class and sometimes school, adding the comment: "Reading is boring and stupid—I'd rather be cycling." He also complained about the amount of reading he had to do—even in math—and commented, "Reading takes so much time. By the time I figure out a word, I can't 'member what I just read and so have to read the stuff again."

Psychologic and psychoeducational assessment included the *Wechsler Intelligence Scale for Children–IV, Clinical Evaluation of Language Fundamentals–IV* (CELF-IV), and the *Wechsler Individual Achievement Test–II*, and self-ratings of anxiety, depression, and self-esteem. Results indicated low-average verbal and above-average performance IQ, poor word attack and word identification skills (below 12th percentile), poor comprehension (below 9th percentile), poor spelling (below 6th percentile), weak comprehension of oral language (below 16th percentile), elevated but subthreshold scores on the *Children's Depression Inventory*, and low self-esteem. Although Jason manifested several marked symptoms of inattention, some restlessness, and oppositional behavior (particularly at school), he did not meet criteria for ADHD or any other internalizing or externalizing disorder. However, he did meet DSM-IV-TR criteria for reading disorder and receptive-expressive language disorders. Comparison with results from the previous psychoeducational assessment revealed that, although he had made some small gains, he had not closed the gap between his reading skills and those of his peers, despite being in special education for 2 years. Recommendations included continuation in special education plus attendance at a summer camp specializing in children with reading disorder as well as ongoing monitoring of self-esteem and depressive traits.

At 1-year follow-up, Jason and his parents reported striking improvements in his reading, overall school performance, mood, and self-esteem, which they attributed to the specialized instruction provided during the summer camp. The program had provided one-on-one focused and explicit instruction for 1 hour a day for a total of 70 hours. Jason explained that he had been taught a set of specific decoding strategies to use in a systematic way ("like a game plan") and challenged the clinician to give him a "really tough long word to read." He demonstrated the strategies that he used to read the word "unconditionally" and also explained what it meant. To boost his fluency in reading and reading comprehension, the clinical team recommended the use of repeated reading, reading along with audiotaped (unabridged) versions of his favorite books, use of graphic organizers to facilitate reading for comprehension, and further participation in the summer camp reading program. (Courtesy of Rosemary Tannock, Ph.D.)

Pathology and Laboratory Examination

No specific physical signs or laboratory measures are helpful in the diagnosis of reading disorder. Psychoeducational testing, however, is critical in determining this diagnosis. The diagnosis of reading disorder is made after collecting data from a standardized intelligence test and an educational assessment of achievement. The diagnostic battery generally includes a standardized spelling test, written composition, processing and using oral language, design copying, and judgment of the adequacy of pencil use. The reading subtests of the *Woodcock-Johnson Psycho-Educational Battery–Revised* and the *Peabody Individual Achievement Test–Revised* are useful in identifying reading disability. A screening projective battery may include human-figure drawings, picture-story tests, and sentence completion. The evaluation should also include systematic observation of behavioral variables.

Course and Prognosis

Many children with reading disorder gain some knowledge of printed language during their first 2 years in grade school, even without any remedial assistance. By the end of the first grade, many children with reading disorder, in fact, have learned how to read a few words; however, by the time a child with a reading disorder reaches the third grade, keeping up with classmates is exceedingly difficult without remedial educational intervention. In the best circumstances, a child is recognized as being at risk for a reading disorder during the kindergarten year or early in the first grade. When remediation is instituted early, in milder cases, it is no longer necessary by the end of the first or second grade. In severe cases and depending on the pattern of deficits and strengths, remediation may be continued into middle and high school.

Differential Diagnosis

Reading disorder is often accompanied by comorbid disorders, such as expressive language disorder, disorder of written expression, and ADHD. A recent study indicates that children with reading disorder consistently present difficulties with linguistic abilities, whereas children with ADHD do not. Children with reading disorder who do not qualify for a diagnosis of ADHD, however, were shown to have some overlapping deficits in the area of cognitive inhibition such that they perform impulsively on continuous performance tasks. Deficits in expressive language and speech discrimination in reading disorder can be sufficiently severe to warrant the additional diagnosis of expressive language disorder or mixed receptive-expressive language disorder. Some children exhibit a discrepancy between scores on verbal and performance intelligence. Visual perceptual deficits occur in only about 10 percent of cases. Reading disorder must be differentiated from mental retardation syndromes in which reading, along with other skills, is below the achievement expected for a child's chronologic age. Intellectual testing helps to differentiate global deficits from more specific reading difficulties.

Poor reading skills resulting from inadequate schooling can be detected by finding out whether other children in the same school have similarly poor reading performances on standardized reading tests. Hearing and visual impairments should be ruled out with screening tests.

Treatment

Most current remediation strategies for children with reading disorder are characterized by direct instruction of the various components of reading that focus a child's attention to the connections between speech sounds and spelling. A recent survey of the efficacy of specific word study with text reading practice or word study tutoring in first graders who scored within the lowest quartile for reading skills indicated that students exposed to either of the aforementioned instructions outperformed those who only received classroom instruction. Improvements were noted on measures of reading accuracy, reading comprehension, reading efficiency, passage reading fluency, and spelling. Many effective remediation programs begin by teaching the child to make accurate associations between letters and sounds. This approach is based on the current consensus that, in most cases, the core deficits in reading disorders are related to difficulty recognizing and remembering the associations between letters and sounds. After individual letter–sound associations have been mastered, remediation can target larger components of reading such as syllables and words.

The exact focus of any reading program can be determined only after accurate assessment of a child's specific deficits and weaknesses. Positive coping strategies include small, structured reading groups that offer individual attention and make it easier for a child to ask for help.

Children and adolescents with reading disorders are entitled to an individual education program (IEP) provided by the public school system. Yet, for high school students with persistent reading disorders and ongoing difficulties with decoding and work identification, however, IEP services may be insufficient to remediate their problems. A recent study of students with reading disorders in 54 schools indicated that, at the high school level, specific goals are not adequately met solely through school remediation. It is likely that high school students with persisting reading difficulties may have greater benefit from individualized reading remediation.

Reading instruction programs, such as the *Orton Gillingham and Direct Instructional System for Teaching and Remediation* (DISTAR) approaches, begin by concentrating on individual letters and sounds, advance to the mastery of simple phonetic units, and then blend these units into words and sentences. Thus, if children are taught to cope with graphemes, they will learn to read. Other reading remediation programs, such as the Merill program, and the *Science Research Associates, Inc. (SRA) Basic Reading Program,* begin by introducing whole words first and then teach children how to break them down and recognize the sounds of the syllables and the individual letters in the word. Another approach teaches children with reading disorders to recognize whole words through the use of visual aids and bypasses the sounding-out process. One such program is called the *Bridge Reading Program.* The Fernald method uses a multisensory approach that combines teaching whole words with a tracing technique so that the child has kinesthetic stimulation while learning to read the words.

As in psychotherapy, the therapist–patient relationship is important to a successful treatment outcome in remedial educational therapy. Children should be placed in a grade as close as possible to their social functional level and given special remedial work in reading. Coexisting emotional and behavioral problems should be treated by appropriate psychotherapeutic means. Parental counseling may also be helpful. Approximately 75 percent of children with learning disorders can be differentiated from comparison samples by lower measures of social competence. It is important, therefore, to include social skills improvement as a therapeutic component of a treatment program for children with reading disorders.

Pharmacotherapy. Pharmacotherapy is not indicated in reading disorder unless there is a comorbid condition (i.e., anxiety or depression) or that is a contributing factor to the disorder or resulting from the disorder as a reaction to it.

MATHEMATICS DISORDER

Children with mathematics disorder have difficulty learning and remembering numerals, cannot remember basic facts about numbers, and are slow and inaccurate in computation. Poor achievement in four groups of skills have been identified in mathematics disorder: linguistic skills (those related to understanding mathematic terms and converting written problems into mathematic symbols), perceptual skills (the ability to recognize and understand symbols and order clusters of numbers), mathematic skills (basic addition, subtraction, multiplication, division, and following sequencing of basic operations), and attentional skills (copying figures correctly and observing operational symbols correctly). A variety of terms over the years, including *dyscalculia, congenital arithmetic disorder, acalculia, Gerstmann syndrome,* and *developmental arithmetic disorder,* have been used to denote the difficulties present in mathematics disorder.

Mathematics disorder can occur in isolation or in conjunction with language and reading disorders. The diagnosis of mathematics disorder consists of deficits in arithmetic skills expected for a child's intellectual capacity and educational level, as measured by standardized, individually administered tests. This lack of expected mathematics ability must interfere with school performance or daily life activities, and the difficulties must exceed impairment associated with any existing neurologic or sensory deficits.

Epidemiology

Mathematics disorder alone is estimated to occur in about 1 percent of school-age children, that is, approximately one of every five children with learning disorder. Epidemiologic studies have indicated that 6 percent of school-age children have some difficulty with mathematics. Mathematics disorder may occur with greater frequency in girls. Many studies of learning disorders in children have grouped several disorders together rather than separating them into individual disorders, which makes it more difficult to ascertain the precise prevalence of mathematics disorder.

Comorbidity

Mathematics disorder is commonly found to be comorbid with reading disorder and disorder of written expression. Children with mathematics disorder may also be at higher risk for expressive language disorder, mixed receptive-expressive language disorder, and developmental coordination disorder.

Etiology

Mathematics disorder, as with other learning disorders, is probably at least partly caused by genetic factors. An early theory proposed a neurologic deficit in the right cerebral hemisphere, particularly in the occipital lobe areas. These regions are responsible for processing visual-spatial stimuli, which are responsible for mathematic skills. This theory, however, has received little support in subsequent neuropsychiatric studies.

Currently, the cause is thought to be multifactorial, so that maturational, cognitive, emotional, educational, and socioeconomic factors account in varying degrees and combinations for mathematics disorder. Compared with reading, arithmetic abilities seem to depend more on the amount and quality of instruction.

Diagnosis

The diagnosis of mathematics disorder is made when a child's skills in mathematics fall significantly below what is expected for that child's age, intellectual ability, and education. Many different skills are needed for mathematics proficiency. These include linguistic skills, conceptual skills, and computational skills. Linguistic skills involve being able to understand mathematic terms, understand word problems, and translate them into the proper mathematic process. Conceptual skills involve recognition of mathematic symbols and being able to use mathematic signs correctly. Computational skills include the ability to line up numbers correctly and to follow the "rules" of the mathematic operation. A definitive diagnosis can be made only after a child takes an individually administered standardized arithmetic test and scores markedly below the level expected in view of the child's schooling and intellectual capacity as measured by a standardized intelligence test. A pervasive developmental disorder and mental retardation should also be ruled out before confirming the diagnosis of mathematics disorder. The DSM-IV-TR diagnostic criteria for mathematics disorder are given in Table 3–2.

Table 3–2
DSM-IV-TR Diagnostic Criteria for Mathematics Disorder

A. Mathematic ability, as measured by individually administered standardized tests, is substantially below that expected given the person's chronologic age, measured intelligence, and age-appropriate education.
B. The disturbance in Criterion A significantly interferes with academic achievement or activities of daily living that require mathematic ability.
C. If a sensory deficit is present, the difficulties in mathematic ability are in excess of those usually associated with it.

Coding note: If a general medical (e.g., neurologic) condition or sensory deficit is present, code the condition on Axis III.

From American Psychiatric Association. *Diagnostic and Statistical Manual of Mental Disorders.* 4th ed. Text rev. Washington, DC: American Psychiatric Association; copyright 2000, with permission.

Clinical Features

Common features of mathematics disorder include difficulty with various components of mathematics, such as learning number names, remembering the signs for addition and subtraction, learning multiplication tables, translating word problems into computations, and doing calculations at the expected pace. Most children with mathematics disorder can be detected during the second and third grades in elementary school. A child with mathematics disorder generally has significant problems with concepts, such as counting and adding even one-digit numbers, compared with classmates of the same age. During the first 2 or 3 years of elementary school, a child with mathematics disorder may just get by in mathematics by relying on rote memory. But soon, as mathematics problems require discrimination and manipulation of spatial and numeric relations, a child with mathematics disorder is overwhelmed.

Some investigators have classified mathematics disorder into the following categories: difficulty learning to count meaningfully, difficulty mastering cardinal and ordinal systems, difficulty performing arithmetic operations, and difficulty envisioning clusters of objects as groups. Children with the disorder may have trouble associating auditory and visual symbols, understanding the conservation of quantity, remembering sequences of arithmetic steps, and choosing principles for problem-solving activities. Children with these problems are presumed to have good auditory and verbal abilities.

Mathematics disorder often coexists with other disorders affecting reading, expressive writing, coordination, and expressive and receptive language. Spelling problems, deficits in memory or attention, and emotional or behavioral problems may be present. Young grade-school children often show other learning disorders first and should be checked for mathematics disorder. Children with cerebral palsy may have mathematics disorder with normal overall intelligence.

The relationship between mathematics disorder and other communication and learning disorders is unclear. Although children with mixed receptive-expressive language disorder and expressive language disorder are not necessarily affected by mathematics disorder, the conditions often coexist because they are associated with impairments in decoding and encoding processes.

K. R., an 8-year-old girl, was referred for evaluation of increasing problems in attention, behavior, and learning, which were first noted in kindergarten, but were now causing difficulty at home and school. At the time of this first assessment, she was enrolled in a regular third-grade class in a local public school, which she had been attending since midway through first grade, when the family had moved into the district.

Clinical interview with her parents revealed a normal pregnancy. K. R. had been slow to talk (e.g., first words at approximately 20 months of age and short sentences at approximately 3 years of age), but otherwise had no major developmental concerns until kindergarten, when the teacher had raised concerns about K. R.'s inattentiveness and difficulty following instructions and mastering basic number concepts (e.g., inaccurate counting of sets of objects). A speech, language, and hearing assessment completed at the end of kindergarten revealed mild receptive and expressive language problems that did not warrant specific intervention. School reports from grade 1 noted ongoing concerns about inattention, some difficulty learning to read, difficulty mastering simple arithmetic facts, and "making careless mistakes in copying numbers from the board and in doing addition and subtraction." These problems continued through grade 2, despite some in-school accommodations (e.g., moving K. R.'s seat closer to the teacher and next to an academically strong student) and modifications (e.g., provision of printed sheets of arithmetic problems to reduce copying errors and reduction in number of assigned problems). Her parents also reported a 3-year history and current problems with losing things, twirling her hair and fiddling with anything in sight, difficulty concentrating on games and schoolwork, and forgetting to bring notes to and from school. Parents also reported that the older sibling (female) was also weak in mathematics and added the comment, "but I guess that is fairly common among girls."

Psychologic assessment included the *Wechsler Intelligence Scale for Children–III, Clinical Evaluation of Language Fundamentals–IV, Comprehensive Test of Phonological Processing,* and the *Woodcock-Johnson Psychoeducational Battery–III.* Results indicated average intelligence, with relatively weaker performance on tests of perceptual organization, weak phonologic awareness, subclinical problems in receptive and expressive language, and reading and arithmetic abilities that were well below grade level. Parent and teacher ratings on a standardized behavior questionnaire (*Conners' Rating Scales–Long Form*) were above clinical threshold for DSM-IV inattention.

The clinical team formulated a diagnosis of ADHD, predominantly inattentive type, and reading disorder, based on the developmental history, clinical picture, and standardized assessment. She did not meet criteria for communication disorder, and it was speculated that her arithmetic difficulties were most likely associated with the reading disorder and ADHD. Recommendations included the following: psychoeducation (primarily bibliotherapy for ADHD and reading disorder), specific educational intervention for reading, and treatment of the marked inattentiveness with psychostimulant medication.

At 1-year follow-up, K. R. and her parents reported a marked lessening of her inattention, but ongoing problems with reading and mathematics, although she had just started to read "chapter books" with the special education teacher who was providing small-group instruction several times a week. Another follow-up appointment was recommended, but no other changes were made in treatment.

Two years later, when K. R. was 11 years old, her parents called for an "urgent reevaluation" because of increasing home and school difficulties. Clinical evaluation revealed persisting ADHD, inattentive type, that was responding well to stimulant treatment and slow but fairly accurate reading albeit with weak comprehension, but marked difficulties with mathematics. The parents reported that K. R. had started lying about having mathematics homework or refused to do it, was suspended from mathematics class twice in the past 3 months because of oppositional behavior, and had failed sixth-grade mathematics. K. R. acknowledged disliking and worrying about math: "whenever the teacher starts asking questions and looks in my direction, my mind just goes blank and I feel sort of shaky—it's so bad in tests that I have to leave class to get myself together." At this point, the clinical team formulated the following diagnoses: ADHD, inattentive type; reading disorder; mathematics disorder; and also noted marked math anxiety. Recommendations were expanded to include specific educational remediation for mathematics.

At follow-up, K. R. reported that the resource teacher had taught her some helpful strategies to address her anxiety about mathematics as well as ways of classifying word problems and differentiating critical information from irrelevant information. The availability of several extended-release formulations of stimulant medication allowed a change from standard to longer-acting stimulant, which addressed K. R.'s concerns about having to go to the school office for her midday dose and difficulties concentrating on homework after school. (Courtesy of Rosemary Tannock, Ph.D.)

Pathology and Laboratory Examination

No physical signs or symptoms indicate mathematics disorder, but educational testing and standardized measurement of intellectual function are necessary to make this diagnosis. The *Keymath Diagnostic Arithmetic Test* measures several areas of mathematics, including knowledge of mathematic content, function, and computation. It is used to assess ability in mathematics of children in grades 1 to 6.

Course and Prognosis

A child with a mathematics disorder can usually be identified by the age of 8 years (third grade). In some children, the disorder is apparent as early as 6 years (first grade); in others, it may not be apparent until age 10 (fifth grade) or later. Too few data are currently available from longitudinal studies to predict clear patterns of developmental and academic progress of children classified as having mathematics disorder in early school grades. On the other hand, children with a moderate mathematics disorder who do not receive intervention may have complications, including continuing academic difficulties, shame, poor self-concept, frustration, and depression. These complications can lead to reluctance to attend school, truancy, and eventual hopelessness about academic success.

Differential Diagnosis

Mathematics disorder must be differentiated from global causes of impaired functioning such as mental retardation syndromes. Arithmetic difficulties in mental retardation are accompanied by generalized impairment in overall intellectual functioning. In unusual cases of mild mental retardation, arithmetic skills may be significantly below the level expected on the basis of a person's schooling and level of mental retardation. In such cases, an additional diagnosis of mathematics disorder should be made. Treatment of the arithmetic difficulties can particularly help a child's chances for employment in adulthood. Inadequate schooling can often affect a child's poor arithmetic performance on a standardized arithmetic test. Conduct disorder or ADHD can occur with mathematics disorder, and, in these cases, both diagnoses should be made.

Treatment

Mathematics difficulties for children has not been shown to be a stable disorder over time, thus early intervention may lead to improved skills in basic computation. The presence of reading disorder along with mathematics difficulties can impede progress, yet children are responsive to remediation in early grade school. For children as early as in kindergarten, indications of mathematics disorder and the need for intervention include lack of mastery in knowledge of which digit in a pair is larger, counting abilities, identification of numbers, and poor working memory for numbers, such as difficulty with reverse digit span.

Currently, the most effective treatments for mathematics disorder combine teaching mathematics concepts with continuous practice in solving math problems. Flash cards, workbooks, and computer games can be a viable part of this treatment. A recent report indicates that mathematics instruction is most helpful when the focus is on problem-solving activities, including word problems, rather than computation only. *Project MATH*, a multimedia self-instructional or group-instructional in-service training program, has been successful for some children with mathematics disorder. Computer programs can be helpful and can increase compliance with remediation efforts.

Social skills deficits can contribute to a child's hesitation in asking for help in math. Thus, a child identified with a mathematics disorder may benefit from gaining positive problem-solving skills in a social arena as well as in mathematics.

Pharmacotherapy. Pharmacotherapy is not indicated in mathematics disorder unless there is a comorbid condition (i.e., anxiety or depression) that is a contributing factor to the disorder or resulting from the disorder as a reaction to it.

DISORDER OF WRITTEN EXPRESSION

Written expression is the most complex skill acquired to convey an understanding of language and to express thoughts and ideas. Writing skills are highly correlated with reading for most children; for some children, however, reading comprehension may far surpass their ability to express complex thoughts. Written expression in some cases is a sensitive index of more subtle, although impairing, deficits in language usage that typically are not detected by standardized reading and language tests.

Disorder of written expression is characterized by writing skills that are significantly below the expected level for a child's age and intellectual capacity. These difficulties impair the child's academic performance and writing in everyday life. The many components of writing disorder include poor spelling, errors in grammar and punctuation, and poor handwriting. Spelling errors are among the most common difficulties for a child with a writing disorder. Spelling mistakes are most often phonetic errors; that is, an erroneous spelling that sounds like the correct spelling. Examples of common types of spelling errors are "fone" for "phone," or "beleeve" for "believe."

Historically, dysgraphia (i.e., poor writing skills) was considered to be a form of reading disorder; however, evidence indicates that disorder of written expression can occur on its own. Terms previously used to describe writing disability include *spelling disorder* and *spelling dyslexia*. Writing disabilities are often associated with other learning disorders, but they may be diagnosed later because expressive writing is acquired later than language and reading.

Epidemiology

The prevalence of disorder of written expression alone has not been studied, but as with reading disorder, it is estimated to occur in approximately 4 percent of school-age children. The gender ratio in writing disorder is believed to be similar that of reading disorder, occurring in about three times as many boys. Disorder of written expression often occurs along with reading disorder, but not always.

Comorbidity

Children with writing disorder are at higher risk for a variety of other learning and language disorders, including reading disorder, mathematics disorder, and expressive and receptive language disorders. ADHD occurs with greater frequency in children with writing disorders than in the general population. Finally, children with writing disorders are believed to be at higher risk for social skills difficulties, and some go on to develop poor self-esteem and depressive symptoms.

Etiology

Causes of writing disorders are believed to be similar to those of reading disorder; that is, a deficit in the use of the components of language related to letter sounds. It is likely that genetic factors are significant in the development of writing disorder. Writing difficulties often accompany language disorders in which a child may have trouble understanding grammatic rules, finding words, and expressing ideas clearly. According to one hypothesis, a disorder of written expression may result from the combined effects of one or more of the following: expressive language disorder, mixed receptive-expressive language disorder, and reading disorder. Hereditary predisposition to the disorder is supported by findings that most children with disorder of written expression have first-degree relatives with the disorder. Children with limited attention spans and high levels of distractibility may find writing an arduous task.

Diagnosis

A diagnosis of disorder of written expression is based on a child's poor performance on composing written text, including handwriting and impaired ability to spell and to place words sequentially in coherent sentences, compared with most other children of the same age and intellectual ability. In addition to spelling mistakes, a child with writing disorder may have serious grammatic mistakes, such as using incorrect tenses, forgetting words in sentences, and placing words in the wrong order. Punctuation may be incorrect, and the child may have poor ability to remember which words begin with capital letters. Poor handwriting may also contribute to writing disorder, including letters that are illegible, inverted letters, and mixtures of capital and lowercase letters in a given word. Other features of writing disorders include poor organization of written stories, which lack critical elements such as "where," "when," and "who," or clear expression of the plot.

Clinical Features

Children with disorder of written expression have difficulties early in grade school in spelling words and expressing their thoughts according to age-appropriate grammatic norms. Their spoken and written sentences contain an unusually large number of grammatic errors and poor paragraph organization. During and after the second grade, these children commonly make simple grammatic errors in writing a short sentence. For example, despite constant reminders, they frequently fail to capitalize the first letter of the first word in a sentence and to end the sentence with a period. Common features of the disorder of written expression are spelling errors, grammatic errors, punctuation errors, poor paragraph organization, and poor handwriting.

As they grow older and progress into higher grades in school, children's spoken and written sentences become more conspicuously primitive, odd, and inferior to what is expected of students at their grade level. Their word choices are erroneous and inappropriate; their paragraphs are disorganized and are not in proper sequence; and spelling errors increase as their vocabulary becomes larger and more abstract. Associated features of disorder of written expression include refusal or reluctance to go to school and to do assigned written homework, poor academic performance in other areas (e.g., mathematics), general avoidance of school work, truancy, attention deficit, and conduct disturbance.

Many children with disorder of written expression become frustrated and angry because of feelings of inadequacy and failure in their academic performance. In severe cases, depressive disorders can result from a growing sense of isolation, estrangement, and despair. Young adults with disorder of written expression who do not receive remedial intervention continue to have difficulties in social adaptation involving writing skills and a continuing sense of incompetence, inferiority, isolation, and estrangement. Some even try to avoid writing a response letter or a simple greeting card for fear of exposing their writing incompetence.

Cole, an 11-year-old boy, was referred for evaluation of increasing problems in school over the past 2 years, including consistent failure to complete assigned schoolwork and homework, some inattention and oppositional behavior, and a pattern of deteriorating grades and test scores. At the time of assessment, he was enrolled in a regular fifth-grade class in a public school, which he had been attending since first grade.

Clinical interview with parents revealed that Cole had a twin brother (monozygotic) and was born at term after an unremarkable pregnancy. His brother has a history of language problems for which he received speech–language therapy in the preschool years and remedial reading in the primary grades. Cole had not exhibited any difficulty in speech or language development, according to parental report and scores on standardized tests of oral language administered in the preschool years. His current and previous school reports indicate that, although Cole participated well in class discussions and had no difficulty in reading or mathematics computation, his written work was so far below grade level that he was at risk for failing the current year. Over the past 2 years, the teachers had expressed increasing concerns about Cole's unwillingness or refusal to complete written work, failure to hand in homework, daydreaming and fidgeting in class, skipping classes, and some defiant behavior.

Cole admitted to an increasing dislike of school and finding writing to be an extremely tedious activity. He explained that he had lots of ideas and that school would be more fun if the teacher would simply allow him to talk about his ideas, rather than writing everything ("It's writing, writing all day long—even in math and science. I know how to do the problems and the experiments, but I hate having to write it all down—my mind just goes blank."). He also admitted to skipping class, but only when he knew that he would have to do a lot of written work ("well, he [the teacher] is always on at me, telling me that I'm lazy and haven't done enough, and that my writing is atrocious. He slings my work back at me to do over again, gives me a detention, and when I try to explain he tells me, I've got a bad attitude—so why should I go to class?"). Both Cole and his parents reported that, over the past year, he exhibited low self-esteem, increasing frustration with, and refusal to do, homework, and a few brief episodes of depressed mood.

Testing by a clinical psychologist revealed average to high-average scores on the verbal and performance scales of the Wechsler Intelligence Scale for Children–III and average scores on the reading and arithmetic subtests of the Wide Range Achievement Test–3 (WRAT-3). However, scores on the WRAT-3 spelling subtest were below the 9th percentile, which was significantly below expectations for age and ability. Examination of his spelling errors revealed that although his spelling was typically phonologically accurate (i.e., could plausibly be pronounced to sound like the target word), it was orthographically unacceptable in that he used letter sequences that did not resemble English orthography, regardless of pronunciation (e.g., "houses" was written as "howssis," "phones" was written as "fones," and "exact" was written as "egszakt"). Further evidence of poor orthographic skills was demonstrated on a timed orthographic choice task, which required him to circle the real word in a pair of printed words that are pronounced the same (same phonologic code), but spelled differently (different orthographic code; e.g., sammon and salmon).

Moreover, his performance was well below age and grade on standardized tests of written expression (TOWL-3) as well as on a brief (5-minute) informal assessment of expository text generation on a favorite topic (e.g., newspaper article on recent sports event). During the 5-minute writing activity, he was observed to frequently stare out the window, to shift positions, to chew on his pencil, to get up to sharpen his pencil, to sigh when he did put pencil to paper, and to write slowly and laboriously. At the end of 5 minutes, he had produced three short sentences without any punctuation or capitalization that were barely legible, containing several misspellings and grammatic errors, and that were not linked semantically. By contrast, later in the assessment, he described the sporting event with detail and enthusiasm. A speech–language evaluation revealed average scores on standard tests of oral language (*Clinical Evaluation of Language Fundamentals–IV*), but he was noted to omit sounds or syllables in a multisyllabic word in a nonword repetition test, which has been found to be sensitive to mild residual language impairments and written language impairments.

The clinical team formulated a diagnosis of disorder of written expression, based on the clinical picture of Cole's inability to compose written text, poor spelling, and grammatic errors in the absence of low intelligence, reading or mathematics disorder, or history of, or current, language impairments. He did not meet diagnostic criteria for any other DSM-IV disorder, including oppositional defiant disorder, ADHD, or mood disorder. Recommendations included the following: psychoeducation (primarily bibliotherapy), the need for educational accommodations (e.g., provision of additional time for test taking and written assignments, specific educational intervention to facilitate written expression and to teach note taking, and use of specific computer software to support written composition and spelling), and counseling or psychotherapy should his depressive episodes continue or worsen. (Courtesy of Rosemary Tannock, Ph.D.)

Pathology and Laboratory Examination

Whereas no physical stigmata of a writing disorder exist, educational testing is used in making a diagnosis of writing disorder. Diagnosis is based on a child's writing performance

Table 3–3
DSM-IV-TR Diagnostic Criteria for Disorder of Written Expression

A. Writing skills, as measured by individually administered standardized tests (or functional assessments of writing skills), are substantially below those expected given the person's chronologic age, measured intelligence, and age-appropriate education.
B. The disturbance in Criterion A significantly interferes with academic achievement or activities of daily living that require the composition of written texts (e.g., writing grammatically correct sentences and organized paragraphs).
C. If a sensory deficit is present, the difficulties in writing skills are in excess of those usually associated with it.

Coding note: If a general medical (e.g., neurologic) condition or sensory deficit is present, code the condition on Axis III.

From American Psychiatric Association. *Diagnostic and Statistical Manual of Mental Disorders.* 4th ed. Text rev. Washington, DC: American Psychiatric Association; copyright 2000, with permission.

being markedly below his or her intellectual capacity, as confirmed by an individually administered standardized expressive writing test (Table 3–3). Currently available tests of written language include the *Test of Written Language* (TOWL), the DEWS, and the *Test of Early Written Language* (TEWL). The presence of a major disorder, such as a pervasive developmental disorder, or mental retardation may obviate the diagnosis of disorder of written expression. Other disorders to be differentiated from disorder of written expression are communication disorders, reading disorder, and impaired vision and hearing. A child suspected of having disorder of written expression should first be given a standardized intelligence test, such as WISC-III or the revised *Wechsler Adult Intelligence Scale* (WAIS-R) to determine the child's overall intellectual capacity.

Course and Prognosis

Because writing, language, and reading disorders often coexist, and because a child normally speaks well before learning to read and learns to read well before writing well, a child with all these disorders has expressive language disorder diagnosed first and disorder of written expression diagnosed last. In severe cases, a disorder of written expression is apparent by age 7 (second grade); in less severe cases, the disorder may not be apparent until age 10 (fifth grade) or later. Most persons with mild and moderate disorder of written expression fare well if they receive timely remedial education early in grade school. Severe disorder of written expression requires continual, extensive remedial treatment through the latter part of high school and even into college.

The prognosis depends on the severity of the disorder, the age or grade when the remedial intervention is started, the length and continuity of treatment, and the presence or absence of associated or secondary emotional or behavioral problems. Those who later become well compensated or who recover from disorder of written expression are often from families with high socioeconomic backgrounds.

Differential Diagnosis

It is important to determine whether another disorder, such as ADHD or a depressive disorder, is preventing a child from being able to concentrate on writing tasks in the absence of writing disorder itself. If this is the case, treatment for the other disorder should improve a child's writing performance. Disorder of written expression can also occur with a variety of other language and learning disorders. Common associated disorders are reading disorder, mixed receptive–expressive language disorder, expressive language disorder, mathematics disorder, developmental coordination disorder, and disruptive behavior disorder and ADHD.

Treatment

Remedial treatment for writing disorder includes direct practice in spelling and sentence writing and a review of grammatic rules. Intensive and continuous administration of individually tailored, one-on-one expressive and creative writing therapy seems to lead to a favorable outcome. Teachers in some special schools devote as much as 2 hours a day to such writing instruction. The effectiveness of a writing intervention largely depends on an optimal relationship between the child and the writing specialist. Success or failure in sustaining the patient's motivation greatly affects the treatment's long-term efficacy. Associated secondary emotional and behavioral problems should be given prompt attention, with appropriate psychiatric treatment and parental counseling.

Pharmacotherapy. Pharmacotherapy is not indicated in disorder of written expression unless there is a comorbid condition (i.e., anxiety or depression) that is a contributing factor to the disorder or resulting from the disorder as a reaction to it.

LEARNING DISORDER NOT OTHERWISE SPECIFIED

Learning disorder not otherwise specified is a new category in DSM-IV-TR for disorders that do not meet the criteria for any specific learning disorder, but cause impairment and reflect learning abilities below those expected for a person's intelligence, education, and age (Table 3–4). An example of a disability that could be placed in this category is a spelling skills deficit.

Table 3–4
DSM-IV-TR Diagnostic Criteria for Learning Disorder Not Otherwise Specified

This category is for disorders in learning that do not meet criteria for any specific learning disorder. This category might include problems in all three areas (reading, mathematics, written expression) that together significantly interfere with academic achievement even though performance on tests measuring each individual skill is not substantially below that expected given the person's chronologic age, measured intelligence, and age-appropriate education.

From American Psychiatric Association. *Diagnostic and Statistical Manual of Mental Disorders.* 4th ed. Text rev. Washington, DC: American Psychiatric Association; copyright 2000, with permission.

4

Motor Skills Disorder: Developmental Coordination Disorder

Children with developmental motor coordination struggle to perform accurately the motor activities of daily life, such as jumping, hopping, running, or catching a ball. Children with coordination problems may also agonize to use utensils correctly, tie their shoelaces, or write. A child with developmental coordination disorder may exhibit delays in achieving motor milestones, such as sitting, crawling, and walking, because of clumsiness, and yet excel at verbal skills.

Developmental coordination disorder, thus, may be characterized by either clumsy gross and/or fine motor skills, resulting in poor performance in sports and even in academic achievement because of poor writing skills. A child with developmental coordination disorder may bump into things more often than siblings or drop things. In the 1930s, the term *clumsy child syndrome* began to be used in the literature to denote a condition of awkward motor behaviors that could not be correlated with any specific neurologic disorder or damage. This term continues to be used to identify imprecise or delayed gross and fine motor behavior in children, resulting in subtle motor inabilities, but often significant social rejection. Currently, certain indications are that perinatal problems, such as prematurity, low birthweight, and hypoxia, may contribute to the emergence of developmental coordination disorders. Children with developmental coordination disorder are at higher risk for language and learning disorders. A strong association is seen between speech and language problems and coordination problems, as well as an association of coordination difficulties with hyperactivity, impulsivity, and poor attention span.

Children with developmental coordination disorder may resemble younger children because of their inability to master motor activities typical for their age group. For example, children with developmental coordination disorder in elementary school may not be adept at bicycle riding, skateboarding, running, skipping, or hopping. In the middle school years, children with this disorder may have trouble in team sports, such as soccer, baseball, or basketball. Fine motor skill manifestations of developmental coordination disorder typically include clumsiness using utensils and difficulty with buttons and zippers in the preschool age group. In older children, using scissors and more complex grooming skills, such as styling hair or putting on makeup, is difficult.

Children with developmental coordination disorder are often ostracized by peers because of their poor skills in many sports, and they often have long-standing difficulties with peer relationships. Developmental coordination disorder is the sole disorder in the text revision of the 4th edition of the *Diagnostic and Statistical Manual of Mental Disorders* (DSM-IV-TR) category motor skills disorder. Gross and fine motor impairment in this disorder cannot be explained on the basis of a medical condition, such as cerebral palsy, muscular dystrophy, or any other neuromuscular disorder.

EPIDEMIOLOGY

The prevalence of developmental coordination disorder has been estimated at about 5 percent of school-age children. The male-to-female ratio in referred populations tends to show increased rates of the disorder in boys, but schools refer boys more often for testing and special education evaluations. Reports in the literature of the male-to-female ratio have ranged from 2:1 to 4:1. These rates may also be inflated because motor behaviors in boys are scrutinized more closely than those in girls.

COMORBIDITY

Developmental coordination disorder is strongly associated with speech and language disorders. Children with coordination difficulties have higher than expected rates of speech and language disorders, and studies of children with speech disorders report very high rates of "clumsiness." Some studies have found associations between fine motor skills in the upper arms and expressive and receptive language disorders, whereas gross motor problems and visual motor coordination problems were not associated with language disturbance. Developmental coordination disorder is also associated with reading disorders, mathematics disorder, and disorder of written expression. Higher than expected rates of attention-deficit/hyperactivity disorder (ADHD) are also associated with developmental coordination disorder. A recent study of children with developmental coordination disorder reported that, although motor ability accounts largely for accuracy in tasks that require speed, the degree of motor incoordination is not correlated with degree of inattention. Therefore, developmental coordination disorder and ADHD appear to be distinct disorders that occur concurrently with greater frequency than chance.

Secondary peer relationship problems are common among children with developmental coordination disorders because of the rejection that occurs along with their poor performance in sports and games that require good motor skill. Adolescents with coordination problems often exhibit poor self-esteem and academic difficulties. Recent studies underscore the importance of attention to both victimization of children and adolescents with developmental motor coordination by peers and the potential resulting damage to self-worth. Children and adolescents with developmental coordination disorder who are bullied have higher rates of poor self-esteem that often deserves clinical attention.

Table 4–1
DSM-IV-TR Diagnostic Criteria for Developmental Coordination Disorder

A. Performance in daily activities that require motor coordination is substantially below that expected given the person's chronologic age and measured intelligence. This may be manifested by marked delays in achieving motor milestones (e.g., walking, crawling, sitting), dropping things, "clumsiness," poor performance in sports, or poor handwriting.

B. The disturbance in Criterion A significantly interferes with academic achievement or activities of daily living.

C. The disturbance is not due to a general medical condition (e.g., cerebral palsy, hemiplegia, or muscular dystrophy) and does not meet criteria for a pervasive developmental disorder.

D. If mental retardation is present, the motor difficulties are in excess of those usually associated with it.

Coding note: If a general medical (e.g., neurologic) condition or sensory deficit is present, code the condition on Axis III.

From American Psychiatric Association. *Diagnostic and Statistical Manual of Mental Disorders.* 4th ed. Text rev. Washington, DC: American Psychiatric Association; copyright 2000, with permission.

ETIOLOGY

The causes of developmental coordination disorder are believed to include both "organic" and "developmental" factors. Risk factors postulated to contribute to this disorder include prematurity, hypoxia, perinatal malnutrition, and low birthweight. Prenatal exposure to alcohol, cocaine, and nicotine has also been hypothesized to contribute to low birthweight and cognitive and behavioral abnormalities. Neurochemical abnormalities and parietal lobe lesions have also been suggested to contribute to coordination deficits. Developmental coordination disorder and communication disorders have strong associations, although the specific causative agents are unknown for both. Coordination problems are also more frequently found in children with hyperactivity syndromes and learning disorders.

Recent studies of postural control (that is, the ability to regain balance after being in motion) indicate that children with developmental coordination disorder who do not have significant difficulties with balance when standing still are unable to accurately correct for movement, resulting in impaired balance compared with other children. A recent study concluded that, in children with developmental coordination disorder, signals from the brain to particular muscles (including the tibialis anterior and peroneus muscles) involved in balance are not being optimally sent or received. These findings have implicated the cerebellum as a contributing origin of dysfunction for developmental coordination disorder.

DIAGNOSIS

The diagnosis of developmental coordination disorder depends on poor performance, for a child's age and intellectual level, in activities requiring coordination. Diagnosis is based on a history of the child's delay in achieving early motor milestones as well as on direct observation of current deficits in coordination. An informal screen for developmental coordination disorder involves asking the child to perform tasks involving gross motor coordination (e.g., hopping, jumping, and standing on one foot), fine motor coordination (e.g., finger-tapping and shoelace tying), and hand-eye coordination (e.g., catching a ball and copying letters). Judgments regarding poor performance must be based on what is expected for a child's age. A child who is mildly clumsy, but whose functioning is not impaired, does not qualify for a diagnosis of developmental coordination disorder.

The diagnosis may be associated with below-normal scores on performance subtests of standardized intelligence tests and by normal or above-normal scores on verbal subtests. Specialized tests of motor coordination can be useful, such as the *Bender Visual Motor Gestalt Test*, the *Frostig Movement Skills Test Battery*, and the *Bruininks-Oseretsky Test of Motor Development*. The child's chronologic age and intellectual capacity must be taken into account, and the disorder cannot be caused by a neurologic or neuromuscular condition. Examination, however, may occasionally reveal slight reflex abnormalities and other soft neurologic signs. The DSM-IV-TR diagnostic criteria are given in Table 4–1.

CLINICAL FEATURES

The clinical signs suggesting the existence of developmental coordination disorder are evident in infancy in some cases, when a child begins to attempt tasks requiring motor coordination. The essential clinical feature is significantly impaired performance in motor coordination. The difficulties in motor coordination may vary with a child's age and developmental stage (Table 4–2).

Table 4–2
Manifestations of Developmental Coordination Disorder

Gross motor manifestations
- Preschool age
  - Delays in reaching motor milestones, such as sitting, crawling, and walking
  - Balance problems: falling, getting bruised frequently, and poor toddling
  - Abnormal gait
  - Knocking over objects, bumping into things, and destructiveness
- Primary-school age
  - Difficulty with riding bikes, skipping, hopping, running, jumping, and doing somersaults
  - Awkward or abnormal gait
- Older
  - Poor at sports, throwing, catching, kicking, and hitting a ball

Fine motor manifestations
- Preschool age
  - Difficulty learning dressing skills (tying, fastening, zipping, and buttoning)
  - Difficulty learning feeding skills (handling knife, fork, or spoon)
- Primary-school age
  - Difficulty assembling jigsaw pieces, using scissors, building with blocks, drawing, or tracing
- Older
  - Difficulty with grooming (putting on makeup, blow-drying hair, and doing nails)
  - Messy or illegible writing
  - Difficulty using hand tools, sewing, and playing piano

In infancy and early childhood, the disorder may be manifested by delays in developmental motor milestones, such as turning over, crawling, sitting, standing, walking, buttoning shirts, and zipping up pants. Between the ages of 2 and 4 years, clumsiness appears in almost all activities requiring motor coordination. Affected children cannot hold objects and drop them easily, their gait may be unsteady, they often trip over their own feet, and they may bump into other children while attempting to go around them. Older children may display impaired motor coordination in table games, such as putting together puzzles or building blocks, and in any type of ball game. Although no specific features are pathognomonic of developmental coordination disorder, developmental milestones are frequently delayed. Many children with the disorder also have speech and language difficulties. Older children may have secondary problems, including academic difficulties, as well as poor peer relationships based on social rejection. It has been reported widely that children with motor coordination problems are more likely to have problems understanding subtle social cues and are often rejected by peers. A recent study indicated that children with motor difficulties were found to perform more poorly on scales that measure recognition of static and changing facial expressions of emotion. This finding is likely to be correlated to the clinical observations that children with motor coordination have difficulties in social behavior and peer relationships.

Peter was brought for evaluation of poor coordination at 8 years of age after complaining to his parents that he was being teased by peers for being "bad" in sports, and he was always picked last for the team. His friends laughed at him because he always dropped the ball even when he could initially catch it, and he looked "funny" while running. He was so upset about ridicule from peers that he no longer wanted to play baseball or basketball with his friends.

A developmental history obtained from his parents revealed that Peter's development had been delayed for sitting, which he did not do until 10 months of age, and he was unable to walk without falling over until 24 months of age. His parents reported an awareness that he was somewhat clumsy, but they believed that he would outgrow that. On questioning about Peter's current motor function, his parents reported that, during meal times, Peter still constantly spilled his drinks and was awkward when he used a fork. His food often fell off of a fork or spoon before it reached his mouth, and he had great difficulty using a knife and a fork.

A comprehensive assessment of fine and gross motor skills yielded the following results: Peter was able to hop, but he could not skip without briefly stopping after each step. Peter could stand with both feet together, but could not stand on tiptoe. Although Peter could catch a ball, he held a ball bounced to him at chest level, and he could not catch a ball bounced to him on the ground from a distance of 15 feet. Peter's agility and coordination were measured with the Bruininks-Oseretsky Test of Motor Development, which revealed functioning levels commensurate with those of an average 6-year-old child.

Peter was referred to a neurologist for a comprehensive evaluation because he appeared to be generally weak, and his muscles seemed floppy. Neurologic evaluation was negative for diagnosable neurologic disorders, and his muscle strength was actually found to be normal, despite his appearance. Based on the negative neurologic examination and the finding of the Bruininks-Oseretsky Test of Motor Development, Peter was given a diagnosis of developmental coordination disorder. Peter's symptoms included mild hypotonia and fine motor clumsiness.

After the diagnosis of developmental motor coordination was made, a treatment plan was developed that included private sessions with an occupational therapist who used perceptual-motor exercises to improve his fine motor skills, targeting particularly writing and use of utensils, and a request for an individualized evaluation from the school with a goal of administering an adaptive physical education program. He was also enrolled in a treatment program using motor imagery training to reduce his clumsiness, administered by a psychologist.

Peter was relieved to be receiving help, especially for his writing and for sports activities because these were the areas in which his peers had teased him. Over a period of 3 months of treatment, Peter showed significant improvement in the legibility of his handwriting, although he remained a slow writer. He felt much better with this improvement because he was receiving more praise from his teachers and parents, and his classmates were teasing him less. As he began to feel better about himself, he began to play sports informally with his peers, although not competitively. He was given a modified physical education program in school, and he was not required to play on teams, but he practiced throwing and catching a ball and playing basketball.

Peter continued to have some degree of clumsiness in his fine motor skills over the next few years, but he was cooperative with the occupational therapy interventions, and he showed continual improvement. (Courtesy of Caroly Pataki, M.D. and Sarah Spence, M.D.)

DIFFERENTIAL DIAGNOSIS

The differential diagnosis includes medical conditions that produce coordination difficulties (e.g., cerebral palsy and muscular dystrophy), pervasive developmental disorders, and mental retardation. In mental retardation and in the pervasive developmental disorders, coordination usually does not stand out as a significant deficit compared with other skills. Children with neuromuscular disorders may exhibit more global muscle impairment, rather than clumsiness and delayed motor milestones. Neurologic examination and workups usually reveal more extensive deficits in neurologic conditions than in developmental coordination disorder. Extremely hyperactive and impulsive children may be physically careless because of their high levels of motor activity. Clumsy gross and fine motor behavior and ADHD seem to be associated.

COURSE AND PROGNOSIS

Few data are available on the prospective longitudinal outcomes of treated and untreated children with developmental coordination disorder. For the most part, although clumsiness may continue, some children can compensate by developing interests in other skills. Some studies suggest a favorable outcome for children who have an average or above-average intellectual capacity, in that they come up with strategies to develop friendships that do not depend on physical activities. Clumsiness generally persists into adolescence and adult life. One study following a group of children with developmental coordination problems over a decade found that the clumsy children remained less dexterous, showed poor balance, and continued to be physically awkward. The affected children were also more likely to have academic problems and poor self-esteem. Commonly associated features include delays in nonmotor milestones, expressive language disorder, and mixed receptive–expressive language disorder.

TREATMENT

Interventions for children with developmental coordination disorder utilize multiple modalities, including visual, auditory, and tactile materials targeting perceptual motor training for specific motor tasks. More recently, motor imagery training has been incorporated into treatment. These approaches are visual imagery exercises using CD-ROM; they have a broad range of foci, including predictive timing for motor tasks, relaxation and mental preparation, visual modeling of fundamental motor skills, and mental rehearsal of various tasks. This type of intervention is based on the notion that improved internal representation of a movement task would improve a child's actual motor behavior.

The treatment of developmental coordination disorder generally includes versions of sensory-integration programs and modified physical education. Sensory integration programs, usually administered by occupational therapists, consist of physical activities that increase awareness of motor and sensory function. For example, a child who bumps into objects often might be given the task of trying to balance on a scooter, under supervision, to improve balance and body awareness. Children who have difficulty writing letters are often given tasks to increase awareness of hand movements. School-based occupational therapies for motor coordination problems in writing include utilizing mechanisms that provide resistance or vibration during writing exercises, to improve grip, and practicing vertical writing on a chalk board to increase arm strength and stability while writing. These programs have been shown to improve legibility of student's writing, but not necessarily speed because students learn to write with greater accuracy and deliberate letter formation. Currently, many schools also allow and may even encourage children with coordination difficulties that affect writing to use computers to aid in writing reports and long papers.

Adaptive physical education programs are designed to help children enjoy exercise and physical activities without the pressures of team sports. These programs generally incorporate certain sports actions, such as kicking a soccer ball or throwing a basketball. Children with coordination disorder may also benefit from social skills groups and other prosocial interventions. The Montessori technique (developed by Maria Montessori) may promote motor skill development, especially with preschool children, because this educational program emphasizes the development of motor skills. Small studies have suggested that exercise in rhythmic coordination, practicing motor movements, and learning to use word processing keyboards may be beneficial. Parental counseling may help reduce parents' anxiety and guilt about their child's impairment, increase their awareness, and facilitate their confidence to cope with the child.

A recent investigation of children with developmental coordination disorder showed positive results using a computer game designed to improve ability to catch a ball. These children were able to improve their game score by practicing virtual catching without specific instructions on how to utilize the visual cues. This has implications for treatment in that certain types of motor task coordination can be positively influenced through the practice of specific motor tasks, even without overt instructions.

Pharmacotherapy. Pharmacotherapy is not indicated in developmental coordination disorder unless there is a comorbid condition (i.e., anxiety or depression) that is a contributing factor to the disorder or resulting from the disorder as a reaction to it.

5

Communication Disorders

Communication disorders are among the most common disorders in childhood. To communicate effectively, children must have a mastery of language—that is, the ability to understand and express ideas—using words and speech, the manner in which words are spoken. Language disorders include expressive and mixed receptive–expressive language disorder, whereas speech disorders include phonologic disorder and stuttering. Children with expressive language disorders have difficulties expressing their thoughts with words and sentences at a level of sophistication expected for their age and developmental level in other areas. These children may struggle with limited vocabularies; speak in sentences that are short or ungrammatical; and often present descriptions of situations that are disorganized, confusing, and infantile. They may be delayed in developing an understanding and a memory of words compared with others their age.

Language and speech are pragmatically intertwined, despite the distinct categories of language disorders and speech disorders within the text revision of the fourth edition of the American Psychiatric Association's *Diagnostic and Statistical Manual of Mental Disorders* (DSM-IV-TR). Language competence spans four domains: phonology, grammar, semantics, and pragmatics. *Phonology* refers to the ability to produce sounds that constitute words in a given language and the skills to discriminate the various phonemes (sounds that are made by a letter or group of letters in a language). To imitate words, a child must be able to produce the sounds of a word. *Grammar* designates the organization of words and the rules for placing words in an order that makes sense in that language. *Semantics* refers to the organization of concepts and the acquisition of words themselves. A child draws from a mental list of words to produce sentences. Children with language impairments exhibit a wide range of difficulties with semantics that include acquiring new words, storage and organization of known words, and word retrieval. Speech and language evaluations that are sufficiently broad to test all of the aforementioned skill levels are more accurate in evaluating a child's remedial needs. *Pragmatics* has to do with skill in the actual use of language and the "rules" of conversation, including pausing so that a listener can answer a question and knowing when to change the topic when a break occurs in a conversation. By age 2 years, toddlers may know up to 200 words, and by age 3 years, most children understand the basic rules of language and can converse effectively. Table 5–1 provides an overview of typical milestones in language and nonverbal development.

EXPRESSIVE LANGUAGE DISORDER

Expressive language disorder is diagnosed when a child demonstrates a selective deficit in expressive language development relative to receptive language skills and nonverbal intelligence. Thus, a child with expressive language disorder may be identified using the *Wechsler Intelligence Scale for Children–III* (WISC-III) in that verbal intellectual level may appear to be depressed compared with the child's overall intelligence quotient (IQ). A child with expressive language disorder is likely to function below the expected levels of acquired vocabulary, correct tense usage, complex sentence constructions, and word recall. Children with expressive language disorder often present verbally as younger than their age.

Language disability can be acquired at any time during childhood (e.g., secondary to a trauma or a neurologic disorder), or it can be developmental; it is usually congenital, without an obvious cause. Most childhood language disorders fall in the developmental category. In either case, deficits in receptive skills (language comprehension) or expressive skills (ability to use language) can occur. Expressive language disturbance often occurs in the absence of comprehension difficulties, whereas receptive dysfunction generally diminishes proficiency in the expression of language. Children with expressive language disorder alone have courses and prognoses that differ from children with mixed receptive–expressive language disorder.

In DSM-IV-TR, the diagnosis of expressive language disorder can be made in the absence of receptive language disorder. Mixed receptive–expressive language disorder is diagnosed according to DSM-IV-TR when both receptive and expressive language syndromes are present, and mixed receptive–expressive language disorder is an exclusionary criterion for expressive language disorder. Generally, whenever receptive skills are sufficiently impaired to warrant a diagnosis, expressive skills are also impaired. In DSM-IV-TR, expressive language disorder and mixed receptive–expressive language disorder are not limited to developmental language disabilities; acquired forms of language disturbances are included. To meet the criteria for expressive language disorder, patients must have scores on standardized

Table 5–1
Normal Development of Speech, Language, and Nonverbal Skills in Children

Speech and Language Development	Nonverbal Development
1 yr	
Recognizes own name	Stands alone
Follows simple directions accompanied by gestures (e.g., bye-bye)	Takes first steps with support
Speaks one or two words	Uses common objects (e.g., spoon, cup)
Mixes words and jargon sounds	Releases objects willfully
Uses communicative gestures (e.g., showing, pointing)	Searches for object in location where last seen
2 yr	
Uses 200 to 300 words	Walks up and down stairs alone, but without alternating feet
Names most common objects	Runs rhythmically, but is unable to stop or start smoothly
Uses two-word or longer phrases	Eats with a fork
Uses a few prepositions (e.g., in, on), pronouns (e.g., you, me), verb endings (e.g., -ing, -s, -ed) and plurals (-s), but not always correctly	Cooperates with adult in simple household tasks
Enjoys play with action toys	Follows simple commands not accompanied by gestures
3 yr	
Uses 900–1,000 words	Rides tricycle
Creates three- to four-word sentences, usually with subject and verb but simple structure	Enjoys simple "make-believe" play
Follows two-step commands	Matches primary colors
Repeats five- to seven-syllable sentences	Balances momentarily on one foot
Speech is usually understood by family members	Shares toys with others for short periods
4 yr	
Uses 1,500 to 1,600 words	Walks up and down stairs with alternating feet
Recounts stories and events from recent past	Hops on one foot
Understands most questions about immediate environment	Copies block letters
Uses conjunctions (e.g., if, but, because)	Role-plays with others
Speech is usually understood by strangers	Categorizes familiar objects
5 years	
Uses 2,100 to 2,300 words	Dresses self without assistance
Discusses feelings	Cuts own meat with knife
Understands most prepositions referring to space (e.g., above, beside, toward) and time (e.g., before, after, until)	Draws a recognizable person
	Plays purposefully and constructively
Follows three-step commands	Recognizes part-whole relationships
Prints own name	
6 yr	
Defines words by function and attributes	Rides a bicycle
Uses a variety of well-formed complex sentences	Throws a ball well
Uses all parts of speech (e.g., verbs, nouns, adverbs, adjectives, conjunctions, prepositions)	Sustains attention to motivating tasks
Understands letter-sound associations in reading	Enjoys competitive games
8 years	
Reads simple books for pleasure	
Enjoys riddles and jokes	Understands conservation of liquid, number, length, and so forth
Verbalizes ideas and problems readily	Knows left and right of others
Understands indirect requests (e.g., "It's hot in here" understood as request to open window)	Knows differences and similarities
Produces all speech sounds in an adult-like manner	Appreciates that others have different perspectives
	Categorizes same object into multiple categories

Adapted from Owens RE. Language Development: An Introduction. 4th ed. Needham Heights, MA: Allyn & Bacon; 1996, with permission.

measures of expressive language markedly below those of standardized nonverbal IQ subtests and standardized tests of receptive language.

Epidemiology

The prevalence of expressive language disorder is estimated to be as high as 6 percent in children between the ages of 5 and 11 years of age. Surveys have indicated rates of expressive language as high as 15 percent in children under age 3 years. In school-age children over the age of 11 years, the estimates are lower, ranging from 3 percent to 5 percent. The disorder is two to three times more common in boys than in girls and is most prevalent among children whose relatives have a family history of phonologic disorder or other communication disorders.

Comorbidity

Children with developmental language disorders, such as expressive language disorder, have above-average rates of comorbid psychiatric disorders. In one large study of children with speech and language disorders by Lorian Baker and Dennis Cantwell, the most common comorbid disorders were attention-deficit/hyperactivity disorder (ADHD) (19 percent), anxiety disorders (10 percent), oppositional defiant disorder, and conduct disorder (7 percent combined). Children with expressive language disorder are also at higher risk for a speech disorder, receptive difficulties, and other learning disorders. Many disorders—such as reading disorder, developmental coordination disorder, and other communication disorders—are associated with expressive language disorder. Children with expressive language disorder often have some receptive impairment, although not always sufficiently significant for the diagnosis of mixed receptive–expressive language disorder.

Delayed motor milestones and a history of enuresis are common in children with expressive language disorder. Phonologic disorder is commonly found in young children with the disorder, and neurologic abnormalities have been reported in many children, including soft neurologic signs, depressed vestibular responses, and electroencephalogram (EEG) abnormalities. On the other hand, a recent study found that boys with serious behavior problems also had high levels of unidentified expressive language disorders, thus it may be important to screen for language dysfunction in children who are extremely behavior disordered.

Etiology

The specific cause of developmental expressive language disorder is likely to be multifactorial. Subtle cerebral damage and maturational lags in cerebral development have been postulated as underlying causes. Some children with language disorders have difficulty processing information in a time-limited manner. Scant data are available on the specific brain structure of children with language disorder, but limited magnetic resonance imaging (MRI) studies suggest that language disorders are associated with a loss of the normal left-right brain asymmetry in the perisylvian and planum temporale regions. Results of one small MRI study suggested possible inversion of brain asymmetry (right > left). Left-handedness or ambilaterality seems to be associated with expressive language problems. Evidence shows that language disorders occur with higher frequency in certain families.

Genetic factors have been suspected to play a role, and several studies of twins show significant concordance for monozygotic twins for developmental language disorders. A recent report described a hypothesis of specific genes at 7q11.23 that appear to be exquisitely sensitive to dosage alterations that can influence human language and visuospatial capabilities. The Williams-Beuren syndrome (WBS) locus at 7q11.23 is susceptible to recurrent chromosomal rearrangements, including the microdeletion that causes WBS. WBS typically presents as a phenotype, including characteristic cardiovascular, cognitive, and behavioral features. It is hypothesized, however, that instead of microdeletions, reciprocal duplications of the WBS could also occur and may be associated with the phenotype of language dysfunction. Some studies have found that some individuals with WBS are at an increased risk of expressive language disorder.

Environmental and educational factors are also postulated to contribute to developmental language disorders. Data suggest that prenatal exposures to substances such as alcohol and cocaine are likely to be associated with delays in language acquisition and expressive language ability.

Diagnosis

Expressive language disorder is present when a child has a selective deficit in language skills and is functioning well in nonverbal areas and in receptive skills. Markedly below-age-level verbal or sign language, accompanied by a low score on standardized expressive verbal tests, is diagnostic of expressive language disorder (Table 5–2). The disorder is not caused by a pervasive developmental disorder, and a child with an expressive language disorder usually develops some nonverbal strategies to aid in socialization. A child with an expressive language disorder exhibits the following features: limited vocabulary, simple grammar, and variable articulation. "Inner language" or the appropriate use of toys and household objects is present. One recent assessment tool, the *Carter Neurocognitive Assessment,* has the capacity to itemize and quantify skills in areas of social awareness, visual attention, auditory comprehension, and vocal communication even when there are compromised expressive language and

Table 5–2
DSM-IV-TR Diagnostic Criteria for Expressive Language Disorder

A. The scores obtained from standardized individually administered measures of expressive language development are substantially below those obtained from standardized measures of both nonverbal intellectual capacity and receptive language development. The disturbance may be manifest clinically by symptoms that include having a markedly limited vocabulary, making errors in tense, or having difficulty recalling words or producing sentences with developmentally appropriate length or complexity.
B. The difficulties with expressive language interfere with academic or occupational achievement or with social communication.
C. Criteria are not met for mixed receptive–expressive language disorder or a pervasive developmental disorder.
D. If mental retardation, a speech–motor or sensory deficit, or environmental deprivation is present, the language difficulties are in excess of those usually associated with these problems.

Coding note: If a speech-motor or sensory deficit or a neurologic condition is present, code the condition on Axis III.

From American Psychiatric Association. *Diagnostic and Statistical Manual of Mental Disorders.* 4th ed. Text rev. Washington, DC: American Psychiatric Association; copyright 2000, with permission.

motor skills in very young children—up to 2 years of age. Such a tool may be able to provide a more positive view of the cognitive potential of children with handicaps including expressive language.

To confirm the diagnosis, a child is given standardized expressive language and nonverbal intelligence tests. Observations of children's verbal and sign language patterns in various settings (e.g., school yard, classroom, home, and playroom) and during interactions with other children help ascertain the severity and specific areas of a child's impairment and aid in early detection of behavioral and emotional complications. Family history should include the presence or absence of expressive language disorder among relatives.

Clinical Features

Children with expressive language disorders may be ostracized by peers because of their poor ability to explain what they are talking about. They may appear vague when telling a story and use many filler words such as "stuff" and "things" instead of naming specific objects.

The essential feature of expressive language disorder is marked impairment in the development of age-appropriate expressive language, which results in the use of verbal or sign language markedly below the expected level in view of a child's nonverbal intellectual capacity. Language understanding (decoding) skills remain relatively intact. When severe, the disorder becomes recognizable by about the age of 18 months, when a child fails to utter spontaneously or even echo single words or sounds. Even simple words, such as "Mama" and "Dada," are absent from the child's active vocabulary, and the child points or uses gestures to indicate desires. The child seems to want to communicate, maintains eye contact, relates well to the mother, and enjoys games such as pat-a-cake and peek-a-boo. The child's vocabulary is severely limited. At 18 months, the child may be limited to pointing to common objects when they are named.

When a child with expressive language disorder begins to speak, the language impairment gradually becomes apparent. Articulation is often immature; numerous articulation errors occur but are inconsistent, particularly with such sounds as *th*, *r*, *s*, *z*, *y*, and *l*, which are either omitted or are substituted for other sounds.

By age 4 years, most children with expressive language disorder can speak in short phrases, but may have difficulty retaining new words. After beginning to speak, they acquire language more slowly than most children. Their use of various grammatic structures is also markedly below the age-expected level, and their developmental milestones may be slightly delayed. Emotional problems involving poor self-image, frustration, and depression may develop in school-age children.

Josh was an alert, energetic 2-year-old whose expressive vocabulary was limited to only four words (*mama*, *daddy*, *hi*, and *more*). He used these words one at a time in appropriate situations. He supplemented his infrequent verbal communications with pointing and other simple gestures to request desired objects or actions. He rarely communicated, however, for other purposes (e.g., commenting or protesting). Josh appeared to be developing normally in all other areas except for expressive language. He sat, stood, and walked at the expected times. He played happily with other children, enjoying activities and toys that were appropriate for 2-year-olds. Although he had a history of frequent ear infections, a recent hearing test revealed normal hearing. Importantly, he showed age-appropriate comprehension for the names of familiar objects and actions and for simple verbal instructions (e.g., "Put that down." "Get your shirt." "Clap your hands."). Of course, at his age, comprehension testing had to be carefully conducted to ensure his attention and motivation.

Despite Josh's slow start in language development, most specialists would be reluctant to diagnose an expressive language disorder at his young age. Prospective research on the development of late talkers such as Josh has demonstrated that most of them spontaneously overcome their initial slow start in language development. A parental report measure of vocabulary comprehension has shown promise as a prognostic indicator that can be used as early as 10 months of age. (Courtesy of Carla J. Johnson, Ph.D., and Joseph H. Beitchman, M.D.)

Amy was a sociable, active 5-year-old who was diagnosed with expressive language disorder. She often played with Lisa, her kindergarten classmate. During pretend play one day, each girl told the story of Little Red Riding Hood to her doll. Lisa's story began: "Little Red Riding Hood was taking a basket of food to her grandmother who was sick. A bad wolf stopped Red Riding Hood in the forest. He tried to get the basket away from her, but she wouldn't give it to him."

By contrast, Amy's story illustrated her marked difficulties in verbal expression: "Riding Hood going to grandma house. Her taking food. Bad wolf in a bed. Riding Hood say, what big ears, grandma? Hear you, dear. What big eyes, grandma? See you, dear. What big mouth, grandma? Eat you all up!"

Amy's story contained many features characteristic of children with expressive disorders at her age, including short, incomplete sentences; simple sentence structures; omission of grammatic function words (e.g., *is* and *the*) and inflectional endings (e.g., possessives and present tense verbs); problems in question formation; and incorrect use of pronouns (e.g., *her* for *she*). Amy, however, performed as well as Lisa in understanding the details and plot of the Riding Hood tale, as long as she was tested with methods that did not involve verbal responding. Amy also demonstrated adequate comprehension skills in her kindergarten classroom, where she readily followed the teacher's complex, multistep verbal instructions (e.g., "After you write your name in the top left corner of your paper, get your crayons and scissors, put your library books under your chair, and line up at the back of the room."). (Courtesy of Carla J. Johnson, Ph.D., and Joseph H. Beitchman, M.D.)

Julio was a quiet, sullen 8-year-old whose expressive language problems were no longer obvious in casual, social conversations. His speech now rarely contained the incomplete sentences and grammatic errors that were so evident when he was younger. His expressive problems, however, still surfaced in tasks involving elaborate or abstract uses of language, such as those required in much of his third-grade academic work. An example was Julio's explanation of the outcome of a recent science experiment: "The teacher had stuff in some jars. He poured it, and it got pink. The other thing made it white." Although each sentence was grammatical, his explanation as a whole was difficult to follow because key ideas and details were omitted or poorly explained. Julio also showed problems in word finding, that is, in using specific words for the concepts and actions he was describing. Instead, he relied on vague, nonspecific terms, such as *thing*, *stuff*, and *got*.

In early elementary grades, Julio had kept pace with his classmates in reading, writing, and other academic skills. By third grade, however, the increasing demands for written work began to have a negative effect his overall academic standing. His written work was characterized by problems similar to those noted in his oral expression, such as poor organization and lack of specificity. Classmates also began to tease him about his difficulties, and he reacted quite aggressively, sometimes to the point of fighting. Nonetheless, Julio continued to show relatively good comprehension of spoken language, including classroom lectures concerning abstract concepts. He also comprehended sentences that were grammatically and conceptually complex (e.g., "The car the truck hit had hubcaps that were stolen. Had it been possible, she would have notified us by mail or by phone.") (Courtesy of Carla J. Johnson, Ph.D., and Joseph H. Beitchman, M.D.)

Differential Diagnosis

Language disorders are associated with many other psychiatric disorders, and the language disorder itself may be difficult to separate from other difficulties. In mental retardation, patients have an overall impairment in intellectual functioning, as shown by below-normal intelligence test scores in all areas, but the nonverbal intellectual capacity and functioning of children with expressive language disorder are within normal limits. In mixed receptive–expressive language disorder, language comprehension (decoding) is markedly below the expected age-appropriate level, whereas in expressive language disorder, language comprehension remains within normal limits.

In pervasive developmental disorders, in addition to the cardinal cognitive characteristics, affected children have no inner language, symbolic or imagery play, appropriate use of gesture, or capacity to form warm and meaningful social relationships. Moreover, children show little or no frustration with the inability to communicate verbally. In contrast, all these characteristics are present in children with expressive language disorder.

Children with acquired aphasia or dysphasia have a history of early normal language development; the disordered language had its onset after a head trauma or other neurologic disorder (e.g., a seizure disorder). Children with selective mutism have a history of normal language development. Often, these children speak only in front of family members (e.g., mother, father, and siblings). Children affected by selective mutism are socially anxious and withdrawn outside the family.

Pathology and Laboratory Examination

Children with speech and language disorders should have an audiogram to rule out hearing loss.

Course and Prognosis

The prognosis for expressive language disorder is related to the severity of the disorder. Studies of "late talkers" concur that 50 to 80 percent of these children master language skills that are within the expected level during the preschool years. Most children who begin to talk later than average but catch up during preschool years are not at high risk to develop further language or learning disorders. Outcome of expressive language disorder is influenced by other comorbid disorders. If children do not develop mood disorders or disruptive behavior problems, the prognosis is better. The rapidity and extent of recovery depend on the severity of the disorder, the child's motivation to participate in therapy, and the timely institution of speech and other therapeutic interventions. The presence or absence of other factors—such as moderate to severe hearing loss, mild mental retardation, and severe emotional problems—also affects the prognosis for recovery. As many as 50 percent of children with mild expressive language disorder recover spontaneously without any sign of language impairment, but children with severe expressive language disorder may later display features of mild to moderate language impairment.

Recent literature has shown that children who demonstrate poor comprehension, poor articulation, or poor academic performance tend to continue to have problems in these areas at follow-up 7 years later. An association is also seen between particular language impairment profiles and persistent mood and behavior problems. Children who have poor comprehension associated with expressive difficulties seem to be the most socially isolated and impaired with respect to peer relationships.

Expressive language level and many nonverbal and communication skills are strongly related in children with language impairment. Expressive language may be seen as an index of general development or as a marker of social and other communication skills. Especially in preschool-age groups, expressive language appears to be related to social and nonverbal communication skills as much as it is simply a measure of knowledge of words.

Treatment

Controversy exists among experts regarding whether intervention for young children with expressive language difficulties should be initiated as soon as it is noted, or whether waiting until age 4 or 5 years is the optimal time to begin treatment. Treatment for expressive language disorder is still generally not initiated unless it persists after the preschool years. Various techniques have been used to help a child improve use of such parts of speech as pronouns, correct tenses, and question forms. Direct interventions use a speech and language pathologist who works directly with the child. Mediated interventions, in which a speech and language professional teaches a child's teacher or parent how to promote therapeutic language techniques, have also been efficacious. Language therapy is often aimed at using words to improve communication strategies as well as social interactions. Such therapy consists of behaviorally reinforced exercises and practice with phonemes (sound units), vocabulary, and sentence construction. The goal is to increase the number of phrases by using block-building methods and conventional speech therapies.

Psychotherapy may be useful for children whose language impairment has affected their self-esteem, insofar as it can be used as a positive model for more effective communication and broadening social skills. Supportive parental counseling may be indicated in some cases. Parents may need help to reduce intrafamilial tensions arising from difficulties in rearing language-disordered children and to increase their awareness and understanding of the disorder.

More research is needed to establish whether early intervention for preschoolers with language deficits has long-term benefits and to develop comprehensive treatment programs that may address the direct language interventions along with interventions for common comorbid communication and learning disorders.

Pharmacotherapy. Pharmacotherapy is not indicated in expressive language disorder unless there is a comorbid condition (i.e., anxiety or depression) that is a contributing factor to the disorder or resulting from the disorder as a reaction to it.

MIXED RECEPTIVE–EXPRESSIVE LANGUAGE DISORDER

Children with mixed receptive–expressive learning disorders exhibit impaired skills in the expression and reception (understanding and comprehension) of spoken language. The expressive difficulties in these children may be similar to those of children with only expressive language disorder, which is characterized by limited vocabulary, use of simplistic sentences, and short sentence usage. Children with receptive language difficulties may be experiencing additional deficits in basic auditory processing skills, such as discriminating between sounds, rapid sound changes, association of sounds and symbols, and the memory of sound sequences. These deficits may lead to a whole host of communication barriers for a child, including a lack of understanding of questions or directives from others, or inability to follow the conversations of peers or family members. Recognition of the disorder in children with mixed expressive-receptive language disorders may be delayed because of early misattribution of their communication by teachers and parents as a behavioral problem rather than a deficit in understanding.

The essential features of mixed receptive-expressive language disorder are shown by scores on standardized tests; receptive (comprehension) and expressive language development scores fall substantially below scores obtained from standardized measures of nonverbal intellectual capacity. Language difficulties must be sufficiently severe to impair academic achievement or daily social communication. A patient with this disorder must not meet the criteria for a pervasive developmental disorder, and the language dysfunctions must exceed those usually associated with mental retardation and other neurologic and sensory-deficit syndromes.

Epidemiology

Mixed receptive–expressive language disorder is believed to occur in about 5 percent of preschoolers and to persist in approximately 3 percent of school-age children. It is less common than expressive language disorder alone. Mixed receptive–expressive language disorder is believed to be at least twice as prevalent in boys as in girls.

Comorbidity

Children with mixed receptive–expressive disorder are at high risk for additional speech and language disorders, learning disorders, and additional psychiatric disorders. About half of children with this disorder also have pronunciation difficulties leading to phonologic disorder, and about half also have reading disorder. These rates are significantly higher than the comorbidity found in children with expressive language disorder alone. ADHD is present in at least one third of children with mixed receptive–expressive language disorder.

Etiology

Language disorders most likely have multiple determinants, including genetic factors, developmental brain abnormalities, environmental influences, neurodevelopmental immaturity, and auditory processing features in the brain. As with expressive language disorder alone, evidence is found of familial aggregation of mixed receptive–expressive language disorder. Genetic contribution to this disorder is implicated by twin studies, but no mode of genetic transmission has been proved. Some studies of children with various speech and language disorders also have shown cognitive deficits, particularly slower processing of tasks involving naming objects and fine motor tasks. Slower myelinization of neural pathways has been hypothesized to account for the slow processing found in children with developmental language disorders. Several studies suggest an underlying impairment of auditory discrimination because most children with the disorder are more responsive to environmental sounds than to speech sounds.

Diagnosis

Children with mixed receptive–expressive language disorder develop language more slowly than their peers and have trouble understanding conversations that peers can follow. In mixed receptive–expressive language disorder, receptive dysfunction coexists with expressive dysfunction. Therefore, standardized tests for receptive and expressive language abilities must be given to anyone suspected of having mixed receptive–expressive language disorder. A markedly below-expected level of comprehension of verbal or sign language with intact age-appropriate nonverbal intellectual capacity, confirmation of language difficulties by standardized receptive language tests, and the absence of pervasive developmental disorders confirm the diagnosis of mixed receptive–expressive language disorder (Table 5–3).

Clinical Features

The essential clinical feature of the disorder is significant impairment in both language comprehension and language expression. In the mixed disorder, the expressive impairments are similar to those of expressive language disorder, but can be more severe.

Table 5–3
DSM-IV-TR Diagnostic Criteria for Mixed Receptive–Expressive Language Disorder

A. The scores obtained from a battery of standardized individually administered measures of both receptive and expressive language development are substantially below those obtained from standardized measures of nonverbal intellectual capacity. Symptoms include those for expressive language disorder as well as difficulty understanding words, sentences, or specific types of words, such as spatial terms.
B. The difficulties with receptive and expressive language significantly interfere with academic or occupational achievement or with social communication.
C. Criteria are not met for a pervasive developmental disorder.
D. If mental retardation, a speech–motor or sensory deficit, or environmental deprivation is present, the language difficulties are in excess of those usually associated with these problems.

Coding note: If a speech–motor or sensory deficit or a neurologic condition is present, code the condition on Axis III.

From American Psychiatric Association. *Diagnostic and Statistical Manual of Mental Disorders.* 4th ed. Text rev. Washington, DC: American Psychiatric Association; copyright 2000, with permission.

The clinical features of the receptive component of the disorder typically appear before the age of 4 years. Severe forms are apparent by the age of 2 years; mild forms may not become evident until age 7 (second grade) or older, when language becomes complex. Children with mixed receptive–expressive language disorder show markedly delayed and below-normal ability to comprehend (decode) verbal or sign language, although they have age-appropriate nonverbal intellectual capacity. In most cases of receptive dysfunction, verbal or sign expression (encoding) of language is also impaired. The clinical features of mixed receptive–expressive language disorder in children between the ages of 18 and 24 months result from a child's failure to utter a single phoneme spontaneously or to mimic another person's words.

Many children with mixed receptive–expressive language disorder have auditory sensory difficulties or cannot process visual symbols, such as explaining the meaning of a picture. They have deficits in integrating auditory and visual symbols—for example, recognizing the basic common attributes of a toy truck and a toy passenger car. Whereas at 18 months, a child with expressive language disorder only can comprehend simple commands and can point to familiar household objects when told to do so, a child of the same age with mixed receptive–expressive language disorder cannot either point to common objects or obey simple commands. A child with mixed receptive–expressive language disorder usually appears to be deaf, but the child can hear. He or she responds normally to nonlanguage sounds from the environment, but not to spoken language. If the child later starts to speak, the speech contains numerous articulation errors, such as omissions, distortions, and substitutions of phonemes. Language acquisition is much slower for children with mixed receptive–expressive language disorder than for children without this disorder.

Children with mixed receptive–expressive language disorder have difficulty recalling early visual and auditory memories and recognizing and reproducing symbols in proper sequence. In some cases, bilateral EEG abnormalities are seen. Some children with mixed receptive–expressive language disorder have a partial hearing defect for true tones, an increased threshold of auditory arousal, and an inability to localize sound sources. Seizure disorders and reading disorder are more common among the relatives of children with mixed receptive–expressive language disorder than they are in the general population.

Most children with mixed receptive–expressive language disorder are impaired socially and in terms of nonverbal communication. This impairment causes a variety of additional difficulties and often results in poor self-esteem and feelings of inferiority, which can further prevent the child from succeeding in the usual developmental tasks.

Pathology and Laboratory Examination

An audiogram is indicated for all children thought to have mixed receptive–expressive language disorder, to rule out or confirm the presence of deafness and to determine the types of auditory deficits. A history of the child and family and observation of the child in various settings help to clarify the diagnosis.

Susan was a pleasant 2-year-old who did not yet use any spoken words. She made her needs known with vocalizations and simple gestures (e.g., showing or pointing) such as those typically used by younger children. She seemed to understand the names for a few familiar people and objects (e.g., *mommy, daddy, cat, bottle*, and *cookie*). Compared with other children her age, she had a small comprehension vocabulary and showed limited understanding of simple verbal directions (e.g., "Get your doll." "Close your eyes."). Nonetheless, her hearing was normal, and her motor and play skills were developing as expected for her age. She showed interest in her environment and in the activities of the other children at her day care. (Courtesy of Carla J. Johnson, Ph.D., and Joseph H. Beitchman, M.D.)

Min was a shy, reserved 5-year-old who grew up in a bilingual home. Min's parents and older siblings spoke English and Cantonese proficiently. Her grandparents, who lived in the same home, spoke only Cantonese. Min began to understand and speak both languages much later than her older siblings had. Throughout her preschool years, Min continued to develop slowly in comprehension and production. At the start of kindergarten, Min understood fewer English words for objects, actions, and relations than her classmates did. She showed difficulties in following classroom instructions, particularly those that involved words for concepts of time (e.g., *tomorrow, before*, or *day*) and space (e.g., *behind, next to*, or *under*). It was also hard for Min to match one of several pictures to a syntactically complex sentence that she had heard (e.g., "It was not the train she was waiting for." "Because he had already completed his work, he was not kept after school.").

Min occasionally tried to speak with other children. These conversations usually broke down, however, because she misinterpreted what others said or could not express her own thoughts clearly. Consequently, her classmates generally ignored her, preferring instead to play with more verbally competent peers. Min's infrequent interactions further limited her opportunities to learn and to practice her already weak language skills. Min also showed limited receptive and expressive skills in Cantonese, as revealed by an assessment conducted with the assistance of a Cantonese interpreter. Nonetheless, her nonverbal cognitive and motor skills were within the normal range for her age. She showed no difficulties in solving spatial, numeric, conceptual, or analogic problems, provided that they were presented nonverbally. (Courtesy of Carla J. Johnson, Ph.D., and Joseph H. Beitchman, M.D.)

Fred received a diagnosis of mixed receptive–expressive language disorder when he was a preschooler. By 8 years of age, he had also received the comorbid diagnoses of reading disorder and ADHD. This combination of language, reading, and attention problems made it virtually impossible for Fred to succeed in school. His comprehension and attention difficulties limited his ability to understand and to learn important information from classroom instructions, discussions, and lectures. Because the unlearned information was critical to the understanding of future academic lessons, Fred fell further and further behind his classmates. He was also disadvantaged because he could read only a few familiar words. This meant that he could not learn other academic information that his classmates acquired by reading textbooks, library books, newspapers, and other written materials. His poor reading ability also limited his opportunities to learn the new vocabulary, complex sentence forms, and sophisticated ideas that other children absorbed from reading. Despite his academic problems, however, Fred continued to show nonverbal intellectual skills within the low normal range, although his scores were somewhat lower than those he had earned as a preschooler. (Courtesy of Carla J. Johnson, Ph.D., and Joseph H. Beitchman, M.D.)

Differential Diagnosis

Children with significant mixed receptive–expressive language disorder have a deficit in language comprehension. This deficit may be overlooked at first because the expressive language deficit may be more obvious. In expressive language disorder alone, comprehension of spoken language (decoding) remains within age norms. Children with phonologic disorder or stuttering have normal expressive and receptive language competence, despite the speech impairments. Hearing impairment should be ruled out.

Most children with mixed receptive–expressive language disorder have a history of variable and inconsistent responses to sounds; they respond more often to environmental sounds than to speech sounds (Table 5–4). Mental retardation, selective mutism, acquired aphasia, and pervasive developmental disorders should also be ruled out. Hearing impairment, pervasive developmental disorders, and severe environmental deprivation can contribute significantly to language impairment.

Course and Prognosis

The overall prognosis for mixed receptive–expressive language disorder is less favorable than that for expressive language disorder alone. When the mixed disorder is identified in a young child, it is usually severe, and the short-term prognosis is poor. Language develops at a rapid rate in early childhood, and young children with the disorder may appear to be falling behind. In view of the likelihood of comorbid learning disorders and other mental disorders, the prognosis is guarded. Young children with

Table 5–4
Differential Diagnosis of Language Disorders

	Hearing Impairment	Mental Retardation	Infantile Autism	Expressive Language Disorder	Mixed Receptive–Expressive Language Disorder	Selective Mutism	Phonologic Disorder
Language comprehension	–	–	–	+	–	+	+
Expressive language	–	–	–	–	–	Variable	+
Audiogram	–	+	+	+	Variable	+	+
Articulation	–	–	– (Variable)	– (Variable)	– (Variable)	+	–
Inner language	+	+ (Limited)	–	+	+ (Slightly limited)	+	+
Uses gestures	+	+ (Limited)	–	+	+	+ (Variable)	+
Echoes	–	+	+ (Inappropriate)	+	+	+	+
Attends to sounds	Loud or low frequency only	+	–	+	Variable	+	+
Watches faces	+	+	–	+	+	+	+
Performance	+	–	+	+	+	+	+

+, normal; –, abnormal.
Courtesy of Lorian Baker, Ph.D., and Dennis Cantwell, M.D.

severe mixed receptive–expressive language disorder are likely to have learning disorders in the future. In children with mild versions, mixed disorder may not be identified for several years, and the disruption in everyday life may be less overwhelming than that in severe forms of the disorder. Over the long run, some children with mixed receptive–expressive language disorder achieve close to normal language functions. The prognosis for children who have mixed receptive–expressive language disorder varies widely and depends on the nature and severity of the damage.

Treatment

A comprehensive speech and language evaluation is recommended for children with mixed receptive–expressive language disorder, before embarking on a speech and language remediation program. Preschoolers with mixed receptive–expressive language disorder optimally receive interventions designed to promote social communication and literacy as well as oral language. For children at the kindergarten level, optimal intervention includes direct teaching of key prereading skills as well as social skills training. An important early goal of interventions for young children with mixed receptive–expressive language disorder is the achievement of rudimentary reading skills because these skills are protective against the academic and psychosocial ramifications of falling behind early on in reading. Some language therapists favor a low-stimuli setting, in which children are given individual linguistic instruction. Others recommend that speech and language instruction be integrated into a varied setting with several children who are taught several language structures simultaneously. Often, a child with mixed receptive–expressive language disorder will benefit from a small, special-educational setting that allows more individualized learning.

Psychotherapy may be helpful for children with mixed receptive–expressive language disorder who have associated emotional and behavioral problems. Particular attention should be paid to evaluating the child's self-image and social skills. Family counseling in which parents and children can develop more effective, less frustrating means of communicating may be beneficial.

Pharmacotherapy. Pharmacotherapy is not indicated in mixed receptive–expressive language disorder unless there is a comorbid condition (i.e., anxiety or depression) that is a contributing factor to the disorder or resulting from the disorder as a reaction to it.

PHONOLOGIC DISORDER

Children with phonologic disorder are unable to produce speech sounds correctly because of omissions of sounds, distortions of sounds, or atypical pronunciation. Typical speech disturbances in this disorder include omitting the last sounds of the word (e.g., saying *mou* for *mouse* or *drin* for *drink*), or substituting one sound for another (saying *bwu* instead of *blue* or *tup* for *cup*). Distortions in sounds can occur when children allow too much air to escape from the side of their mouths while saying sounds like *sh* or producing sounds like *s* or *z* with their tongue protruded. Speech sound errors can also occur in patterns because a child has an interrupted airflow instead of a steady airflow preventing the entire word to be pronounced (e.g., *pat* for *pass* or *bacuum* for *vacuum*). Children with a phonologic disorder can be mistaken for younger children because of their difficulties in producing speech sounds correctly.

The diagnosis of a phonologic disorder is made by comparing the skills of a child with the expected skill level of others of the same age. The disorder results in errors in whole words because of incorrect pronunciation of consonants, substitution of one sound for another, omission of entire phonemes, and, in some cases, dysarthria (slurred speech because of incoordination of speech muscles) or dyspraxia (difficulty planning and executing speech). Speech sound development is believed to be based on linguistic and motor development that must be integrated to produce sounds. According to DSM-IV-TR, if mental retardation, a speech–motor or sensory deficit, or environmental deprivation is present, the language dysfunction must exceed that associated with those problems.

Components of phonologic disorder, such as dysarthria and dyspraxia, are more likely to have a neurologic basis. Developmental articulation disorder, however, is the most common phonologic disorder in children. Developmental phonologic disorder, characterized by frequent misarticulation, sound substitution, and speech sound omission, gives the impression of "baby talk." The developmental form of this disorder is not caused by anatomic, structural, physiologic, auditory, or neurologic abnormalities. It varies from mild to severe and results in speech that ranges from completely intelligible to unintelligible.

Epidemiology

Surveys indicate that the prevalence of phonologic disorder is at least 3 percent in preschoolers, 2 percent in children 6 to 7 years of age, and 0.5 percent in adolescents 17 years old. Approximately 7 to 8 percent of 5-year-old children in one large community sample had speech sound production problems of developmental, structural, or neurologic origins. Another study found that 7.5 percent of children between the ages of 7 and 11 years had phonologic disorders. Of those, 2.5 percent had speech delay (deletion and substitution errors past the age of 4 years) and 5 percent had residual articulation errors beyond the age of 8 years. Developmental phonologic disorders occur much more frequently than disorders with known structural or neurologic origin. The disorder is approximately two to three times more common in boys than in girls. It is also more common among first-degree relatives of patients with the disorder than in the general population. According to DSM-IV-TR, the prevalence decreases to 0.5 percent by mid to late adolescence.

Comorbidity

More than half of children with developmental phonologic disorder have some difficulty with expressive language. Disorders that commonly present with phonologic disorder are expressive language disorder, mixed receptive–expressive language disorder, reading disorder, and developmental coordination disorder. Enuresis may also accompany the disorder. A delay in reaching speech milestones (e.g., first word and first sentence) has been reported in some children with phonologic disorder, but most children with the disorder begin speaking at the appropriate age. Children with phonologic disorder who also have language disorders are at greatest risk for attentional problems and learning disorders. Children with phonologic disorder who do not have language dysfunction have lower risk of comorbid psychiatric or behavioral problems.

Etiology

The likely causes of phonologic disturbance include multiple variables—perinatal problems, genetic factors, auditory processing problems, hearing impairment, and structural abnormalities related to speech. A developmental lag or maturational delay in the neurologic process underlying speech has been postulated in some cases. The likelihood of a subtle brain abnormality is supported by the observation that children with phonologic disorder are also more likely to manifest "soft neurologic signs" as well as additional disorders, including receptive and expressive language difficulties and a higher-than-expected rate of reading disorder. Genetic factors are implicated by data from twin studies that show concordance rates for monozygotic twins that are higher than chance.

Articulation disorders caused by structural or mechanical problems are rare. Phonologic disorders caused by neurologic impairment can be divided into dysarthria and apraxia or dyspraxia. Dysarthria results from an impairment in the neural mechanisms regulating the muscular control of speech. This can occur in congenital conditions, such as cerebral palsy, muscular dystrophy, or head injury or because of infectious processes. Apraxia or dyspraxia is characterized by difficulty in the execution of speech even when no obvious paralysis or weakness of the muscles used in speech exists.

Environmental factors may play a role in developmental phonologic disorder, but constitutional factors seem to make the most significant contribution. The high proportion of phonologic disorder in certain families implies a genetic component in the development of this disorder. Poor motor coordination, laterality, and handedness are not associated with phonologic disorder.

Diagnosis

The essential feature of phonologic disorder is a child's delay or failure to produce developmentally expected speech sounds, especially consonants, resulting in sound omissions, substitutions, and distortions of phonemes. A rough guideline for clinical assessment of children's articulation is that normal 3-year-olds correctly articulate *m, n, ng, b, p, h, t, k, q,* and *d*; normal 4-year-olds correctly articulate *f, y, ch, sh,* and *z*; and normal 5-year-olds correctly articulate *th, s, and r*.

Phonologic disorder cannot be attributed to structural or neurologic abnormalities, and it is accompanied by normal language

Table 5–5
DSM-IV-TR Diagnostic Criteria for Phonologic Disorder

A. Failure to use developmentally expected speech sounds that are appropriate for age and dialect (e.g., errors in sound production, use, representation, or organization such as, but not limited to, substitutions of one sound for another [use of /t/ for target /k/ sound] or omissions of sounds such as final consonants).
B. The difficulties in speech sound production interfere with academic or occupational achievement or with social communication.
C. If mental retardation, a speech–motor or sensory deficit, or environmental deprivation is present, the speech difficulties are in excess of those usually associated with these problems.

Coding note: If a speech–motor or sensory deficit or a neurologic condition is present, code the condition on Axis III.

From American Psychiatric Association. *Diagnostic and Statistical Manual of Mental Disorders.* 4th ed. Text rev. Washington, DC: American Psychiatric Association; copyright 2000, with permission.

development. The DSM-IV-TR diagnostic criteria for phonologic disorder are given in Table 5–5.

Clinical Features

Children with phonologic disorder are delayed in, or incapable of, producing speech sounds that are expected for their age, intelligence, and dialect. The sounds are often substitutions—for example, the use of *t* instead of *k*—and omissions, such as leaving off the final consonants of words. Phonologic disorder can be recognized in early childhood. In severe cases, the disorder is first recognized at about 3 years of age. In less severe cases, the disorder may not be apparent until the age of 6 years. A child's articulation is judged disordered when it is significantly behind that of most children at the same age level, intellectual level, and educational level.

In very mild cases, a single speech sound (i.e., phoneme) may be affected. When a single phoneme is affected, it is usually one that is acquired late in normal language acquisition. The speech sounds most frequently misarticulated are also those acquired late in the developmental sequence, including *r, sh, th, f, z, l,* and *ch*. In severe cases and in young children, sounds such as *b, m, t, d, n,* and *h* may be mispronounced. One or many speech sounds may be affected, but vowel sounds are not among them.

Children with phonologic disorder cannot articulate certain phonemes correctly and may distort, substitute, or even omit the affected phonemes. With omissions, the phonemes are absent entirely—for example, "bu" for "blue," "ca" for "car," or "whaa?" for "what's that?" With substitutions, difficult phonemes are replaced with incorrect ones—for example, "wabbit" for "rabbit," "fum" for "thumb, or "whath dat?" for "what's that?" With distortions, the correct phoneme is approximated, but is articulated incorrectly. Rarely, additions (usually of the vowel "uh") occur—for example, "puhretty" for "pretty," "what's uh that uh?" for "what's that?"

Omissions are thought to be the most serious type of misarticulation, with substitutions the next most serious, and distortions the least serious type. Omissions, which are most frequent in the speech of young children, usually occur at the ends of words or in clusters of consonants ("ka" for "car," "scisso" for "scissors"). Distortions, which are found mainly in the speech of older children, result in a sound that is not part of the speaker's dialect. Distortions may be the last type of misarticulation remaining in the speech of children whose articulation problems have mostly remitted. The most common types of distortions are the lateral slip—in which a child pronounces *s* sounds with the air stream going across the tongue, producing a whistling effect—and the palatal or lisp—in which the *s* sound, formed with the tongue too close to the palate, produces a *ssh* sound effect.

The misarticulations of children with phonologic disorder are often inconsistent and random. A phoneme may be pronounced correctly one time and incorrectly another time. Misarticulations are most common at the ends of words, in long and syntactically complex sentences, and during rapid speech.

Omissions, distortions, and substitutions also occur normally in the speech of young children learning to talk. But, whereas young, normally speaking children soon replace these misarticulations, children with phonologic disorder do not. Even as children with phonologic disorder grow and finally acquire the correct phoneme, they may use it only in newly acquired words and may not correct the words learned earlier that they have been mispronouncing for some time.

Most children eventually outgrow phonologic disorder, usually by the third grade. After the fourth grade, however, spontaneous recovery is unlikely, and so it is important to try to remediate the disorder before the development of complications. Often, beginning kindergarten or school precipitates the improvement when recovery from phonologic disorder is spontaneous. Speech therapy is clearly indicated for children who have not shown spontaneous improvement by the third or fourth grade. Speech therapy should be initiated at an early age for children whose articulation is significantly unintelligible and who are clearly troubled by their inability to speak clearly.

Children with phonologic disorder may have various concomitant social, emotional, and behavioral problems, particularly when comorbid expressive language problems are present. Children with expressive language disorder and severe articulation impairment and children whose disorder is chronic and nonremitting are the ones most likely to suffer from psychiatric problems.

Ramon was a talkative, likeable 3-year-old with virtually unintelligible speech, despite his normal hearing and language comprehension skills. Ramon's level of expressive language development could not be determined because his speech was so difficult to understand. The rhythm and melody of his speech, however, suggested that he was trying to produce multiword utterances, as would be expected at his age.

Ramon produced only a few vowels (/ee/, /ah/, and /oo/), some early-developing consonants (/m/, /n/, /d/, /t/, /p/, /b/, /h/, and /w/), and limited syllables. This reduced sound repertoire made many of his spoken words indistinguishable from one another (e.g., he said *bahbah* for *bottle*, *baby*, and *bubble*, and he used *nee* for *knee*, *need*, and *Anita* [his sister]). Moreover, he consistently omitted consonant sounds at the end of words and in consonant cluster sequences (e.g., /tr-/, /st-/, /-nt/, and /-mp/). On occasion, Ramon reacted with frustration and tantrums to his difficulties in making his needs understood. (Courtesy of Carla J. Johnson, Ph.D., and Joseph H. Beitchman, M.D.)

Kent was a pleasant, cooperative 5-year-old who had been diagnosed with a developmental phonologic disorder when he was a preschooler. His hearing and language comprehension skills were within normal limits. He showed some mild expressive language problems, however, in the use of certain grammatic features (e.g., pronouns, auxiliary verbs, and past-tense word endings) and in the formulation of complex sentences. He correctly produced all vowel sounds and most of the early-developing consonants, but was inconsistent in his attempts to produce later-developing consonants (e.g., /r/, /l/, /s/, /z/, /sh/, /th/, and /ch/). Sometimes, he omitted them; sometimes, he substituted other sounds for them (e.g., /w/ for /r/ or /f/ for /th/); occasionally, he even produced them correctly. Kent had particular problems in correctly producing consonant cluster sequences and multisyllabic words. Cluster sequences had omitted or incorrect sounds (e.g., "*blue*" might be produced as "*bue*" or "*bwue*," and "*hearts*" might be said as "*hots*" or "*hars*"). Multisyllabic words had syllables omitted (e.g., "*effant*" for "*elephant*" and "*getti*" for "spaghetti") and sounds mispronounced or even transposed (e.g., "aminal" for "animal" and "lemon" for melon"). Strangers were unable to understand approximately 80% of Kent's speech. Kent often spoke more slowly and clearly than usual, however, when he was asked to repeat something, as he often was. (Courtesy of Carla J. Johnson, Ph.D., and Joseph H. Beitchman, M.D.)

Natasha was a shy, reserved 8-year-old, with a history of significant speech delay. During her preschool and early school years, she had overcome many of her earlier speech errors. A few late-developing sounds ("/r/," "/l/," and "/th/"), however, continued to pose a challenge for her. Natasha often substituted /f/ or /d/ for /th/ and produced /w/ for /r/ and /l/. Overall, her speech was easily understood, despite these minor errors. Nonetheless, she was often reluctant to speak in front of others because of the teasing she received from her classmates about her speech. (Courtesy of Carla J. Johnson, Ph.D., and Joseph H. Beitchman, M.D.)

Differential Diagnosis

The differential diagnosis of phonologic disorder includes a careful determination of symptoms severity and possible medical conditions that might be producing the symptoms. First, the clinician must determine that the misarticulations are sufficiently severe to be considered impairing, rather than a normative developmental process of learning to speak. Second, the clinician must determine that no physical abnormalities account for the articulation errors and must rule out neurologic disorders that may cause dysarthria, hearing impairment, mental retardation, and pervasive developmental disorders. Third, the clinician must obtain an evaluation of receptive and expressive language to determine that the speech difficulty is not solely attributable to the above mentioned disorders.

Neurologic, oral structural, and audiometric examinations may be necessary to rule out physical factors that cause certain types of articulation abnormalities. Children with dysarthria, a disorder caused by structural or neurologic abnormalities, differ from children with developmental phonologic disorder in that dysarthria is less likely to remit spontaneously and may be more difficult to remediate. Drooling, slow, or uncoordinated motor behavior; abnormal chewing or swallowing; and awkward or slow protrusion and retraction of the tongue indicate dysarthria. A slow rate of speech also indicates dysarthria (Table 5–6).

Course and Prognosis

Spontaneous remission of symptoms is common in children whose misarticulations involve only a few phonemes. Children who persist in exhibiting articulation problems after the age of 5 years may be experiencing a myriad of other speech and language impairments, so that a comprehensive evaluation may be indicated at this time. Children older than age 5 with articulation problems are at higher risk for auditory perceptual problems. Spontaneous recovery is rare after the age of 8 years.

Treatment

Treatment is typically recommended for children with moderate to severe developmental phonologic disorders. Two main approaches have been used successfully to improve phonologic difficulties. The first one, the *phonologic approach,* is usually chosen for children with extensive patterns of multiple speech sound errors that may include final consonant deletion, or consonant cluster reduction. Exercises in this approach to treatment focus on guided practice of specific sounds, such as final consonants, and when that skill is mastered, practice is extended to use in meaningful words and sentences. The other approach, the *traditional approach,* is utilized for children who produce substitution or distortion errors in just a few sounds. In this approach, the child practices the production of the problem sound while the clinician provides immediate feedback and cues concerning

Table 5–6
Differential Diagnosis of Phonologic Dysfunctions

Criteria	Phonologic Dysfunction Due to Structural or Neurologic Abnormalities (Dysarthria)	Phonologic Dysfunction Due to Hearing Impairment	Phonologic Disorder	Phonologic Dysfunction Associated with Mental Retardation, Infantile Autism, Developmental Dysphasia, Acquired Aphasia, or Deafness
Language development	Within normal limits	Within normal limits unless hearing impairment is serious	Within normal limits	Not within normal limits
Examination	Possible abnormalities of lips, tongue, or palate; muscular weakness, incoordination, or disturbance of vegetative functions, such as sucking or chewing	Hearing impairment shown on audiometric testing	Normal	
Rate of speech	Slow; marked deterioration of articulation with increased rate	Normal	Normal; possible deterioration of articulation with increased rate	
Phonemes affected	Any phonemes, even vowels	*f*, *th*, *sh*, and *s*	*r*, *sh*, *th*, *ch*, *dg*, *j*, *f*, *v*, *s*, and *z* are most commonly affected	

Courtesy of Lorian Baker, Ph.D., and Dennis Cantwell, M.D.

the correct placement of the tongue and mouth for improved articulation. Children who have errors in articulation because of an abnormal swallowing resulting in tongue thrust and lisps are treated with exercises that improve swallowing patterns and improve speech.

Speech therapy is typically provided by a speech–language pathologist, but parents can be taught to provide adjunctive help by practicing techniques used in the treatment. Early intervention can be helpful because for many children with mild articulation difficulties, even several months of intervention may be helpful in early elementary school. Generally, when a child's articulation and intelligibility is noticeably different than peers by the age of 8 years, speech deficits often lead to problems with peers, learning, and self-image, especially when the disorder is so severe that many consonants are misarticulated, and when errors involve omissions and substitutions of phonemes, rather than distortions.

Children with persistent articulation problems are likely to be teased or ostracized by peers and may become isolated and demoralized. Therefore, it is important to give support to children with phonologic disorders and, whenever possible, to support prosocial activities and social interactions with peers. Parental counseling and monitoring of child–peer relationships and school behavior can help minimize the social impairment with speech and language disorder.

Pharmacotherapy. Pharmacotherapy is not indicated in phonologic disorder unless there is a comorbid condition (i.e., anxiety or depression) that is a contributing factor to the disorder or resulting from the disorder as a reaction to it.

STUTTERING

Stuttering is a condition in which the normal flow of speech is disrupted by involuntary speech motor events. Stuttering can include a variety of specific disruptions of fluency, including sound or syllable repetitions, sound prolongations, dysrhythmic phonations, and complete blocking or unusual pauses between sounds and syllables of words. In severe cases, the stuttering may be accompanied by accessory or secondary attempts to compensate, such as respiratory, abnormal voice phonations, or tongue clicks. Associated behaviors, such as eye blinks, facial grimacing, head jerks, and abnormal body movements, may be observed before or during the disrupted speech. The disorder usually originates in childhood.

Controversy is found among speech and language experts as to whether stuttering should be considered an independent entity or part of a broader speech and language disorder. Some question whether stuttering should be considered a psychiatric condition at all. Many children who stutter do endure significant psychologic distress, and stuttering does cause impairment in everyday life for many children with this condition.

Epidemiology

Surveys conducted mainly in the United States and Europe indicate the prevalence of stuttering is about 1 percent in the general population. Stuttering tends to be most common in young children and has often resolved spontaneously by the time the child is older. The typical age of onset is 2 to 7 years of age with a peak at age 5 years. Estimates are that up to 3 to 4 percent of individuals may have stuttered at some time in their lives.

Approximately 80 percent of young children who stutter are likely to have a spontaneous remission over time. According to DSM-IV-TR, this likelihood decreases to 0.8 percent by adolescence. Stuttering affects about three to four males for every female. The disorder is significantly more common among family members of affected children than in the general population. According to DSM-IV-TR, for men who stutter, 20 percent of their male children and 10 percent of their female children will also stutter.

Comorbidity

Very young children who stutter typically show some delay in the development of language and articulation without additional disorders of speech and language. Preschoolers and school-age children who stutter exhibit an increased incidence of social anxiety, school refusal, and other anxiety symptoms. Older children who stutter also do not necessarily have comorbid speech and language disorders, but often manifest anxiety symptoms and disorders. When stuttering persists into adolescence, social isolation occurs at higher rates than in the general adolescent population. Stuttering is also associated with a variety of abnormal motor movements, upper body tics, and facial grimaces. Other disorders that coexist with stuttering include phonologic disorder, expressive language disorder, mixed receptive–expressive language disorder, and ADHD.

Etiology

Converging evidence indicates that cause of stuttering is multifactorial, including genetic, neurophysiologic, and psychologic factors that predispose a child to have poor speech fluency. Although research evidence does not indicate that anxiety or conflicts cause stuttering or that persons who stutter have more psychiatric disturbances than those with other forms of speech and language disorders, stuttering can be exacerbated by certain stressful situations.

Other theories about the cause of stuttering include organic models and learning models. Organic models include those that focus on incomplete lateralization or abnormal cerebral dominance. Several studies using EEG found that stuttering males had right-hemispheric alpha suppression across stimulus words and tasks; nonstutterers had left-hemispheric suppression. Some studies of stutterers have noted an overrepresentation of left-handedness and ambidexterity. Twin studies and striking gender differences in stuttering indicate that stuttering has some genetic basis.

Learning theories about the cause of stuttering include the semantogenic theory, in which stuttering is basically a learned response to normative early childhood dysfluencies. Another learning model focuses on classic conditioning, in which the stuttering becomes conditioned to environmental factors. In the cybernetic model, speech is viewed as a process that depends on appropriate feedback for regulation; stuttering is hypothesized to occur because of a breakdown in the feedback loop. The observations that stuttering is reduced by white noise and that delayed auditory feedback produces stuttering in normal speakers lend support to the feedback theory.

The motor functioning of some children who stutter appears to be delayed or slightly abnormal. The observation of difficulties in speech planning exhibited by some children who stutter suggests that higher-level cognitive dysfunction may contribute to stuttering. Although children who stutter do not routinely exhibit other speech and language disorders, family members of these children often exhibit an increased incidence of a variety of speech and language disorders. Stuttering is most likely to be caused by a set of interacting variables that include genetic and environmental factors.

Diagnosis

The diagnosis of stuttering is not difficult when the clinical features are apparent and well developed, and each of the four phases (described in the next section) can be readily recognized. Diagnostic difficulties can arise when trying to determine the existence of stuttering in young children because some preschool children experience transient dysfluency. It may not be clear whether the nonfluent pattern is part of normal speech and language development, or whether it represents the initial stage in the development of stuttering. If incipient stuttering is suspected, referral to a speech pathologist is indicated. Table 5–7 presents the DSM-IV-TR diagnostic criteria for stuttering.

Table 5–7
DSM-IV-TR Diagnostic Criteria for Stuttering

A. Disturbance in the normal fluency and time patterning of speech (inappropriate for the individual's age), characterized by frequent occurrences of one or more of the following:
   (1) sound and syllable repetitions
   (2) sound prolongations
   (3) interjections
   (4) broken words (e.g., pauses within a word)
   (5) audible or silent blocking (filled or unfilled pauses in speech)
   (6) circumlocutions (word substitutions to avoid problematic words)
   (7) words produced with an excess of physical tension
   (8) monosyllabic whole-word repetitions (e.g., "I-I-I-I see him")

B. The disturbance in fluency interferes with academic or occupational achievement or with social communication.

C. If a speech–motor or sensory deficit is present, the speech difficulties are in excess of those usually associated with these problems.

Coding note: If a speech–motor or sensory deficit or a neurologic condition is present, code the condition on Axis III.

From American Psychiatric Association. *Diagnostic and Statistical Manual of Mental Disorders.* 4th ed. Text rev. Washington, DC: American Psychiatric Association; copyright 2000, with permission.

Clinical Features

Stuttering usually appears between the ages of 18 months and 9 years, with two sharp peaks of onset between 2 to 3.5 years and 5 to 7 years. Some, but not all, stutterers have other speech and language problems, such as phonologic disorder and expressive language disorder. Stuttering does not begin suddenly; it typically develops over weeks or months with a repetition of initial consonants, whole words that are usually the first words of a phrase, or long words. As the disorder progresses, the repetitions become more frequent, with consistent stuttering on the most important words or phrases. Even after it develops, stuttering may be absent during oral readings, singing, and talking to pets or inanimate objects.

Four gradually evolving phases in the development of stuttering have been identified:

- **Phase 1** occurs during the preschool period. Initially, the difficulty tends to be episodic and appears for weeks or months between long interludes of normal speech. A high percentage of recovery from these periods of stuttering occurs. During this phase, children stutter most often when excited or upset, when they seem to have a great deal to say, and under other conditions of communicative pressure.
- **Phase 2** usually occurs in the elementary school years. The disorder is chronic, with few, if any, intervals of normal speech. Affected children become aware of their speech difficulties and regard themselves as stutterers. In phase 2, the stuttering occurs mainly with the major parts of speech—nouns, verbs, adjectives, and adverbs.
- **Phase 3** usually appears after the age of 8 years and up to adulthood, most often in late childhood and early adolescence. During phase 3, stuttering comes and goes largely in response to specific situations, such as reciting in class, speaking to strangers, making purchases in stores, and using the telephone. Some words and sounds are regarded as more difficult than others.
- **Phase 4** typically appears in late adolescence and adulthood.

Stutterers show a vivid, fearful anticipation of stuttering. They fear words, sounds, and situations. Word substitutions and circumlocutions are common. Stutterers avoid situations requiring speech and show other evidence of fear and embarrassment.

Stutterers may have associated clinical features: vivid, fearful anticipation of stuttering, with avoidance of particular words, sounds, or situations in which stuttering is anticipated; and eye blinks, tics, and tremors of the lips or jaw. Frustration, anxiety, and depression are common among those with chronic stuttering.

Differential Diagnosis

Normal speech dysfluency in preschool years is difficult to differentiate from incipient stuttering. In stuttering occurs more nonfluencies, part-word repetitions, sound prolongations, and disruptions in voice airflow through the vocal track. Children who stutter appear to be tense and uncomfortable with their speech pattern, in contrast to young children who are nonfluent in their speech, but seem to be at ease. Spastic dysphonia is a stuttering-like speech disorder distinguished from stuttering by the presence of an abnormal breathing pattern.

Cluttering is a speech disorder characterized by erratic and dysrhythmic speech patterns of rapid and jerky spurts of words and phrases. In cluttering, those affected are usually unaware of the disturbance, whereas after the initial phase of the disorder, stutterers are aware of their speech difficulties. Cluttering is often an associated feature of expressive language disorder.

Course and Prognosis

The course of stuttering is usually long-term, with some periods of partial remission lasting for weeks or months and exacerbations occurring most frequently when a stutterer is under pressure to communicate. Of all children who stutter, mostly those with mild cases, 50 to 80 percent recover spontaneously. School-age children who stutter chronically may have impaired peer relationships as a result of testing and social ostracism. The children may face academic difficulties if they avoid speaking in class. Later major complications include an affected person's limitations in occupational choice and advancement.

Treatment

Two distinct forms of intervention have been used in the treatment of stuttering. Direct speech therapy typically targets modification of the stuttering response to fluent-sounding speech by systematic steps and rules of speech mechanics that the person can practice. Another form of therapy for stuttering targets diminishing tension and anxiety during speech. These treatments utilize breathing exercises and relaxation techniques, to help children slow the rate of speaking and modulate speech volume. Until the end of the 19th century, the most common treatments for stuttering were distraction, suggestion, and relaxation. Recent approaches using distraction include teaching stutterers to talk in time to rhythmic movements of the arm, hand, or fingers. Stutterers are also advised to speak slowly in a sing-song or monotone manner. These approaches, however, remove stuttering only temporarily. Suggestion techniques, such as hypnosis, also stop stuttering but, again, only temporarily. Relaxation techniques are based on the premise that it is nearly impossible to be relaxed and stutter in the usual manner at the same time. Current interventions for stuttering use individualized combinations of behavioral distraction, relaxation techniques, and directed speech modification.

Stutterers who have poor self-image, comorbid anxiety disorders, or depressive disorders are likely to require additional treatments. Most modern treatments of stuttering include components that target stuttering as, in part, a learned behavior that can be modified through behavioral techniques regardless of the complexity of how they emerged. These approaches work directly with the speech difficulty to minimize stuttering responses, to modify or decrease the severity of stuttering by eliminating the secondary symptoms, and to encourage stutterers to speak, even when stuttering, in a relatively easy and effortless fashion that aims to eliminate fear and blocks.

One example of this approach is the self-therapy proposed by the Speech Foundation of America. Self-therapy is based on the premise that stuttering is not a symptom, but a behavior that can be modified. Stutterers are told that they can learn to control their difficulty partly by modifying their feelings about stuttering and attitudes toward it and partly by modifying the deviant behaviors associated with their stuttering blocks. The approach includes desensitizing; reducing the emotional reaction to, and fears of, stuttering; and substituting positive action to control the moment of stuttering.

Recently developed therapies focus on restructuring fluency. The entire speech production pattern is reshaped, with emphasis on a variety of target behaviors, including rate reduction; easy or gentle onset of voicing; and smooth transitions between sounds, syllables, and words. The approaches have met with substantial success in establishing perceptually fluent speech in adults, but fluency maintenance over long periods and relapses remain problems for all involved in adult-stuttering treatment.

Pharmacotherapy. Psychopharmacologic intervention, such as treatment with benzodiazepines (e.g., clonazepam [Klonopin]), have been used to promote relaxation; no data exist to assess the efficacy of this approach. Whichever therapeutic approach is used, individual and family assessments and supportive interventions may be helpful. A team assessment of a child or adolescent and his or her family should be made before any approaches to treatment are begun.

COMMUNICATION DISORDER NOT OTHERWISE SPECIFIED

Disorders that do not meet the diagnostic criteria for any specific communication disorder fall into the category of communication disorder not otherwise specified. An example is voice disorder, in which the patient has an abnormality in pitch, loudness, quality, tone, or resonance. To be coded as a disorder, the voice abnormality must be sufficiently severe to impair academic achievement or social communication (Table 5–8). Operationally, speech production can be broken down into five interacting subsystems, including respiration (airflow from the lungs), phonation (sound generation in the larynx), resonance (shaping of the sound quality in the pharynx and nasal cavity), articulation (modulation of the sound stream into consonant and vowel sounds with the tongue, jaw, and lips), and suprasegmentalia (speech rhythm, loudness, and intonation). Altogether, these systems work together to convey information, and, as importantly, voice quality conveys information about the speaker's emotional, psychologic, and physical status. Thus, voice abnormalities can cover a broad area of communication as well as indicate many different types of abnormalities.

Table 5–8
DSM-IV-TR Diagnostic Criteria for Communication Disorder Not Otherwise Specified

This category is for disorders in communication that do not meet criteria for any specific communication disorder; for example, a voice disorder (i.e., an abnormality of vocal pitch, loudness, quality, tone, or resonance).

From American Psychiatric Association. *Diagnostic and Statistical Manual of Mental Disorders.* 4th ed. Text rev. Washington, DC: American Psychiatric Association; copyright 2000, with permission.

Cluttering is not listed as a disorder in DSM-IV-TR, but it is an associated speech abnormality in which the disturbed rate and rhythm of speech impair intelligibility. Speech is erratic and dysrhythmic and consists of rapid, jerky spurts that are inconsistent with normal phrasing patterns. The disorder usually occurs in children between 2 and 8 years of age; in two thirds of cases, the patient recovers spontaneously by early adolescence. Cluttering is associated with learning disorders and other communication disorders.

J. K. was a 14-year-old boy with a repaired unilateral complete cleft lip and palate who presented at his cleft palate center for a follow-up examination. Approximately 4 years had passed since his last appointment with the cleft palate team, partly because his family had moved. J. K. was still mildly hypernasal, but did not exhibit any of the common cleft-type compensatory articulations. For the hypernasality, he was having speech–language therapy in his new hometown. It became immediately obvious during the interview that the pitch of his voice was too high. J. K. was of regular height and build for his age, and, when the clinician palpated his larynx, it had an age-appropriate size.

During the interview, the patient and his family reported that he had experienced teasing at school because of his high-pitched voice. The patient and his family attributed the voice quality to the repaired cleft lip and palate. During a brief course of diagnostic voice therapy, J. K. could immediately be stimulated to lower his pitch to a physiologic level. The diagnosis of postmutational falsetto was made. This condition usually has a strong psychogenic component, so the speech–language pathologist recommended an additional psychiatric consultation as a standard procedure. The patient and his family, however, declined further psychiatric evaluations at this time. The speech–language pathologist in J. K.'s hometown was informed about the diagnosis. She was instructed to change her focus of therapy and treat the voice disorder on its own merits. When the patient came back to the cleft center 1 year later, the problem had been resolved, and the patient had an age-appropriate pitch. (Courtesy of Tim Bressmann, Ph.D., and Joseph H. Beitchman, M.D.)

Because the patient and the family in the case study had refused a psychiatric evaluation, the exact causes of the postmutational falsetto could not be determined. Research shows, however, that psychopathology is not higher in persons with cleft lip and palate than in the normal population. The postmutational falsetto was probably an independent condition that was mistakenly assumed to be caused by the cleft lip and palate by the patient, as well as by professionals involved with his care.

6

Pervasive Developmental Disorders

Pervasive developmental disorders include several that are characterized by impaired reciprocal social interactions, aberrant language development, and restricted behavioral repertoire. Pervasive developmental disorders typically emerge in young children before the age of 3 years, and parents often become concerned about a child by 18 months as language development does not occur as expected. In about 25 percent of cases, some language develops and is subsequently lost. Some children with pervasive developmental disorders are not identified with problems until school age because they make relatively few demands and have minimal conflicts with others owing to their infrequent social engagement. Children with pervasive developmental disorders often exhibit idiosyncratic intense interest in a narrow range of activities, resist change, and are not appropriately responsive to the social environment. These disorders affect multiple areas of development, are manifested early in life, and cause persistent dysfunction. Autistic disorder, the best known of these disorders, is characterized by sustained impairment in comprehending and responding to social cues, aberrant language development and usage, and restricted, stereotypical behavioral patterns. According to the text revision of the fourth edition of the *Diagnostic and Statistical Manual of Mental Disorders* (DSM-IV-TR), to meet criteria for autistic behavior, abnormal functioning in at least one of the previously mentioned areas must be present by age 3 years. More than two thirds of children with autistic disorder have mental retardation, although it is not required for the diagnosis.

The DSM-IV-TR includes five pervasive developmental disorders: autistic disorder, Rett's disorder, childhood disintegrative disorder, Asperger's disorder, and pervasive developmental disorder not otherwise specified. Rett's disorder appears to occur exclusively in girls; it is characterized by normal development for at least 6 months, stereotyped hand movements, a loss of purposeful motions, diminishing social engagement, poor coordination, and decreasing language use. In childhood disintegrative disorder, development progresses normally for the first 2 years, after which the child shows a loss of previously acquired skills in two or more of the following areas: language use, social responsiveness, play, motor skills, and bladder or bowel control. Asperger's disorder is a condition in which the child is markedly impaired in social relatedness and shows repetitive and stereotyped patterns of behavior without a delay in language development. In Asperger's disorder, a child's cognitive abilities and adaptive skills are normal. A recent survey revealed that the average age of diagnosis for children with pervasive developmental disorders was 3.1 years for autistic disorder, 3.9 years for pervasive developmental disorder not otherwise specified, and 7.2 years for Asperger's disorder. Children with severe language deficits received a diagnosis an average of 1 year earlier than other children. Children with behaviors such as hand-flapping, toe-walking, and odd play were identified with disorders at a younger age.

AUTISTIC DISORDER

Autistic disorder (historically called *early infantile autism*, *childhood autism*, or *Kanner's autism*) is characterized by symptoms from each of the following three categories: qualitative impairment in social interaction, impairment in communication, and restricted repetitive and stereotyped patterns of behavior or interests.

History

As early as 1867, Henry Maudsley, a psychiatrist, noted a group of very young children with severe mental disorders who had marked deviation, delay, and distortion in development. In that era, most serious disturbance in young children was believed to fall within the category of psychoses. In 1943 Leo Kanner, in his classic paper "Autistic Disturbances of Affective Contact," coined the term *infantile autism* and provided a clear, comprehensive account of the early childhood syndrome. He described children who exhibited extreme autistic aloneness; failure to assume an anticipatory posture; delayed or deviant language development with echolalia and pronominal reversal (using "you" for "I"); monotonous repetitions of noises or verbal utterances; excellent rote memory; limited range of spontaneous activities, stereotypies, and mannerisms; anxiously obsessive desire for the maintenance of sameness and dread of change; poor eye contact; abnormal relationships with persons; and a preference for pictures and inanimate objects. Kanner suspected that the syndrome was more frequent than it seemed and suggested that some children with this disorder had been misclassified as mentally retarded or schizophrenic. Before 1980, children with pervasive developmental disorders were generally diagnosed with childhood schizophrenia. Over time, it became evident that autistic disorder and schizophrenia were two distinct psychiatric entities. In some cases, however, a child with autistic disorder may develop a comorbid schizophrenic disorder later in childhood.

Epidemiology

Prevalence. Autistic disorder is believed to occur at a rate of about 8 cases per 10,000 children (0.08 percent). Multiple epidemiologic surveys, mainly in Europe, have resulted in variable rates of autistic disorder ranging from 2 to 30 cases per 10,000. By definition, the onset of autistic disorder is before the age of 3 years, although in some cases, it is not recognized until a child is much older.

Some recent studies have shown an apparent increase in the prevalence of autistic disorder. One study reported a prevalence of 19.5 per 10,000 in California, which was also accompanied by a decreased prevalence of mental retardation. Other studies reported rates of up to 60 per 10,000 for autism. The evidence suggests that the majority, if not all, of the reported rise in incidence and prevalence is due to changes in diagnostic criteria; whether there has been a true increase in incidence is under investigation.

Sex Distribution. Autistic disorder is four to five times more frequent in boys than in girls. Girls with autistic disorder are more likely to have more severe mental retardation.

Socioeconomic Status. Early studies suggested that a high socioeconomic status was more common in families with autistic children; however, these findings were probably based on referral bias. Over the last 25 years, no epidemiologic studies have demonstrated an association between autistic disorder and any socioeconomic status.

Etiology and Pathogenesis

Genetic Factors. Current evidence supports a genetic basis for the development of autistic disorder in most cases, with a contribution of up to four or five genes. Family studies have demonstrated a 50 to 200 times increase in the rate of autism in siblings of an index child with autistic disorder. In addition, even when not affected with autism, siblings are at increased risk for a variety of developmental disorders often related to communication and social skills. These difficulties in the nonautistic relatives of persons with autistic disorder are also known by researchers as the "broad phenotype." The specific modes of inheritance are not yet clear. Hypotheses include genetic inheritance of a more general predisposition to developmental difficulties and specific genetic etiology of autistic disorder.

Current research has revealed promising leads on candidate genes likely to underlie the development of autistic disorder. Linkage analyses have demonstrated that regions of chromosomes 7, 2, 4, 15, and 19 are likely to contribute to the genetic basis of autism. It appears that multiple genes are involved in the development of autism. Researchers hypothesize that some genetic forms of autism may be identified in the near future.

The concordance rate of autistic disorder in the two largest twin studies was 36 percent in monozygotic pairs versus 0 percent in dizygotic pairs in one study and about 96 percent in monozygotic pairs versus about 27 percent in dizygotic pairs in the second study. High rates of cognitive difficulties, even in the nonautistic twin in monozygotic twins with perinatal complications, suggest that contributions of perinatal insult along with genetic vulnerability may lead to autistic disorder.

Fragile X syndrome, a genetic disorder in which a portion of the X chromosome fractures, appears to be associated with autistic disorder. Approximately 1 percent of children with autistic disorder also have fragile X syndrome. Children with fragile X syndrome tend to show gross motor and fine motor difficulties and relatively poorer expressive language compared with children with autism without fragile X syndrome. Tuberous sclerosis, a genetic disorder with autosomal dominant transmission characterized by multiple benign tumors, is found with greater frequency among children with autistic disorder. Up to 2 percent of children with autistic disorder may also have tuberous sclerosis.

Recently, researchers screened the DNA of more than 150 pairs of siblings with autism. They found extremely strong evidence that two regions on chromosomes 2 and 7 contain genes involved with autism. Likely locations for autism-related genes were also found on chromosomes 16 and 17, although the strength of the correlation was somewhat weaker. Historically, Kanner, in 1943, described 11 cases of developmentally disordered people and hypothesized that their autistic features were caused by emotionally unresponsive "refrigerator" mothers, but no validity exists to this hypothesis. On the other hand, much evidence supports a biological substrate for this disorder.

Biological Factors. The high rate of mental retardation among children with autistic disorder and the higher-than-expected rates of seizure disorders further support the biological basis for autistic disorder. Approximately 70 percent of children with autistic disorder have mental retardation. About one third of these children have mild to moderate mental retardation, and close to half of these children have severe or profound mental retardation. Children with autistic disorder and mental retardation typically show more-marked deficits in abstract reasoning, social understanding, and verbal tasks than in performance tasks, such as block design and digit recall, in which details can be remembered without reference to the "gestalt" meaning.

Of persons with autism, 4 to 32 percent have grand mal seizures at some time, and about 20 to 25 percent show ventricular enlargement on computed tomography (CT) scans. Various electroencephalogram (EEG) abnormalities are found in 10 to 83 percent of autistic children, and although no EEG finding is specific to autistic disorder, there is some indication of failed cerebral lateralization. Recently, one magnetic resonance imaging (MRI) study revealed hypoplasia of cerebellar vermal lobules VI and VII, and another MRI study revealed cortical abnormalities, particularly polymicrogyria, in some autistic patients. Those abnormalities may reflect abnormal cell migrations in the first 6 months of gestation. An autopsy study revealed fewer Purkinje cells, and another study found increased diffuse cortical metabolism during positron emission tomography (PET) scanning.

Autistic disorder is also associated with neurologic conditions, notably congenital rubella, phenylketonuria (PKU), and tuberous sclerosis. Autistic children have higher-than-expected histories of perinatal complications compared with the general population and also compared with children with other psychiatric disorders. The finding that autistic children have significantly more minor congenital physical anomalies than expected suggests abnormal development within the first trimester of pregnancy.

Immunologic Factors. Several reports have suggested that immunologic incompatibility (i.e., maternal antibodies directed at the fetus) may contribute to autistic disorder. The lymphocytes of some autistic children react with maternal antibodies, which raises the possibility that embryonic neural or extraembryonic tissues may be damaged during gestation.

Perinatal Factors. A higher-than-expected incidence of perinatal complications seems to occur in infants who are later diagnosed with autistic disorder. Maternal bleeding after the first trimester and meconium in the amniotic fluid have been reported in the histories of autistic children more often than in the general population. In the neonatal period, autistic children have a high incidence of respiratory distress syndrome and neonatal anemia. Males with autism, as a group, have been found to be the products of longer gestational age and were heavier at birth than babies in the general population. Females with autism are more likely to be the product of postterm pregnancies than babies in the general population.

Neuroanatomic Factors. The neuroanatomic basis of autism is unknown; however, recent evidence suggests that enlargement of gray and white matter cerebral volumes, but not cerebellar volumes, is present in children with autistic disorder at 2 years of age. Head circumference appears normal at birth, and the increased rate of head circumference growth appears to emerge at about 12 months of age. MRI studies comparing autistic patients and normal controls revealed total brain volume was larger in those with autism, although autistic children with severe mental retardation generally have smaller heads. The greatest average percentage increase in size occurred in the occipital lobe, parietal lobe, and temporal lobe. No differences were found in the frontal lobes. Specific origins of this enlargement are unknown. The increased volume can arise from three possible mechanisms: increased neurogenesis, decreased neuronal death, and increased production of nonneuronal brain tissue, such as glial cells or blood vessels. Brain enlargement has been suggested as a possible biological marker for autistic disorder.

The temporal lobe is believed to be one of the critical areas of brain abnormality in autistic disorder. This suggestion is based on reports of autistic-like syndromes in some persons with temporal lobe damage. When the temporal region of animals is damaged, normal social behavior is lost, and restlessness, repetitive motor behavior, and a limited behavioral repertoire are seen. Some brains of autistic individuals exhibit a decrease in cerebellar Purkinje cells, which is believed to account potentially for abnormalities of attention, arousal, and sensory processes.

Interesting reports of differences between male and female brains are hypothesized to have possible implications for understanding autism insofar as the traits of "empathy" and "systemizing" are involved. Empathizing, the capacity to predict and respond to feelings and behavior of others by inferring their emotional states, is a stronger trait in females than in males at a population level. Males, on the other hand, at a population level, are stronger at systemizing, that is, inferring rules that govern "cause and effect" relationships of behaviors. People with pervasive developmental disorders are characterized by deficits in empathizing, and those with high intellectual capacity have been reported to have relative strengths in rule-bound thinking.

Biochemical Factors. A number of studies in the last few decades have demonstrated that about one third of patients with autistic disorder have high plasma serotonin concentrations. This finding, however, is not specific to autistic disorder, and persons with mental retardation without autistic disorder also display this trait. Several studies have reported that autistic individuals without mental retardation have a high incidence of hyperserotonemia. In some autistic children, a high concentration of homovanillic acid (the major dopamine metabolite) in cerebrospinal fluid (CSF) is associated with increased withdrawal and stereotypes. Some evidence indicates that symptom severity decreases as the ratio of 5-hydroxyindoleacetic acid (5-HIAA, metabolite of serotonin) to homovanillic acid in CSF increases. The 5-HIAA concentration in CSF may be inversely proportional to blood serotonin concentrations, which are increased in one third of autistic disorder patients, a nonspecific finding that also occurs in persons with mental retardation.

Psychosocial and Family Factors. Studies comparing parents of autistic children with parents of nonautistic children have shown no significant differences in child-rearing skills.

Children with autistic disorder, like children with other disorders, can respond with exacerbated symptoms to psychosocial stressors, including family discord, the birth of a new sibling, or a family move. Some children with autistic disorder may be excruciatingly sensitive to even small changes in their families and immediate environment.

Table 6–1
DSM-IV-TR Diagnostic Criteria for Autistic Disorder

A. A total of six (or more) items from (1), (2), and (3), with at least two from (1), and one each from (2) and (3):
(1) qualitative impairment in social interaction, as manifested by at least two of the following:
(a) marked impairment in the use of multiple nonverbal behaviors such as eye-to-eye gaze, facial expression, body postures, and gestures to regulate social interaction
(b) failure to develop peer relationships appropriate to developmental level
(c) a lack of spontaneous seeking to share enjoyment, interests, or achievements with other people (e.g., by a lack of showing, bringing, or pointing out objects of interest)
(d) lack of social or emotional reciprocity
(2) qualitative impairments in communication as manifested by at least one of the following:
(a) delay in, or total lack of, the development of spoken language (not accompanied by an attempt to compensate through alternative modes of communication such as gesture or mime)
(b) in individuals with adequate speech, marked impairment in the ability to initiate or sustain a conversation with others
(c) stereotyped and repetitive use of language or idiosyncratic language
(d) lack of varied, spontaneous make-believe play or social imitative play appropriate to developmental level
(3) restricted repetitive and stereotyped patterns of behavior, interests, and activities, as manifested by at least one of the following:
(a) encompassing preoccupation with one or more stereotyped and restricted patterns of interest that is abnormal either in intensity or focus
(b) apparently inflexible adherence to specific, nonfunctional routines or rituals
(c) stereotyped and repetitive motor mannerisms (e.g., hand or finger flapping or twisting, or complex whole-body movements)
(d) persistent preoccupation with parts of objects

B. Delays or abnormal functioning in at least one of the following areas, with onset prior to age 3 years: (1) social interaction, (2) language as used in social communication, or (3) symbolic or imaginative play.

C. The disturbance is not better accounted for by Rett's disorder or childhood disintegrative disorder.

From American Psychiatric Association. *Diagnostic and Statistical Manual of Mental Disorders.* 4th ed. Text rev. Washington, DC: American Psychiatric Association; copyright 2000, with permission.

Diagnosis and Clinical Features

The DSM-IV-TR diagnostic criteria for autistic disorder are given in Table 6–1.

Physical Characteristics. On first glance, children with autistic disorder do not show any physical signs indicating the disorder. These children do have high rates of minor physical anomalies, such as ear malformations and others that may reflect abnormalities in fetal development of those organs along with parts of the brain.

A greater-than-expected number of autistic children do not show lateralization and remain ambidextrous at an age when cerebral dominance is established in most children. Autistic children also have a higher incidence of abnormal dermatoglyphics (e.g., fingerprints) than those in the general population. This finding may suggest a disturbance in neuroectodermal development.

Behavioral Characteristics

QUALITATIVE IMPAIRMENTS IN SOCIAL INTERACTION. Autistic children do not exhibit the expected level of subtle reciprocal social skills that demonstrate relatedness to parents and peers. As infants, many lack a social smile and anticipatory posture for being picked up as an adult approaches. Less frequent or poor eye contact is common. The social development of autistic children is characterized by impaired but not usually totally absent attachment behavior. Autistic children often do not acknowledge or differentiate the most important persons in their lives—parents, siblings, and teachers—and may show extreme anxiety when their usual routine is disrupted, but they may not react overtly to being left with a stranger. When autistic children have reached school age, their withdrawal may have diminished and be less obvious, particularly in higher-functioning children. A notable deficit is seen in ability to play with peers and to make friends; their social behavior is awkward and may be inappropriate. Cognitively, children with autistic disorder are more skilled in visual-spatial tasks than in tasks requiring skill in verbal reasoning.

One description of the cognitive style of children with autism is that they cannot infer the feelings or mental state of others around them. That is, they cannot make attributions about the motivation or intentions of others and, thus, cannot develop empathy. This lack of a "theory of mind" leaves them unable to interpret the social behavior of others and leads to a lack of social reciprocation.

In late adolescence, autistic persons often desire friendships, but their difficulties in responding to another's interests, emotions, and feelings are major obstacles in developing them. They are often shunned by peers and behave in awkward ways that alienate them from others. Autistic adolescents and adults experience sexual feelings, but their lack of social competence and skills prevents many of them from developing sexual relationships.

DISTURBANCES OF COMMUNICATION AND LANGUAGE. Deficits in language development and difficulty in using language to communicate ideas are among the principal criteria for diagnosing autistic disorder. Autistic children are not simply reluctant to speak, and their speech abnormalities do not result from lack of motivation. Language deviance, as much as language delay, is characteristic of autistic disorder. In contrast to normal children and children with mental retardation, autistic children have significant difficulty putting meaningful sentences together even when they have large vocabularies. When children with autistic disorder do learn to converse fluently, their conversations may impart information without providing a sense of acknowledging how the other person is responding. In children with autism and nonautistic children with language disorders, nonverbal communication skills may also be impaired when significant difficulty with expressive language exists.

In the first year of life, an autistic child's pattern of babbling may be minimal or abnormal. Some children emit noises—clicks, sounds, screeches, and nonsense syllables—in a stereotyped fashion without a seeming intent of communication. Unlike normal young children, who generally have better receptive language skills than expressive ones, verbal autistic children may say more than they understand. Words and even entire sentences may drop in and out of a child's vocabulary. It is not atypical for a child with autistic disorder to use a word once and then not use it again for a week, a month, or years. Children with autistic disorder typically exhibit speech that contains echolalia, both immediate and delayed, or stereotyped phrases that seem out of context. These language patterns are frequently associated with pronoun reversals. A child with autistic disorder might say, "You want the toy" when she means that she wants it. Difficulties in articulation are also common. Many children with autistic disorder use peculiar voice quality and rhythm. About 50 percent of autistic children never develop useful speech. Some of the brightest children show a particular fascination with letters and numbers. Children with autistic disorder sometimes excel in certain tasks or have special abilities; for example, a child may learn to read fluently at preschool age (hyperlexia), often astonishingly well. Very young autistic children who can read many words, however, have little comprehension of the words read.

STEREOTYPED BEHAVIOR. In the first years of an autistic child's life, much of the expected spontaneous exploratory play is absent. Toys and objects are often manipulated in a ritualistic manner, with few symbolic features. Autistic children generally do not show imitative play or use abstract pantomime. The activities and play of these children are often rigid, repetitive, and monotonous. Ritualistic and compulsive phenomena are common in early and middle childhood. Children often spin, bang, and line up objects and may exhibit an attachment to a particular inanimate object. Many autistic children, especially those with severe mental retardation, exhibit movement abnormalities. Stereotypies, mannerisms, and grimacing are most frequent when a child is left alone and may decrease in a structured situation. Autistic children are generally resistant to transition and change. Moving to a new house, moving furniture in a room, or being faced with a change, such as having breakfast before a bath when the reverse was the routine, may evoke panic, fear, or temper tantrums.

INSTABILITY OF MOOD AND AFFECT. Some children with autistic disorder exhibit sudden mood changes, with bursts of laughing or crying without an obvious reason. It is difficult to learn more about these episodes if the child cannot express the thoughts related to the affect.

RESPONSE TO SENSORY STIMULI. Autistic children have been observed to overrespond to some stimuli and underrespond to other sensory stimuli (e.g., to sound and pain). It is not uncommon for a child with autistic disorder to appear deaf, at times showing little response to a normal speaking voice; on the other hand, the same child may show intent interest in the sound of a wristwatch. Some children with autistic disorder have a heightened pain threshold or an altered response to pain. Indeed, some autistic children do not respond to an injury by crying or seeking comfort. Many autistic children seem to enjoy music. They frequently hum a tune or sing a song or commercial jingle before saying words or using speech. Some particularly enjoy vestibular stimulation—spinning, swinging, and up-and-down movements.

ASSOCIATED BEHAVIORAL SYMPTOMS. Hyperkinesis is a common behavior problem in young autistic children. Hypokinesis is less frequent; when present, it often alternates with hyperactivity. Aggression and temper tantrums are observed, often prompted by change or demands. Self-injurious behavior includes head banging, biting, scratching, and hair pulling. Short attention span, poor ability to focus on a task, insomnia, feeding and eating problems, and enuresis are also common among children with autism.

ASSOCIATED PHYSICAL ILLNESS. Young children with autistic disorder have been reported to have a higher-than-expected incidence of upper respiratory infections and other minor infections. Gastrointestinal symptoms commonly found among children with autistic disorder include excessive burping, constipation, and loose bowel movements. Also seen is an increased incidence of febrile seizures in children with autistic disorder. Some autistic children do not show temperature elevations with minor infectious illnesses and may not show the typical malaise of ill children. In some children, behavior problems and relatedness seem to improve noticeably during a minor illness, and in some, such changes are a clue to physical illness.

A standardized instrument that can be very helpful in eliciting comprehensive information regarding developmental disorders is the *Autism Diagnostic Observation Schedule-Generic* (ADOS-G).

> John was the second of two children born to middle-class parents after normal pregnancy, labor, and delivery. As an infant, John appeared undemanding and relatively placid; motor development proceeded appropriately, but language development was delayed. Although his parents indicated that they were first concerned about his development when he was 18 months of age and still not speaking, in retrospect, they noted that, in comparison to their previous child, he had seemed relatively uninterested in social interaction and the social games of infancy. Stranger anxiety had never really

developed, and John did not exhibit differential attachment behaviors toward his parents. Their pediatrician initially reassured John's parents that he was a "late talker," but they continued to be concerned. Although John seemed to respond to some unusual sounds, the pediatrician obtained a hearing test when John was 24 months old. Levels of hearing appeared adequate for development of speech, and John was referred for developmental evaluation. At 24 months, motor skills were age appropriate, and John exhibited some nonverbal problem-solving skills close to age level. His language and social development, however, were severely delayed, and he was noted to be resistant to changes in routine and unusually sensitive to aspects of the inanimate environment. His play skills were quite limited, and he used play materials in unusual and idiosyncratic ways. His older sister had a history of some learning difficulties, but the family history was otherwise negative. A comprehensive medical evaluation revealed a normal EEG and CT scan; genetic screening and chromosome analysis were normal as well.

John was enrolled in a special education program in which he gradually began to speak. His speech was characterized by echolalia, extreme literalness, a monotonic voice quality, and pronoun reversal. He rarely used language in interaction and remained quite isolated. By school age, John had developed some evidence of differential attachments to family members; he also had developed a number of self-stimulatory behaviors and engaged in occasional periods of head banging. Extreme sensitivity to change continued. Intelligence testing revealed marked scatter, with a full-scale intelligence quotient (IQ) in the moderately retarded range. As an adolescent, John's behavioral functioning deteriorated, and he developed a seizure disorder. Now an adult, he lives in a group home and attends a sheltered workshop. He has a rather passive interactional style but exhibits occasional outbursts of aggression and self-abuse. (Courtesy of Fred Volkmar, M.D.)

Intellectual Functioning. About 70 to 75 percent of children with autistic disorder function in the mental retardation range of intellectual function. About 30 percent of children function in the mild to moderate range, and about 45 to 50 percent have severe to profound mental retardation. Epidemiologic and clinical studies show that the risk for autistic disorder increases as the IQ decreases. About one fifth of all autistic children have a normal nonverbal intelligence. The IQ scores of autistic children tend to reflect most severe problems with verbal sequencing and abstraction skills, with relative strengths in visuospatial or rote memory skills. This finding suggests the importance of defects in language-related functions.

Unusual or precocious cognitive or visuomotor abilities occur in some autistic children. The abilities, which may exist even in the overall retarded functioning, are referred to as *splinter functions* or *islets of precocity*. Perhaps the most striking examples are idiot or autistic savants, who have prodigious rote memories or calculating abilities, usually beyond the capabilities of their normal peers. Other precocious abilities in young autistic children include hyperlexia, an early ability to read well (although they cannot understand what they read), memorizing and reciting, and musical abilities (singing or playing tunes or recognizing musical pieces).

Differential Diagnosis

Autism must first be differentiated from one of the other pervasive developmental disorders such as Asperser's disorder and pervasive developmental disorder not otherwise specified. Furthermore, it must be differentiated from other developmental disorders, including mental retardation syndromes and developmental language disorders. Other disorders in the differential diagnosis are schizophrenia with childhood onset, congenital deafness or severe hearing disorder, psychosocial deprivation, and disintegrative (regressive) psychoses. It is sometimes difficult to make the diagnosis of autism because of its overlapping symptoms with childhood schizophrenia, mental retardation syndromes with behavioral symptoms, mixed receptive-expressive language disorder, and hearing disorders. Because children with a pervasive developmental disorder usually have many concurrent problems, Michael Rutter and Lionel Hersov suggested a stepwise approach to the differential diagnosis (Table 6–2).

Schizophrenia with Childhood Onset. Although a wealth of literature on autistic disorder is available, few data exist on children younger than age 12 years who meet the diagnostic criteria for schizophrenia. Schizophrenia is rare in children younger than the age of 5 years. It is accompanied by hallucinations or delusions, with a lower incidence of seizures and mental retardation and a more even IQ than autistic children exhibit. Table 6–3 compares autistic disorder and schizophrenia with childhood onset.

Mental Retardation with Behavioral Symptoms. About 40 percent of autistic children have moderate, severe,

Table 6–2
Procedure for Differential Diagnosis on a Multiaxial System

1. Determine intellectual level
2. Determine level of language development
3. Consider whether child's behavior is appropriate for
   (a) chronologic age
   (b) mental age
   (c) language age
4. If not appropriate, consider differential diagnosis of psychiatric disorder according to
   (a) pattern of social interaction
   (b) pattern of language
   (c) pattern of play
   (d) other behaviors
5. Identify any relevant medical conditions
6. Consider whether there are any relevant psychosocial factors

From Rutter M, Hersov I. *Child and Adolescent Psychiatry: Modern Approaches.* 2nd ed. Oxford: Blackwell; 1985:73, with permission.

Table 6–3
Autistic Disorder versus Schizophrenia with Childhood Onset

Criteria	Autistic Disorder	Schizophrenia (with Onset before Puberty)
Age of onset	Before 38 months	Not younger than 5 years of age
Incidence	2–5 in 10,000	Unknown, possibly same or even rarer
Sex ratio (M:F)	3–4:1	1.67:1 (nearly equal, or slight preponderance of males)
Family history of schizophrenia	Not raised or probably not raised	Raised
Socioeconomic status (SES)	Overrepresentation of upper-SES groups (artifact)	More common in lower-SES groups
Prenatal and perinatal complications and cerebral dysfunction	More common in autistic disorder	Less common in schizophrenia
Behavioral characteristics	Failure to develop relatedness; absence of speech or echolalia; stereotyped phrases; language comprehension absent or poor; insistence on sameness and stereotypies	Hallucinations and delusions; thought disorder
Adaptive functioning	Usually always impaired	Deterioration in functioning
Level of intelligence	In most cases subnormal, frequently severely impaired (70%)	Usually within normal range, mostly dull normal (15%–70%)
Pattern of intelligence quotient	Marked unevenness	More even
Grand mal seizures	4%–32%	Absent or lower incidence

Courtesy of Magda Campbell, M.D., and Wayne Green, M.D.

or profound retardation, and children with retardation may have behavioral symptoms that include autistic features. When both disorders are present, both should be diagnosed. The main differentiating features between autistic disorder and mental retardation are that children with mental retardation usually relate to adults and other children in accordance with their mental age, use the language they do have to communicate with others, and exhibit a relatively even profile of impairments without splinter functions.

Mixed Receptive-Expressive Language Disorder. Some children with mixed receptive-expressive language disorder have mild autistic-like features and may present a diagnostic problem. Table 6–4 summarizes the major differences between autistic disorder and mixed receptive-expressive language disorder.

Acquired Aphasia with Convulsion. Acquired aphasia with convulsion is a rare condition that is sometimes difficult to differentiate from autistic disorder and childhood disintegrative disorder. Children with the condition are normal for several years before losing both their receptive and their expressive language over a period of weeks or months. Most have a few seizures and generalized EEG abnormalities at the onset, but these signs

Table 6–4
Autistic Disorder versus Mixed Receptive-Expressive Language Disorder

Criteria	Autistic Disorder	Mixed Receptive-Expressive Language Disorder
Incidence	2–5 of 10,000	5 of 10,000
Sex ratio (M:F)	3–4:1	Equal or almost equal sex ratio
Family history of speech delay or language problems	Present in about 25% of cases	Present in about 25% of cases
Associated deafness	Very infrequent	Not infrequent
Nonverbal communication (e.g., gestures)	Absent or rudimentary	Present
Language abnormalities (e.g., echolalia, stereotyped phrases out of context)	More common	Less common
Articulatory problems	Less frequent	More frequent
Level of intelligence	Often severely impaired	Although may be impaired, less frequently severe
Patterns of intelligence quotient (IQ) tests	Uneven, lower on verbal scores than dysphasic patients, lower on comprehension subtest than dysphasic patients	More even, although verbal IQ lower than performance IQ
Autistic behaviors, impaired social life, stereotypies, and ritualistic activities	More common and more severe	Absent or, if present, less severe
Imaginative play	Absent or rudimentary	Usually present

Adapted from Magda Campbell, M.D., and Wayne Green, M.D.

usually do not persist. A profound language comprehension disorder then follows, characterized by deviant speech pattern and speech impairment. Some children recover but with considerable residual language impairment.

Congenital Deafness or Severe Hearing Impairment. Because autistic children are often mute or show a selective disinterest in spoken language, they are often believed to be deaf. Differentiating factors include the following: Autistic infants may babble only infrequently, whereas deaf infants have a history of relatively normal babbling that then gradually tapers off and may stop at 6 months to 1 year of age. Deaf children respond only to loud sounds, whereas autistic children may ignore loud or normal sounds and respond to soft or low sounds. Most important, audiogram or auditory-evoked potentials indicate significant hearing loss in deaf children. Unlike autistic children, deaf children usually relate to their parents, seek their affection, and enjoy being held as infants.

Psychosocial Deprivation. Severe disturbances in the physical and emotional environment (e.g., maternal deprivation, psychosocial dwarfism, hospitalism, and failure to thrive) can cause children to appear apathetic, withdrawn, and alienated. Language and motor skills can be delayed. Children with these signs almost always improve rapidly when placed in a favorable and enriched psychosocial environment, but such improvement is not the case with autistic children.

Course and Prognosis

Autistic disorder is generally a lifelong disorder with a guarded prognosis. Autistic children with IQs above 70 and those who use communicative language by age 5 to 7 years tend to have the best prognoses. Recent follow-up data comparing high-IQ autistic children at the age of 5 years with their current symptomatology at ages 13 through young adulthood found that a small proportion no longer met criteria for autism, although they still exhibited some features of the disorder. Most demonstrated positive changes in communication and social domains over time.

The symptom areas that did not seem to improve over time were those related to ritualistic and repetitive behaviors. In general, adult-outcome studies indicate that about two thirds of autistic adults remain severely handicapped and live in complete dependence or semidependence either with their relatives or in long-term institutions. Only 1 to 2 percent acquire a normal, independent status with gainful employment, and 5 to 20 percent achieve a borderline normal status. The prognosis is improved if the environment or home is supportive and capable of meeting the extensive needs of such a child. Although symptoms decrease in many cases, severe self-mutilation or aggressiveness and regression may develop in others. About 4 to 32 percent have grand mal seizures in late childhood or adolescence, and the seizures adversely affect the prognosis.

Treatment

The goals of treatment for children with autistic disorder are to target behaviors that will improve their abilities to integrate into schools and develop meaningful peer relationships and increase their likelihood of maintaining independent living as adults. To do this, treatment interventions aim to increase socially acceptable and prosocial behavior, decrease odd behavioral symptoms, and improve verbal and nonverbal communication. Both language and academic remediation are often required. In addition, treatment goals generally include reduction of disruptive behaviors that may be exacerbated especially during transitions and in school. Children with mental retardation need intellectually appropriate behavioral interventions to reinforce socially acceptable behaviors and encourage self-care skills. In addition, parents, often distraught, need support and counseling. Insight-oriented individual psychotherapy has proved ineffective. Educational and behavioral interventions are currently considered the treatments of choice. Structured classroom training, in combination with behavioral methods, is the most effective treatment for many autistic children.

Well-controlled studies indicate that gains in the areas of language and cognition and decreases in maladaptive behaviors are achieved by consistent behavioral programs. Careful training of parents in the concepts and skills of behavior modification and resolution of the parents' concerns may yield considerable gains in children's language, cognitive, and social areas of behavior. These training programs, however, are rigorous and require much parental time. An autistic child requires as much structure as possible, and a daily program for as many hours as feasible is desirable.

Facilitated communication is a technique by which an autistic child or a child with mental retardation with some language is aided in communication by a teacher who helps the child pick out letters on a computer or letter board. Some facilitators have reported success in eliciting language to produce messages demonstrating a child's ability to read and write, do mathematics, express feelings, and even write poetry. Although these techniques are risky, because the facilitator may need to inject much interpretation to produce typical communication, some families of autistic children support this technique and continue to use it.

Psychopharmacologic trials are under way to investigate efficacy of a variety of classes of agents in promoting social interactions and reducing disruptive behaviors in children and adolescents with autism and other pervasive developmental disorders. No specific medications with proved efficacy in the treatment of the core symptoms of autistic disorder are available; however, medications have been shown to be promising in reducing hyperactivity, obsessions and compulsive behaviors, irritability, aggression, and self-injurious behaviors.

A recent open trial of escitalopram (Lexapro) in children with pervasive developmental disorders showed a trend toward improvement in 61 percent of subjects on the following subscales of the Aberrant Behavior Checklist-Community Version

(ABC-CV): Irritability, Lethargy, Stereotypy, Hyperactivity, and Inappropriate Speech. Although irritability was the main outcome variable, the other domains were also rated as improved.

A recent randomized, controlled, crossover trial of methylphenidate (Ritalin) in 72 children between the ages of 5 and 14 years with pervasive developmental disorders and hyperactivity revealed that methylphenidate was superior to placebo in the treatment of hyperactivity in 49 percent of the subjects. Although this response rate is substantially lower than for children with attention-deficit/hyperactivity disorder (ADHD) without pervasive developmental disorders, response rate was significant in almost half of the sample. Adverse effects led to discontinuation of medication in 18 percent of the children, which is higher than expected for children with ADHD without pervasive developmental disorders.

The administration of antipsychotic medication has been shown to be efficacious in the reduction of aggressive and self-injurious behavior. One early study indicated that haloperidol (Haldol) reduced behavioral symptoms such as hyperactivity, stereotypies, withdrawal, fidgetiness, irritability, and labile affect and accelerated learning. Given its potentially serious adverse effects, haloperidol is no longer the antipsychotic agent of choice in the treatment of self-injurious behaviors in children with autistic disorder.

The atypical antipsychotic agents are known to have a lower risk of causing extrapyramidal adverse effects, although some sensitive individuals cannot tolerate the extrapyramidal or anticholinergic adverse effects of the atypical antipsychotic agents. The atypical antipsychotic agents include risperidone (Risperdal), olanzapine (Zyprexa), quetiapine (Seroquel), clozapine (Clozaril), and ziprasidone (Geodon).

Risperidone, a high-potency antipsychotic with combined dopamine D_2– and serotonin 5-HT_2–receptor antagonist properties, has been used to subdue aggressive or self-injurious behaviors. Several reports suggested that risperidone is effective in diminishing aggressiveness, hyperactivity, and self-injurious behavior in children with autistic disorder. In some cases, it reportedly encouraged socially acceptable behaviors. Studies of risperidone use in the treatment of adult and adolescent psychosis indicate that a dose of up to 4 to 6 mg per day may be necessary for optional effect. For children with autism, lower doses, ranging from 0.5 to 4 mg per day, are used in clinical practice. Extrapyramidal effects and akathisia have been reported as adverse effects, as have sedation, dizziness, and weight gain. A recent report on acute and long-term safety and tolerability of risperidone in children with autism documented the following side effects as moderate or higher in children on placebo versus risperidone: somnolence (12 percent vs. 37 percent), excessive appetite (10 percent vs. 33 percent), and rhinitis (8 percent vs. 16 percent). Drooling was reported more in the risperidone group than with the placebo group. In this sample, extrapyramidal symptoms were not reported more commonly in the risperidone group. The side effects that caused the most concern were somnolence and weight gain.

Olanzapine specifically blocks 5-HT_{2A} and D_2 receptors and also blocks muscarinic receptors. No studies provide specific guidelines regarding the use of olanzapine in children with autism. Doses that have been used clinically to target aggression and self-injurious behaviors range from 2.5 to about 10 mg per day. Among olanzapine's most common adverse effects are sedation, orthostatic hypotension, and (over time) weight gain.

Quetiapine is an antipsychotic with more potent 5-H_2– than D_2–receptor blocking properties. Although no data on its effectiveness on aggression in children with autism exist, it is sometimes tried when risperidone and olanzapine are not efficacious or well tolerated. No guidelines exist about the best dose; it has been used in clinical practice at doses ranging from 50 to 200 mg per day. Adverse effects include drowsiness, tachycardia, agitation, and weight gain.

Clozapine has a heterocyclic chemical structure that is related to certain conventional antipsychotics, such as loxapine (Loxitane), although clozapine carries a lower risk of extrapyramidal symptoms. It is not generally used in the treatment of aggression and self-injurious behavior unless those behaviors coexist with psychotic symptoms. Its most serious adverse effect is agranulocytosis, which necessitates monitoring white blood cell count weekly during clozapine's use. Its use is generally limited to treatment-resistant psychotic patients.

Ziprasidone has receptor-blocking properties at the 5-HT_{2A} and D_2 receptor sites and carries little risk of extrapyramidal and antihistaminic effects. No guidelines exist for its use in autistic children with aggressive and self-injurious behaviors, but it has been used clinically to treat the latter behaviors in children who are treatment resistant. In studies of its use in adults with schizophrenia, doses in the range of 40 to 160 mg were found to be effective. Adverse effects include sedation, dizziness, and lightheadedness. An electrocardiogram (ECG) is generally obtained before use of this medication.

Aripiprazole is the newest atypical antipsychotic and has been shown to improve behaviors including aggression, self-injurious behavior, and irritability. In two small trials with mean doses of 7.5 to 12 mg per day it showed significant improvement with less weight gain and extrapyramidal symptoms. Patients experienced mild sedation and mean weight gain of 2.7 pounds.

Lithium (Eskalith) can be administered in the treatment of aggressive or self-injurious behaviors when antipsychotic medications fail.

A recent double-blind study investigated the efficacy of amantadine (Symmetrel), which blocks *N*-methyl-D-aspartate (NMDA) receptors, in the treatment of behavioral disturbance, such as irritability, aggression, and hyperactivity, in children with autism. Some researchers have suggested that abnormalities of the glutamatergic system may contribute to the emergence of pervasive developmental disorders. High glutamate levels have been found in children with Rett's syndrome. In the amantadine study, 47 percent of children on amantadine were rated "improved" by their parents, and 37 percent of children on placebo were rated "improved" by parents in irritability and hyperactivity, although this difference was not statistically significant. Investigators rated the children on amantadine "significantly improved" with respect to hyperactivity. A double-blind, placebo-controlled study of the efficacy of the anticonvulsant lamotrigine (Lamictal) on hyperactivity in children with autism showed high rates of placebo improvement in ratings of hyperactivity.

Clomipramine (Anafranil) has been used in autistic disorders but without positive results. Fenfluramine (Pondimin), which reduces blood serotonin levels, has also been used unsuccessfully in the treatment of autism. Improvement does not seem to be associated with a reduction in blood serotonin level. Naltrexone (ReVia), an opioid-receptor antagonist, has been investigated without much success, based on the notion that blocking endogenous opioids would reduce autistic symptoms.

Tetrahydrobiopterin, a coenzyme that enhances the action of enzymes, has recently been used in a double-blind, placebo-controlled, crossover study of 12 children with autistic disorder and low concentrations of spinal tetrahydrobiopterin. The children received a daily dose of 3 mg tetrahydrobiopterin per kilogram during a 6-month period alternating with placebo. Results indicated small, nonsignificant changes in the total scores on the Childhood Autism Rating Scale after 3- and 6-month treatment. Post hoc analysis of the three core symptoms of autism—social interaction, communication, and stereotyped behaviors—revealed a significant improvement in social interaction score after 6 months of active treatment. A positive correlation was noted between social response and IQ. These results suggest that there is a possible effect of tetrahydrobiopterin on the social functioning of children with autism.

A recent case report suggested that low-dose venlafaxine (Effexor) was efficacious in three adolescents and young adults with autistic disorder with self-injurious behavior and hyperactivity. The dose of venlafaxine used was 18.75 mg per day, and efficacy was reported to be sustained over a 6-month period. Some reports have suggested the use of clonidine, guanefacine, and atomoxetine to reduce symptoms of irritability and stereotypies.

RETT'S DISORDER

In 1965, Andreas Rett, an Austrian physician, identified a syndrome in 22 girls who appeared to have developed normally for at least 6 months followed by devastating developmental deterioration. Rett's disorder is a progressive condition that has its onset after some months of what appears to be normal development. Head circumference is normal at birth, and developmental milestones are unremarkable in early life. Between 5 and 48 months of age, generally between 6 months and 1 year, head growth begins to decelerate.

Data indicate a prevalence of 6 to 7 cases of Rett's disorder per 100,000 girls. Originally, it was believed that Rett's disorder occurred only in females, but males with the disorder or syndromes that are very close to this disorder have now been described.

Etiology

The cause of Rett's disorder is unknown, although the progressive deteriorating course after an initial normal period is compatible with a metabolic disorder. In some patients with Rett's disorder, the presence of hyperammonemia has led to the hypothesis that an enzyme metabolizing ammonia is deficient, but hyperammonemia has not been found in most patients with Rett's disorder. It is likely that Rett's disorder has a genetic basis. It has been seen primarily in girls, and case reports indicate complete concordance in monozygotic twins.

Diagnosis and Clinical Features

During the first 5 months after birth, infants have age-appropriate motor skills, normal head circumference, and normal growth. Social interactions show the expected reciprocal quality. At 6 months to 2 years of age, however, these children develop progressive encephalopathy with a number of characteristic features. The signs often include the loss of purposeful hand movements, which are replaced by stereotypic motions, such as hand-wringing; the loss of previously acquired speech; psychomotor retardation; and ataxia. Other stereotypical hand movements may occur, such as licking or biting the fingers and tapping or slapping. The head circumference growth decelerates, and microcephaly results. All language skills are lost, and both receptive and expressive communicative and social skills seem to plateau at developmental levels between 6 months and 1 year. Poor muscle coordination and an apraxic gait with an unsteady and stiff quality develop. All of these clinical features are diagnostic criteria for the disorder (Table 6–5).

Table 6–5
DSM-IV-TR Diagnostic Criteria for Rett's Disorder

A. All of the following:
  (1) apparently normal prenatal and perinatal development
  (2) apparently normal psychomotor development through the first 5 months after birth
  (3) normal head circumference at birth

B. Onset of all of the following after the period of normal development:
  (1) deceleration of head growth between ages 5 and 48 months
  (2) loss of previously acquired purposeful hand skills between ages 5 and 30 months with the subsequent development of stereotyped hand movements (e.g., hand wringing or hand washing)
  (3) loss of social engagement early in the course (although often social interaction develops later)
  (4) appearance of poorly coordinated gait or trunk movements
  (5) severely impaired expressive and receptive language development with severe psychomotor retardation

From American Psychiatric Association. *Diagnostic and Statistical Manual of Mental Disorders.* 4th ed. Text rev. Washington, DC: American Psychiatric Association; copyright 2000, with permission.

Associated features include seizures in up to 75 percent of affected children and disorganized EEGs with some epileptiform discharges in almost all young children with Rett's disorder, even in the absence of clinical seizures. An additional associated feature is irregular respiration, with episodes of hyperventilation, apnea, and breath-holding. The disorganized breathing occurs in most patients while they are awake; during sleep, the breathing usually normalizes. Many patients with Rett's disorder also have scoliosis. As the disorder progresses, muscle tone seems to change from an initial hypotonic condition to spasticity to rigidity.

Although children with Rett's disorder may live for well more than a decade after the onset of the disorder, after 10 years, many patients are wheelchair bound, with muscle wasting, rigidity, and virtually no language ability. Long-term receptive and expressive communication and socialization abilities remain at a developmental level of less than 1 year.

> Darla was born at term after an uncomplicated pregnancy. An amniocentesis had been obtained because of maternal age and was normal. At birth, Darla was in good condition; weight, height, and head circumference were all near the 50th percentile. Her development during the first months of life was within normal limits. At approximately 8 months of age, her development seemed to stagnate and her interest in the environment, including the social environment, waned. Her developmental milestones then became markedly delayed; she was just starting to walk at her second birthday and had no spoken language. Evaluation at that time revealed that head growth had decelerated. Some self-stimulatory behaviors were present. Marked cognitive and communicative delays were noted on formal testing. Darla began to lose purposeful hand movements and developed unusual hand-washing stereotyped behaviors. By age 6, her EEG was abnormal and purposeful hand movements were markedly impaired. Subsequently, she developed truncal ataxia and breath-holding spells, and motor skills deteriorated further. (Courtesy of Fred Volkmar, M.D.)

Differential Diagnosis

Some children with Rett's disorder receive initial diagnoses of autistic disorder because of the marked disability in social interactions in both disorders, but the two disorders have some predictable differences. In Rett's disorder, a child shows deterioration of developmental milestones, head circumference, and overall growth; in autistic disorder, aberrant development is usually present early. In Rett's disorder, specific and characteristic hand motions are always present; in autistic disorder, hand mannerisms may or may not appear. Poor coordination, ataxia, and apraxia are predictably part of Rett's disorder; many persons with autistic disorder have unremarkable gross motor function. In Rett's disorder, verbal abilities are usually lost completely; in autistic disorder, patients use characteristically aberrant language. Respiratory irregularity is characteristic of Rett's disorder, and seizures often appear early; in autistic disorder, no respiratory disorganization is seen, and seizures do not develop in most patients; when seizures do develop, they are more likely in adolescence than in childhood.

Course and Prognosis

Rett's disorder is progressive. The prognosis is not fully known, but patients who live into adulthood remain at a cognitive and social level equivalent to that in the first year of life.

Treatment

Treatment is symptomatic. Physiotherapy has been beneficial for the muscular dysfunction, and anticonvulsant treatment is usually necessary to control the seizures. Behavior therapy, along with medication, may help to control self-injurious behaviors, as it does in the treatment of autistic disorder, and it may help to regulate the breathing disorganization.

CHILDHOOD DISINTEGRATIVE DISORDER

Childhood disintegrative disorder is characterized by marked regression in several areas of functioning after at least 2 years of apparently normal development. Childhood disintegrative disorder, also called *Heller's syndrome* and *disintegrative psychosis*, was described in 1908 as a deterioration over several months of intellectual, social, and language function occurring in 3- and 4-year-olds with previously normal functions. After the deterioration, the children closely resembled children with autistic disorder.

Epidemiology

Epidemiological data have been complicated by the variable diagnostic criteria used, but childhood disintegrative disorder is estimated to be at least one tenth as common as autistic disorder, and the prevalence has been estimated to be about 1 case in 100,000 boys. The ratio of boys to girls is estimated to be between 4 and 8 boys to 1 girl.

Etiology

The cause of childhood disintegrative disorder is unknown, but it has been associated with other neurologic conditions, including seizure disorders, tuberous sclerosis, and various metabolic disorders.

Diagnosis and Clinical Features

The diagnosis is made on the basis of features that fit a characteristic age of onset, clinical picture, and course. Cases reported have ranged in onset from ages 1 to 9 years, but in most, the onset is between 3 and 4 years; according to DSM-IV-TR, the

Table 6–6
DSM-IV-TR Diagnostic Criteria for Childhood Disintegrative Disorder

A. Apparently normal development for at least the first 2 years after birth as manifested by the presence of age-appropriate verbal and nonverbal communication, social relationships, play, and adaptive behavior.
B. Clinically significant loss of previously acquired skills (before age 10 years) in at least two of the following areas:
 (1) expressive or receptive language
 (2) social skills or adaptive behavior
 (3) bowel or bladder control
 (4) play
 (5) motor skills
C. Abnormalities of functioning in at least two of the following areas:
 (1) qualitative impairment in social interaction (e.g., impairment in nonverbal behaviors, failure to develop peer relationships, lack of social or emotional reciprocity)
 (2) qualitative impairments in communication (e.g., delay or lack of spoken language, inability to initiate or sustain a conversation, stereotyped and repetitive use of language, lack of varied make-believe play)
 (3) restricted, repetitive, and stereotyped patterns of behavior, interests, and activities, including motor stereotypies and mannerisms
D. The disturbance is not better accounted for by another specific pervasive developmental disorder or by schizophrenia.

From American Psychiatric Association. *Diagnostic and Statistical Manual of Mental Disorders.* 4th ed. Text rev. Washington, DC: American Psychiatric Association; copyright 2000, with permission.

minimum age of onset is 2 years (Table 6–6). The onset may be insidious over several months or relatively abrupt, with abilities diminishing in days or weeks. In some cases, a child displays restlessness, increased activity level, and anxiety before the loss of function. The core features of the disorder include loss of communication skills, marked regression of reciprocal interactions, and the onset of stereotyped movements and compulsive behavior. Affective symptoms are common, particularly anxiety, as is the regression of self-help skills, such as bowel and bladder control.

To receive the diagnosis, a child must exhibit loss of skills in two of the following areas: language, social, or adaptive behavior; bowel or bladder control; play; and motor skills. Abnormalities must be present in at least two of the following categories: reciprocal social interaction, communication skills, and stereotyped or restricted behavior. The main associated neurologic feature is seizure disorder.

Bob's early history was within normal limits. By age 2, he was speaking in sentences, and his development appeared to be proceeding appropriately. At age 40 months he abruptly exhibited a period of marked behavioral regression shortly after the birth of a sibling. He lost previously acquired skills in communication and was no longer toilet trained. He became uninterested in social interaction, and various unusual self-stimulatory behaviors became evident. Comprehensive medical examination failed to reveal any conditions that might account for this developmental regression. Behaviorally, he exhibited features of autistic disorder. At follow-up at age 12 he spoke only an occasional single word and was severely retarded. (Courtesy of Fred Volkmar, M.D.)

Differential Diagnosis

The differential diagnosis of childhood disintegrative disorder includes autistic disorder and Rett's disorder. In many cases, the clinical features overlap with autistic disorder, but childhood disintegrative disorder is distinguished from autistic disorder by the loss of previously acquired development. Before the onset of childhood disintegrative disorder (occurring at 2 years or older), language has usually progressed to sentence formation. This skill is strikingly different from the premorbid history of even high-functioning patients with autistic disorder, in whom language generally does not exceed single words or phrases before diagnosis of the disorder. Once the disorder occurs, however, those with childhood disintegrative disorder are more likely to have no language abilities than are high-functioning patients with autistic disorder. In Rett's disorder, the deterioration occurs much earlier than in childhood disintegrative disorder, and the characteristic hand stereotypies of Rett's disorder do not occur in childhood disintegrative disorder.

Course and Prognosis

The course of childhood disintegrative disorder is variable, with a plateau reached in most cases, a progressive deteriorating course in rare cases, and some improvement in occasional cases to the point of regaining the ability to speak in sentences. Most patients are left with at least moderate mental retardation.

Treatment

Because of the clinical similarity to autistic disorder, the treatment of childhood disintegrative disorder includes the same components available in the treatment of autistic disorder.

ASPERGER'S DISORDER

Asperger's disorder is characterized by impairment and oddity of social interaction and restricted interest and behavior reminiscent of those seen in autistic disorder. Unlike autistic disorder, in Asperger's disorder no significant delays occur in language, cognitive development, or age-appropriate self-help skills. In 1944, Hans Asperger, an Austrian physician, described a syndrome that he named "autistic psychopathy." His original description of the syndrome applied to persons with normal intelligence who exhibit a qualitative impairment in reciprocal social interaction and behavioral oddities without delays in language development. Asperger's disorder occurs in a wide variety of severities, including cases in which very subtle social cues are missed but overall social interactions are mastered.

Etiology

The cause of Asperger's disorder is unknown, but family studies suggest a possible relationship to autistic disorder. The similarity of Asperger's disorder to autistic disorder supports the presence of genetic, metabolic, infectious, and perinatal contributing factors.

Diagnosis and Clinical Features

The clinical features include at least two of the following indications of qualitative social impairment: markedly abnormal nonverbal communicative gestures, failure to develop peer relationships, lack of social or emotional reciprocity, and impaired ability to express pleasure in other persons' happiness. Restricted interests and patterns of behavior are always present, but when they are subtle, they may not be immediately identified or singled out as different from those of other children. According to DSM-IV-TR, the patient shows no language delay, clinically significant cognitive delay, or adaptive impairment (Table 6–7).

Tom was an only child. Birth, medical, and family histories were unremarkable. His motor development was somewhat delayed, but communicative milestones were within normal limits. His parents became concerned about him at age 4 when he was enrolled in a nursery school and was noted to have marked difficulties in peer interaction that were so pronounced that he could not continue in the program. In grade school, he was enrolled in special education classes and was noted to have some learning problems. His greatest difficulties arose in peer interaction—he was viewed as markedly eccentric and had no friends. His preferred activity, watching the weather channel on television, was pursued with great interest and intensity. On examination at age 13, he had markedly circumscribed interests and exhibited pedantic and odd patterns of communication with a monotonic voice quality. Psychological testing revealed an IQ within the normal range, with marked scatter evident. Formal communication examination revealed age-appropriate skills in receptive and expressive language but marked impairment in pragmatic language skills. (Courtesy of Fred Volkmar, M.D.)

Table 6–7
DSM-IV-TR Diagnostic Criteria for Asperger's Disorder

A. Qualitative impairment in social interaction, as manifested by at least two of the following:
   (1) marked impairment in the use of multiple nonverbal behaviors such as eye-to-eye gaze, facial expression, body postures, and gestures to regulate social interaction
   (2) failure to develop peer relationships appropriate to developmental level
   (3) a lack of spontaneous seeking to share enjoyment, interests, or achievements with other people (e.g., by a lack of showing, bringing, or pointing out objects of interest to other people)
   (4) lack of social or emotional reciprocity

B. Restricted repetitive and stereotyped patterns of behavior, interests, and activities, as manifested by at least one of the following:
   (1) encompassing preoccupation with one or more stereotyped and restricted patterns of interest that is abnormal either in intensity or focus
   (2) apparently inflexible adherence to specific, nonfunctional routines or rituals
   (3) stereotyped and repetitive motor mannerisms (e.g., hand or finger flapping or twisting, or complex whole-body movements)
   (4) persistent preoccupation with parts of objects

C. The disturbance causes clinically significant impairment in social, occupational, or other important areas of functioning.

D. here is no clinically significant general delay in language (e.g., single words used by age 2 years, communicative phrases used by age 3 years).

E. There is no clinically significant delay in cognitive development or in the development of age-appropriate self-help skills, adaptive behavior (other than in social interaction), and curiosity about the environment in childhood.

F. Criteria are not met for another specific pervasive developmental disorder or schizophrenia.

From American Psychiatric Association. *Diagnostic and Statistical Manual of Mental Disorders.* 4th ed. Text rev. Washington, DC: American Psychiatric Association; copyright 2000, with permission.

Differential Diagnosis

The differential diagnosis includes autistic disorder, pervasive developmental disorder not otherwise specified, and, in patients approaching adulthood, schizoid personality disorder. According to DSM-IV-TR, the most obvious distinctions between Asperger's disorder and autistic disorder are the absence of language delay and dysfunction. The lack of language delay and impaired use of language are requirements for Asperger's disorder, whereas language impairment is a core feature in autistic disorder. Recent studies comparing children with Asperger's disorder and autistic disorder found that children with Asperger's disorder were more likely to look for social interaction and sought more vigorously to make friends. Although significant general delay in language is an exclusionary criterion in the diagnosis of Asperger's disorder, some delay in the acquisition of language has been seen in more than one third of clinical samples.

Course and Prognosis

Although little is known about the cohort described by the DSM-IV-TR diagnostic criteria, past case reports showed variable courses and prognoses for patients who received diagnoses of Asperger's disorder. The factors associated with a good prognosis are a normal IQ and high-level social skills. Anecdotal reports of some adults diagnosed with Asperger's disorder as children show them to be verbal and intelligent; however, they relate in an awkward way to other adults, appear socially uncomfortable and shy, and often exhibit illogical thinking.

Treatment

Treatment of Asperger's disorder is supportive, and goals are to promote social behaviors and peer relationships. Interventions are initiated with the goal of shaping interactions so that they better match those of peers. Very often children with Asperger's disorder are highly verbal and have excellent academic achievement. The tendency of children and adolescents with Asperger's disorder to rely on rigid rules and routines can become a source of difficulty for them and be an area that requires therapeutic intervention. A comfort with routines, however, can be used to foster positive habits that may enhance the social life of a child with Asperger's disorder. Self-sufficiency and problem-solving techniques are often helpful for these individuals in social situations and in a work setting. Some of the same techniques used for autistic disorder are likely to benefit patients with Asperger's disorder with severe social impairment.

Pharmacotherapy. Psychopharmacologic therapy can also be used and is similar to that of autism discussed previously.

PERVASIVE DEVELOPMENTAL DISORDER NOT OTHERWISE SPECIFIED

The DSM-IV-TR defines pervasive disorder not otherwise specified as severe, pervasive impairment in communication skills or the presence of stereotyped behavior, interests, and activities with associated impairment in social interactions. The criteria for a specific pervasive developmental disorder, schizophrenia, and schizotypal and avoidant personality disorders are not met, however (Table 6–8). Some children who receive the diagnosis exhibit a markedly restricted repertoire of activities and interest. The condition usually shows a better outcome than autistic disorder.

Table 6–8
DSM-IV-TR Diagnostic Criteria for Pervasive Developmental Disorder Not Otherwise Specified (Including Atypical Autism)

This category should be used when there is a severe and pervasive impairment in the development of reciprocal social interaction associated with impairment in either verbal or nonverbal communication skills or with the presence of stereotyped behavior, interests, and activities, but the criteria are not met for a specific pervasive developmental disorder, schizophrenia, schizotypal personality disorder, or avoidant personality disorder. For example, this category includes "atypical autism"—presentations that do not meet the criteria for autistic disorder because of late age at onset, atypical symptomatology, or subthreshold symptomatology, or all of these.

From American Psychiatric Association. *Diagnostic and Statistical Manual of Mental Disorders.* 4th ed. Text rev. Washington, DC: American Psychiatric Association; copyright 2000, with permission.

Leslie was the older of two children. She had been a difficult baby who was not easy to console but whose motor and communicative development seemed appropriate. She was socially related and sometimes enjoyed interaction, but was easily overstimulated. She exhibited some hand flapping. Her parents sought evaluation when she was 4 years of age because of difficulties in nursery school. Leslie had problems with peer interaction. She was often preoccupied with possible adverse events. At evaluation she displayed both communicative and cognitive functions within the normal range. Although differential social relatedness was present, Leslie had difficulty using her parents as sources of support and comfort. She displayed behavioral rigidity and a tendency to impose routines on social skills. Subsequently, she was placed in a transitional kindergarten and did well academically, although problems in peer interactions and unusual affective responses persisted. As an adolescent, she describes herself as a "loner" who has difficulties with social interaction and tends to enjoy solitary activities. (Courtesy of Fred Volkmar, M.D.)

Treatment

The treatment approach—both pharmacologically and psychosocially—is basically the same as in autistic disorder. Mainstreaming in school may be possible. Compared with autistic children, those with pervasive developmental disorder not otherwise specified generally have better language skills and more self-awareness, and so they are better candidates for psychotherapy.

7 Attention-Deficit Disorders

ATTENTION-DEFICIT/HYPERACTIVITY DISORDER

Attention-deficit/hyperactivity disorder (ADHD) is characterized by a pattern of diminished sustained attention and higher levels of impulsivity in a child or adolescent than expected for someone of that age and developmental level. Whereas in the past, hyperactivity was believed to be the underlying impairing symptom in this disorder, the current consensus is that hyperactivity is often secondary to poor impulse control. Impulsivity and hyperactivity share one dimension in today's diagnostic criteria for ADHD. Currently, the diagnosis of ADHD is based on the consensus of experts that three observable subtypes—*inattentive*, *hyperactive/impulsive*, and *combined*—are all manifestations of the same disorder. To meet the criteria for the diagnosis of ADHD, some symptoms must be present before the age of 7 years, although ADHD is not diagnosed in many children until they are older than 7 years when their behaviors cause problems in school and other places. To confirm a diagnosis of ADHD, impairment from inattention and/or hyperactivity-impulsivity must be observable in at least two settings and interfere with developmentally appropriate functioning socially, academically, or in extracurricular activities. ADHD is not diagnosed when symptoms occur in a child, adolescent, or adult with a pervasive developmental disorder, schizophrenia, or other psychotic disorder.

The disorder has been identified in the literature for many years under a variety of terms. In the early 1900s, impulsive, disinhibited, and hyperactive children—many of whom had neurologic damage caused by encephalitis—were grouped under the label *hyperactive syndrome*. In the 1960s, a heterogeneous group of children with poor coordination, learning disabilities, and emotional lability but without specific neurologic damage were described as having minimal brain damage. Since then, other hypotheses have been put forth to explain the origin of the disorder, such as genetically based condition involving abnormal arousal and poor ability to modulate emotions. This theory was initially supported by the observation that stimulant medications help to produce sustained attention and improve these children's ability to focus on a given task. Currently, no single factor is believed to cause the disorder, although many environmental variables may contribute to it and many predictable clinical features are associated with it.

Epidemiology

Reports on the incidence of ADHD in the United States have varied from 2 to 20 percent of grade-school children. A conservative figure is about 3 to 7 percent of prepubertal elementary school children. In Great Britain a lower incidence is reported than in the United States, less than 1 percent. ADHD is more prevalent in boys than in girls, with the ratio ranging from 2:1 to as much as 9:1. First-degree biological relatives (e.g., siblings of probands with ADHD) are at high risk to develop it, as well as to develop other disorders, including disruptive behavior disorders, anxiety disorders, and depressive disorders. Siblings of children with ADHD are also at higher risk than the general population to have learning disorders and academic difficulties. The parents of children with ADHD show an increased incidence of hyperkinesis, sociopathy, alcohol use disorders, and conversion disorder. Symptoms of ADHD are often present by age 3 years, but the diagnosis is generally not made until the child is in a structured school setting, such as preschool or kindergarten, when teacher information is available comparing the attention and impulsivity of the child in question with peers of the same age.

Etiology

Consensus that the etiology of ADHD involves complex interactions of neuroanatomic and neurochemical systems is based on twin and adoption family genetic studies, dopamine transport gene studies, neuroimaging studies, and neurotransmitter data. Most children with ADHD have no evidence of gross structural damage in the central nervous system (CNS). Despite the lack of a specific neurophysiologic or neurochemical basis for the disorder, it is predictably associated with a variety of other disorders that affect brain function, such as learning disorders. The suggested contributory factors for ADHD include prenatal toxic exposures, prematurity, and prenatal mechanical insult to the fetal nervous system. Food additives, colorings, preservatives, and sugar have also been proposed as possible causes of hyperactive behavior. No scientific evidence indicates that these factors cause ADHD.

Genetic Factors. Evidence for a genetic contribution to the emergence of ADHD includes greater concordance in monozygotic than in dizygotic twins. In addition, siblings of hyperactive children have about twice the risk of having the disorder as those in the general population. One sibling may have predominantly hyperactivity symptoms, and others may have predominantly inattention symptoms. Biological parents of children with the disorder have a higher risk for ADHD than adoptive parents. Children with ADHD are at higher risk of developing conduct disorders, and alcohol use disorders and antisocial personality disorder are more common in their parents than in those in the general population.

Developmental Factors. Reports in the literature state that September is the peak month for births of children with ADHD with and without comorbid learning disorders. The implication is that prenatal exposure to winter infections during the first trimester may contribute to the emergence of ADHD symptoms in some susceptible children.

BRAIN DAMAGE. It has been speculated that some children affected by ADHD had subtle damage to the CNS and brain development during their fetal and perinatal periods. The hypothesized brain damage may potentially be associated with circulatory, toxic, metabolic, mechanical, or physical insult to the brain during early infancy caused by infection, inflammation, and trauma. Children with ADHD exhibit nonfocal (soft) neurologic signs at higher rates than those in the general population.

Neurochemical Factors. Many neurotransmitters have been associated with ADHD symptoms. Animal studies have shown that the locus ceruleus, consisting of mainly noradrenergic neurons, plays a major role in attention. The noradrenergic system consists of the central system (originating in the locus ceruleus) and the peripheral sympathetic system. The peripheral noradrenergic system may be more important in ADHD. Thus, a dysfunction in peripheral epinephrine that causes the hormone to accumulate peripherally could potentially feed back to the central system and "reset" the locus ceruleus to a lower level. In part, hypotheses about the neurochemistry of the disorder have arisen from the impact of many medications that exert a positive effect on it. The most widely studied drugs in the treatment of ADHD—the stimulants—affect both dopamine and norepinephrine, leading to neurotransmitter hypotheses that include possible dysfunction in both the adrenergic and dopaminergic systems. Stimulants increase catecholamine concentrations by promoting their release and blocking their uptake. Stimulants and some tricyclic drugs—for example, desipramine (Norpramin)—reduce levels of urinary 3-methoxy-4-hydroxyphenylglycol (MHPG), a metabolite of norepinephrine. Clonidine (Catapres), a norepinephrine agonist, has been helpful in treating hyperactivity. Other drugs that have reduced hyperactivity include tricyclic drugs and monoamine oxidase inhibitors (MAOIs). Overall, no clear-cut evidence implicates a single neurotransmitter in the development of ADHD, but many neurotransmitters may be involved in the process.

Neurophysiologic Factors. The human brain normally undergoes major growth spurts at several ages: 3 to 10 months, 2 to 4 years, 6 to 8 years, 10 to 12 years, and 14 to 16 years. Some children have a maturational delay in the sequence and manifest symptoms of ADHD that appear to normalize by about age 5 years. A physiologic correlate is the presence of a variety of nonspecific abnormal electroencephalogram (EEG) patterns that are disorganized and characteristic of young children. In some cases, the EEG findings normalize over time. A recent study of quantitative EEGs in children with ADHD, in children with undifferentiated attentional problems, and in normal controls indicated that both groups with attentional problems evince increased beta-band relative percentages and decreased rare tone P3000 amplitudes. Increased beta-band percentage or decreased delta-band percentage is associated with increased arousal.

Computed tomographic (CT) head scans of children with ADHD showed no consistent findings. Studies using positron emission tomography (PET) found lower cerebral blood flow and metabolic rates in the frontal lobe areas of children with ADHD than in controls. PET scans also showed that adolescent females with the disorder had globally lower glucose metabolism than both normal control females and males with the disorder. One theory explains these findings by supposing that the frontal lobes in children with ADHD are not adequately performing their inhibitory mechanism on lower structures, an effect leading to disinhibition.

Psychosocial Factors. Children in institutions are frequently overactive and have poor attention spans. These signs result from prolonged emotional deprivation, and they disappear when deprivational factors are removed, such as through adoption or placement in a foster home. Stressful psychic events, disruption of family equilibrium, and other anxiety-inducing factors contribute to the initiation or perpetuation of ADHD. Predisposing factors may include the child's temperament, genetic-familial factors, and the demands of society to adhere to a routinized way of behaving and performing. Socioeconomic status does not seem to be a predisposing factor.

Diagnosis

The principal signs of inattention, impulsivity, and hyperactivity are based on a detailed history of a child's early developmental patterns along with direct observation of the child, especially in situations that require sustained attention. Hyperactivity may be more severe in some situations (e.g., school) and less marked in others (e.g., one-on-one interviews), and it may be less obvious in pleasant structured activities (sports). The diagnosis of ADHD requires persistent, impairing symptoms of either hyperactivity/impulsivity or inattention that cause impairment in at least two different settings. For example, many children with ADHD have difficulties in school and at home. The diagnostic criteria for ADHD are outlined in Table 7–1.

Table 7–1
DSM-IV-TR Diagnostic Criteria for Attention-Deficit/Hyperactivity Disorder

A. Either (1) or (2):
1. six (or more) of the following symptoms of inattention have persisted for at least 6 months to a degree that is maladaptive and inconsistent with developmental level:
Inattention
(a) often fails to give close attention to details or makes careless mistakes in schoolwork, work, or other activities
(b) often has difficulty sustaining attention in tasks or play activities
(c) often does not seem to listen when spoken to directly
(d) often does not follow through on instructions and fails to finish schoolwork, chores, or duties in the workplace (not due to oppositional behavior or failure to understand instructions)
(e) often has difficulty organizing tasks and activities
(f) often avoids, dislikes, or is reluctant to engage in tasks that require sustained mental effort (such as schoolwork or homework)
(g) often loses things necessary for tasks or activities (e.g., toys, school assignments, pencils, books, or tools)
(h) is often easily distracted by extraneous stimuli
(i) is often forgetful in daily activities
2. six (or more) of the following symptoms of **hyperactivity-impulsivity** have persisted for at least 6 months to a degree that is maladaptive and inconsistent with developmental level:
Hyperactivity
(a) often fidgets with hands or feet or squirms in seat
(b) often leaves seat in classroom or in other situations in which remaining seated is expected
(c) often runs about or climbs excessively in situations in which it is inappropriate (in adolescents or adults, may be limited to subjective feelings of restlessness)
(d) often has difficulty playing or engaging in leisure activities quietly
(e) is often "on the go" or often acts as if "driven by a motor"
(f) often talks excessively
Impulsivity
(g) often blurts out answers before questions have been completed
(h) often has difficulty awaiting turn
(i) often interrupts or intrudes on others (e.g., butts into conversations or games)

B. Some hyperactive-impulsive or inattentive symptoms that caused impairment were present before age 7 years.

C. Some impairment from the symptoms is present in two or more settings (e.g., at school [or work] and at home).

D. There must be clear evidence of clinically significant impairment in social, academic, or occupational functioning.

E. The symptoms do not occur exclusively during the course of a pervasive developmental disorder, schizophrenia, or other psychotic disorder and are not better accounted for by another mental disorder (e.g., mood disorder, anxiety disorder, dissociative disorder, or a personality disorder).

Code based on type:
Attention-deficit/hyperactivity disorder, combined type: if both Criteria A1 and A2 are met for the past 6 months
Attention-deficit/hyperactivity disorder, predominantly inattentive type: if Criterion A1 is met but Criterion A2 is not met for the past 6 months
Attention-deficit/hyperactivity disorder, predominantly hyperactive-impulsive type: if Criterion A2 is met but Criterion A1 is not met for the past 6 months
Coding note: For individuals (especially adolescents and adults) who currently have symptoms that no longer meet full criteria, "in partial remission" should be specified.

From American Psychiatric Association. *Diagnostic and Statistical Manual of Mental Disorders.* 4th ed. Text rev. Washington, DC: American Psychiatric Association; copyright 2000, with permission.

Other distinguishing features of ADHD are short attention span and easy distractibility. In school, children with ADHD cannot follow instructions and often demand extra attention from their teachers. At home, they often do not comply with their parents' requests. They act impulsively, show emotional lability, and are explosive and irritable.

Children who have hyperactivity as a predominant feature are more likely to be referred for treatment than are children with primarily symptoms of attention deficit. Children with the predominantly hyperactive-impulsive type are more likely to have a stable diagnosis over time and to have concurrent conduct disorder than are children with the predominantly inattentive type without hyperactivity. Disorders involving reading, arithmetic, language, and coordination skills can occur in association with ADHD. A child's history may give clues to prenatal (including genetic), natal, and postnatal factors that may have affected the CNS structure or function. Rates of development, deviations in development, and parental reactions to significant or stressful behavioral transitions should be ascertained because they may help clinicians to determine the degree to which parents contributed or reacted to a child's inefficiencies and dysfunctions.

School history and teachers' reports are important in evaluating whether a child's difficulties in learning and school behavior are primarily caused by the child's inability to sustain attention or compromised understanding of the academic material. Additional school difficulties can result from attitudinal or maturational problems, social rejection, and poor self-image because of felt inadequacies. These reports may also reveal how the child has handled these problems. How the child has related to siblings, peers, adults, and free and structured activities gives valuable diagnostic clues to the presence of ADHD and helps to identify the complications of the disorder.

The mental status examination may show a secondarily depressed mood but no thought disturbance, impaired reality testing, or inappropriate affect. A child may show great distractibility, perseveration, and a concrete and literal mode of thinking. Indications of visual-perceptual, auditory-perceptual, language, or cognition problems may be present. Occasionally, evidence appears of a basic, pervasive, organically based anxiety, often referred to as *body anxiety*. A neurologic examination may reveal visual, motor, perceptual, or auditory discriminatory immaturity or impairments without overt signs of visual or auditory acuity disorders. Children may have problems with motor coordination and difficulty copying age-appropriate figures, rapid alternating movements, right–left discrimination, ambidexterity, reflex asymmetries, and a variety of subtle nonfocal neurologic signs (soft signs).

Clinicians should obtain an EEG to recognize the child with frequent bilaterally synchronous discharges resulting in short absence spells. Such a child may react in school with hyperactivity out of sheer frustration. The child with an unrecognized temporal lobe seizure focus can have a secondary behavior disorder. In these instances, several features of ADHD are often present. Identification of the focus requires an EEG obtained during drowsiness and during sleep.

Clinical Features

Attention-deficit/hyperactivity disorder can have its onset in infancy, although it is rarely recognized until a child is at least of toddler age. Infants with the disorder are unduly sensitive to stimuli and are easily upset by noise, light, temperature, and other environmental changes. At times, the reverse occurs, and the children are placid and limp, sleep much of the time, and appear to develop slowly in the first months of life. More commonly, however, infants with ADHD are active in the crib, sleep little, and cry a great deal. They are far less likely than normal children to reduce their locomotor activity when their environment is structured by social limits.

In school, children with ADHD may attack a test rapidly but answer only the first two questions. They may be unable to wait to be called on in school and may respond before everyone else. At home, they cannot be put off for even a minute. Children with ADHD are often explosive or irritable. The irritability may be set off by relatively minor stimuli, which may puzzle and dismay the child. They are frequently emotionally labile and easily set off to laughter or to tears; their mood and performance are apt to be variable and unpredictable. Impulsiveness and an inability to delay gratification are characteristic. Children are often susceptible to accidents.

Concomitant emotional difficulties are frequent. The resulting negative self-concept and reactive hostility are worsened by the children's recognition that they have problems.

The most-cited characteristics of children with ADHD, in order of frequency, are hyperactivity, perceptual motor impairment, emotional lability, general coordination deficit, attention deficit (short attention span, distractibility, perseveration, failure to finish tasks, inattention, poor concentration), impulsivity (action before thought, abrupt shifts in activity, lack of organization, jumping up in class), memory and thinking deficits, specific learning disabilities, speech and hearing deficits, and equivocal neurologic signs and EEG irregularities. About 75 percent of children with ADHD show behavioral symptoms of aggression and defiance fairly consistently. Whereas defiance and aggression are generally associated with adverse intrafamily relationships, however, hyperactivity is more closely related to impaired performance on cognitive tests requiring concentration.

School difficulties, both learning and behavioral, commonly coexist with ADHD. They sometimes come from concomitant communication disorders or learning disorders or from the child's distractibility and fluctuating attention, which hamper the acquisition, retention, and display of knowledge. These difficulties are noted especially on group tests. The adverse reactions of school personnel to the behavior characteristics of ADHD and the lowering of self-regard because of felt inadequacies may combine with the adverse comments of peers to make school a place of unhappy defeat. This situation can lead to acting-out antisocial behavior and self-defeating, self-punitive behaviors.

Anthony was first referred to a child psychiatric clinic at age 7. Reasons for referral included the following:

- Severe restlessness and hyperactivity since he began to walk
- Poor concentration
- Disobedient, not listening (teachers "liked" Anthony but wanted him out of the class)
- Poor speech articulation
- Repeating grade 1
- Very untidy and disorganized

Anthony's birth history was uneventful, and his EEG and neurologic examination findings were normal. Anthony's Wechsler Intelligence Scale for Children (WISC) (Full Scale) was 115, with marked scatter. He was found to have body image and visuomotor difficulties. Psychiatric evaluation revealed a friendly, good-looking, 7-year-old boy with speech (i.e., articulation) difficulties who was restless and hyperactive. The parents stated they were happily married and there were two older sisters, both doing well. The father was a sales executive and traveled a great deal, the mother a homemaker. Their ethnic origin was Anglo-Saxon. A diagnosis of ADHD was made.

FIVE-YEAR FOLLOW-UP: 14 YEARS OF AGE

This evaluation was delayed because Anthony had been away at boarding school for 3 years, and we had to wait until he was on holiday. He had received stimulants for only a short period because he was noncompliant, because he hated the dampening effects. At 14 years, Anthony seemed very immature and was still restless and distractible. His learning difficulties made school success in a regular classroom almost impossible, but Anthony had a "happy-go-lucky" attitude about his failures. There was no stealing or other indication of antisocial behavior, but Anthony had no close friends. His mother believed he was worse because he did not accept responsibility and had no goals for the future. He was very poor at spelling and behind in reading and found schoolwork boring. Although he lacked any insight into his difficulties, he was found to be friendly and likable. Repeat WISC IQ (Full Scale) was unchanged.

TEN-YEAR FOLLOW-UP: 20 YEARS OF AGE

Anthony was seen late also for the 10-year follow-up study because his parents had moved overseas, where his father had started a business. We wrote to Anthony there, sending him numerous self-rating scales and a history for him to complete. The former included the California Personality Inventory (CPI), a self-rating scale that all subjects completed. We did not hear from Anthony for 2 years after the forms were mailed and gave up on him as a lost subject. One day, Anthony knocked at G. W.'s office door and announced himself and his girlfriend, Sally. He said he had come from New Zealand to see us with Sally to let us know that the CPI was a truly crazy test and there was no way that he could ever complete "500 dumb questions." When asked what he was really doing here, he said he had told us the truth, then gave a report of his past 5 years and agreed to complete the whole 10-year follow-up evaluation.

While still living with his parents overseas, Anthony had refused to continue schooling, but he had completed grade 9 in Montreal. He worked intermittently at various menial jobs and lived with his parents. (His last job was collecting stray cats and dogs for the local Society for the Prevention of Cruelty to Animals.) He believed his father looked down on this job even though he had told Anthony that any honest job is OK. "He obviously didn't mean it," Anthony added. "Anyway, I got laid off, and since I have ants in my pants, I went to New Zealand." He planned to go perhaps to find work, perhaps for a holiday. But there he met Sally, who suggested that he could try mowing people's lawns for some income. Sally and Anthony soon lived together, and she helped Anthony settle down. She encouraged him to work hard, and soon he had saved $1,500. They borrowed another $1,000 and bought a few second-hand lawnmowers. They then employed younger boys to mow lawns, and a year later had saved $5,500 and paid back the debts. "I gave up the lawnmower business because one day I just found it boring and tense, and I wanted to quit and travel. Also, I wanted to see you to show you how crazy this test that you sent me is."

Anthony appeared happy and as impulsive as ever and had great charm. He had succeeded in getting Sally a job in Montreal, which was extremely difficult at the time, by telling the immigration department that if they did not give her a work permit, he would marry her, and then they would have to give her one anyway. They would feel sorry to have made him marry so young (Sally got her work permit). Sally turned out to be a bright, quite delightful, stable young woman who appreciated Anthony's qualities and had a strong influence on him. She made subsequent appointments for him and made sure he was on time for them. They planned to return to New Zealand after a few months in Montreal but see the world on the way back.

FIFTEEN-YEAR-FOLLOW-UP: 25 YEARS OF AGE

We could not go to New Zealand to interview Anthony, but we were able to meet with his parents, who were visiting Montreal. They had recently visited Anthony in New Zealand and were in close touch with him and with Sally. Anthony was now taking a university degree in communications. It seemed that where he ended up, he could enter university as a mature student without completing high school (he had completed only grade 9). He was pursuing his courses with some difficulties but was passing in spite of concentration problems. He was interested in what he was doing. Anthony and Sally were still living together and were planning on getting married. During this time, Sally had had a malignant lump removed from her breast. Anthony's parents stated that he and Sally "had an excellent relationship" and that they had dealt with their grief and anxiety over her diagnosis well. Sally, they stated, still takes charge of organizational family matters and helps Anthony with his writing assignments. The friends they have are made by Sally, as Anthony lets her take all the initiative with friends; however, he is well liked by them. His parents believe that in the past year, partly as a result of Sally's medical problems, Anthony has matured greatly. He was described as still impulsive, still very restless, but he listens to Sally. He still talks too much and "has a big mouth." He has occasionally lost part-time jobs because of this. The couple has no debts, and Anthony plans to start an advertising business when he receives his university degree. His father stated he would help him financially but still would not trust him to handle money responsibly. Anthony himself is not close to the friends the couple has, but he feels close to Sally. Although Sally has obviously done a great deal for Anthony, it was believed that the relationship is complementary rather than neurotic.

We asked Anthony's parents what they believed were the reasons for Anthony's good outcome because they were extremely happy about his progress. His father stated, "Even while Anthony was hyperactive and a discipline problem as a child, he was very lovable. In school, he couldn't learn because he felt so inferior. At 17 years, we sent him to Switzerland to learn a trade, but this did not work out. At 18 years, we gave him a one-way ticket to New Zealand and said to him, if you want to come back you have to earn the money for your ticket. Sally was the turning point for Anthony. She gave him what we couldn't, confidence in himself and a sense of direction. She had always loved him and even way back believed in his future when we frankly did not. Sally and Anthony are now saving to buy a house, and we send them money toward this, but we always send it to Sally. She keeps the books."

It seemed clear to us that Anthony without his fiancée would not be functioning as well as he is and would still be having many life difficulties related to the ADHD disorder. (Courtesy of G. Weiss, M.D.)

Pathology and Laboratory Examination

No specific laboratory measures are pathognomonic of ADHD. Several laboratory measures often yield nonspecific abnormal results in hyperactive children, such as a disorganized, immature result on an EEG, and PET may show decreased cerebral blood flow in the frontal regions. Cognitive testing that helps to confirm a child's inattention and impulsivity includes a continuous performance task in which a child is asked to press a button each time a particular sequence of letters or numbers is flashed on a screen. Children with poor attention make errors of omission—that is, they fail to press the button, even when the sequence has flashed. Impulsivity is manifested by errors of commission, in which children cannot resist pushing the button, although the desired sequence has not yet appeared on the screen.

Differential Diagnosis

A temperamental constellation consisting of high activity level and short attention span but in the normal range of expectation for a child's age should be considered first. Differentiating these temperamental characteristics from the cardinal symptoms of ADHD before the age of 3 years is difficult, mainly because of the overlapping features of a normally immature nervous system and the emerging signs of visual-motor-perceptual impairments frequently seen in ADHD. Anxiety in a child needs to be evaluated. Anxiety can accompany ADHD as a secondary feature, and anxiety alone can be manifested by overactivity and easy distractibility.

It is not uncommon for a child with ADHD to become demoralized or, in some cases, to develop depressive symptoms in reaction to persistent frustration with academic difficulties and resulting low self-esteem. Mania and ADHD share many core features, such as excessive verbalization, motoric hyperactivity, and high levels of distractibility. In addition, in children with mania, irritability seems to be more common than euphoria. Although mania and ADHD can coexist, children with bipolar I disorder exhibit more waxing and waning of symptoms than those with ADHD. Recent follow-up data for children who met the criteria for ADHD and subsequently developed bipolar disorder suggest that certain clinical features occurring during the course of ADHD predict future mania. Children with ADHD who had developed bipolar I disorder at 4-year follow-up had a greater co-occurrence of additional disorders and a greater family history of bipolar disorders and other mood disorders than children without bipolar disorder.

Frequently, conduct disorder and ADHD coexist, and both must be diagnosed. Learning disorders of various kinds must also be distinguished from ADHD; a child may be unable to read or do mathematics because of a learning disorder rather than because of inattention. ADHD often coexists with one or more learning disorders, including reading disorder, mathematics disorder, and disorder of written expression.

Course and Prognosis

The course of ADHD is variable. Symptoms have been shown to persist into adolescence or adult life in approximately 50 percent of cases. In the remaining 50 percent, they may remit at puberty or in early adulthood. In some cases, the hyperactivity may disappear, but the decreased attention span and impulse-control problems persist. Overactivity is usually the first symptom to remit, and distractibility is the last. ADHD does not usually remit during middle childhood. Persistence is predicted by a family history of the disorder, negative life events, and comorbidity with conduct symptoms, depression, and anxiety disorders. Remission is unlikely before the age of 12 years. When remission does occur, it is usually between the ages of 12 and 20 years. Remission can be accompanied by a productive adolescence and adult life, satisfying interpersonal relationships, and few significant sequelae. Most patients with the disorder, however, undergo partial remission and are vulnerable to antisocial behavior, substance use disorders, and mood disorders. Learning problems often continue throughout life.

In about 40 to 50 percent of cases, symptoms persist into adulthood. Those with the disorder may show diminished hyperactivity but remain impulsive and accident-prone. Although their educational attainments as a group are lower than those of people without ADHD, their early employment histories do not differ from those of people with similar educations.

Children with the disorder whose symptoms persist into adolescence are at risk for developing conduct disorder. Children with both ADHD and conduct disorder are also at risk for developing a substance-related disorder. The development of substance abuse disorders during adolescence appears to be related to the presence of conduct disorder rather than to ADHD alone.

Most children with ADHD have some social difficulties. Socially dysfunctional children with ADHD have significantly higher rates of comorbid psychiatric disorders and experience more problems with behavior in school as well as with peers and family members. Overall, the outcome of ADHD in childhood seems to be related to the degree of persistent comorbid psychopathology, especially conduct disorder, social disability, and chaotic family factors. Optimal outcomes may be promoted by ameliorating children's social functioning, diminishing aggression, and improving family situations as early as possible.

Table 7–2
Stimulant Medications in the Treatment of Attention-Deficit/Hyperactivity Disorder (ADHD)

Medication	Preparation (mg)	Approximate Duration (hr)	Recommended Dose
Methylphenidate preparations			
Ritalin	5, 10, 15, 20	3–4	0.3–1 mg/kg t.i.d; up to 60 mg/day
Ritalin-SR	20	8	Up to 60 mg/day
Concerta	18, 36, 54	12	Up to 54 mg/q AM
Metadate ER	10, 20	8	Up to 60 mg/day
Metadate CD	20	12	Up to 60 mg/q AM
Ritalin LA	5, 10, 15, 20	8	
Dexmethylphenidate preparation			
Focalin	2.5, 5, 10	3–4	Up to 10 mg
Focalin XR	5, 10, 20	6–8	Up to 20 mg
Dextroamphetamine preparations			
Dexedrine	5, 10	3–4	0.15–0.5 mg/kg b.i.d.; up to 40 mg/day
Dexedrine Spansule	5, 10, 15	8	Up to 40 mg/day
Dextroamphetamine and amphetamine salt preparations			
Adderall	5, 10, 20, 30	4–6	0.15–0.5 mg/kg b.i.d.; up to 40 mg/day
Adderall XR	10, 20, 30	12	Up to 40 mg q AM
Proamphetamine preparation			
Lisdexamfetamine (Vyvanse)	30, 50, 70	8	30–70 mg/day

b.i.d, twice daily; q, every; t.i.d., three times daily.

Treatment

Pharmacotherapy. Pharmacologic treatment is considered to be the first line of treatment for ADHD. Central nervous system stimulants are the first choice of agents, in that they have been shown to have the greatest efficacy with generally mild, tolerable side effects. Although excellent safety records are documented for short- and sustained-release preparations of methylphenidate (Ritalin, Ritalin-SR, Concerta, Metadate CD, Metadate ER [the U.S. Food and Drug Administration (FDA) approved the first skin patch, called Daytrana, designed to be worn for 9 hours, which contains methylphenidate]), dextroamphetamine (Dexedrine, Dexedrine Spansule), and dextroamphetamine and amphetamine salt combinations (Adderall, Adderall XR), current strategies favor once-a-day sustained-release preparations for their convenience and diminished rebound side effects. A newer preparation of methylphenidate, containing only the D-enantiomer dexmethylphenidate (Focalin), was recently placed on the market, aimed at maximizing the target effects and minimizing the adverse effects in individuals with ADHD who obtained partial response from methylphenidate but for whom adequate dosing was limited by side effects. Advantages of the sustained-release preparations for children are that one dose in the morning sustains the effects all day and the child is no longer required to interrupt his or her school day and that, physiologically, the medication is sustained at an approximately even level in the body throughout the day, so that periods of rebound and irritability are avoided. Table 7–2 contains comparative information on the foregoing medications. Second-line agents with evidence of efficacy for some children and adolescents with ADHD include atomoxetine (Stratera), a norepinephrine uptake inhibitor shown to be effective in the treatment of children with ADHD; antidepressants, such as bupropion (Wellbutrin, Wellbutrin SR) and venlafaxine (Effexor, Effexor XR); and the α-adrenergic receptor agonists clonidine (Catapres) and guanfacine (Tenex). (Table 7–3 contains comparative information on the nonstimulant medications.) The FDA approved the use of dextroamphetamine in children 3 years of age and older and methylphenidate in children 6 years of age and older. These are the two most commonly used pharmacologic agents for the treatment of children with ADHD.

Table 7–3
Nonstimulant Medications for Attention-Deficit/Hyperactivity Disorder (ADHD)

Medication	Preparation (mg)	Recommended Dose
Atomoxetine HCl		
Strattera	10, 18, 25, 40	(0.5–1.8 mg/kg) 40–80 mg/day; may use b.i.d. dosing
Bupropion preparations		
Wellbutrin	75, 100	(3–6 mg/kg) 150–300 mg/day; up to 150 mg/dose b.i.d.
Wellbutrin SR	100, 150	(3–6 mg/kg) 150–300 mg/day; up to 150 mg q AM; greater than 150 mg/day, use b.i.d. dosing
Venlafaxine		
Effexor	25, 37.5, 50, 75, 100	25–150 mg/day; use b.i.d. dosing
Effexor XR	37.5, 75, 150	37.5–150 mg q AM
α-Adrenergic agonists		
Clonidine (Catapres)	0.1, 0.2, 0.3	3–10 μg/kg/day divided t.i.d.; up to 0.1 mg t.i.d.
Guanfacine (Tenex)	1, 2	0.5–1.5 mg/day

b.i.d, twice daily; q, every; t.i.d., three times daily.

STIMULANT MEDICATIONS. Methylphenidate and amphetamine preparations are dopamine agonists; however, the precise mechanism of the stimulant's central action is unknown. The idea of paradoxical response by hyperactive children is no longer accepted. Methylphenidate has been shown to be highly effective in up to three fourths of all children with ADHD, with relatively few adverse effects. Methylphenidate is a short-acting medication that is generally used to be effective during school hours so that children with the disorder can attend to tasks and remain in the classroom. The drug's most common adverse effects include headaches, stomachaches, nausea, and insomnia. Some children experience a rebound effect in which they become mildly irritable and appear to be slightly hyperactive for a brief period when the medication wears off. In children with a history of motor tics, some caution must be used; in some cases, methylphenidate can exacerbate the tic disorder. Another common concern about methylphenidate is whether it causes some growth suppression. During periods of use, methylphenidate is associated with growth suppression, but children tend to make up the growth when they are given drug holidays in the summer or on weekends. An important question about using methylphenidate is how much it normalizes school performance. A recent study found that about 75 percent of a group of hyperactive children exhibited significant improvement in their ability to pay attention in class and on measures of academic efficiency when treated with methylphenidate. The drug has been shown to improve hyperactive children's scores on tasks of vigilance, such as the continuous-performance task and paired associations. Dextroamphetamine and dextroamphetamine/amphetamine salt combinations are usually the second drugs of choice when methylphenidate is not effective.

A transdermal delivery system has recently been developed for administering methylphenidate, the methylphenidate transdermal system (MTS), which is designed to release methylphenidate continuously on application of the patch to the skin. Advantages of this form of administration of methylphenidate include an alternate mode of receiving the medication for children who have difficulties swallowing pills and the fact that the patch continues to deliver the medication until it is removed. A recent double-blind, randomized study of MTS use in children with ADHD who wore the patch for 12 hours at a time showed efficacy at doses ranging from patches delivering 0.45 mg per hour of methylphenidate to those delivering 1.8 mg per hour of methylphenidate. The effectiveness of the patch reached a plateau without much further improvement as dose was increased, but intensive behavioral interventions were also being administered. The delay in the onset of effect of the transdermal medication was approximately 1 hour. Side effects were similar to those of oral preparations of methylphenidate. Approximately half of the children exhibited at least minor erythematous reactions to the patch, although none of the study patients discontinued the MTS because of severe skin reactions. It is not clear how long the effect of methylphenidate remains after the patch is removed. The MTS provides a new strategy for administering a medication well established in the treatment of ADHD and is likely to be on the market within the next year.

A prodrug of amphetamine called lisdexamfetamine (Vyvnase) was recently approved for ADHD. It has a similar side effect profile to amphetamine and is prescribed once a day. In children 6 to 12 years of age, the recommended dose is 30 mg per day given in the morning. If required, the dose may be increased incrementally by 20 mg per day at weekly intervals to a maximum of 70 mg per day. It is available in 30-, 50-, or 70-mg extended-release capsules.

NONSTIMULANT MEDICATIONS. Atomoxetine HCl (Strattera) is a norepinephrine uptake inhibitor approved by the FDA in the treatment of ADHD for children age 6 years and older. The mechanism of action is not well understood, but it is believed to involve selective inhibition of presynaptic norepinephrine transporter. Atomoxetine is well absorbed by the gastrointestinal tract, and maximal plasma levels are reached 1 to 2 hours after ingestion. It has been shown to be effective for inattention as well as impulsivity in children and in adults with ADHD. Its half-life is approximately 5 hours, and it is usually administered twice daily. Most common side effects include diminished appetite, abdominal discomfort, dizziness, and irritability. In some cases, increases in blood pressure and heart rate have been reported. Atomoxetine is metabolized by the cytochrome P450 (CYP) 2D6 hepatic enzyme system. A small fraction of the population are poor metabolizers of CYP 2D6–metabolized drugs, and, for those individuals, plasma concentrations of the drug may rise as much as fivefold for a given dose of medication. Drugs that inhibit CYP 2D6, including fluoxetine, paroxetine, and quinidine, may lead to increased plasma levels of this medication. Despite its short half-life, atomoxetine has been shown in a recent study to be effective in reducing symptoms of ADHD in children during the school day when administered once daily. Another recent study of a combination of atomoxetine alone and combined with fluoxetine in the treatment of 127 children with ADHD and symptoms of anxiety or depression suggested that atomoxetine alone can lead to improvements in mood and anxiety. Children who received combined atomoxetine and fluoxetine experienced greater increases in blood pressure and pulse than those who were treated with atomoxetine only. Some cases of hepatotoxicity have been reported with atomoxetine.

Bupropion has been shown to be an effective antidepressant and is effective for some children and adolescents in the treatment of ADHD. A recent multisite, double-blind, placebo-controlled study confirmed the efficacy of bupropion. No further studies have compared bupropion with other stimulants. The risk of seizure development while on this drug is similar to that of other antidepressant medications when dose does not exceed 450 mg per day. Venlafaxine has been used in clinical practice, especially for children and adolescents with combinations of ADHD and depression or anxiety features. No clear empirical evidence supports the use of venlafaxine in the treatment of ADHD. Clonidine has also been used in the treatment of ADHD with some success, according to case reports. It may be helpful when patients also have tic disorders. Few data confirm the efficacy of selective serotonin reuptake inhibitors (SSRIs) in the treatment of ADHD, but because of the comorbidity of depression and anxiety with the disorder, these drugs are sometimes considered.

Tricyclic drugs and pemoline (Cylert), previously used to treat ADHD, are no longer recommended because of potential adverse effects on liver function (pemoline) and potential cardiac arrhythmia effects (tricyclic drugs). The report of sudden death in at least four children with ADHD who were being treated with desipramine (Norpramin, Pertofrane) has made the tricyclic antidepressants a less likely choice. Why the deaths occurred is unclear, but they reinforce the need for close follow-up of any child receiving a tricyclic drug. Antipsychotics are occasionally used to treat refractory hyperactivity in children and adolescents who are severely impaired and do not respond to other treatments. Antipsychotics may be efficacious for some children with the disorder, but with the alternative medications available and the risk for tardive dyskinesia, withdrawal dyskinesia, and neuroleptic malignant syndrome, they are less desirable.

Modafinil (Provigil), another type of CNS stimulant, was originally developed to reduce daytime sleepiness in patients with narcolepsy and has been tried clinically in the treatment of adults with ADHD. A recent randomized, double-blind, placebo-controlled study of the efficacy and safety of modafinil film-coated tablets in approximately 250 adolescents with ADHD showed that 48 percent of those on active treatment were rated as "much" or "very much" improved, compared with 17 percent of patients receiving placebo. The dose range was from 170 to 425 mg administered once daily, titrated to optimal doses based on efficacy and tolerability. The most common side effects included insomnia, headache, and decreased appetite. This study concluded that modafinil once daily is a viable treatment for adolescents with ADHD based on its safety and effectiveness in this sample of adolescents. Although stimulants remain the drugs of choice in the pharmacologic treatment of ADHD, a body of evidence now supports the use of nonstimulants, including atomoxetine, and modafinil.

A recent open-label report on the use of reboxetine, a selective norepinephrine reuptake inhibitor, in 31 children and adolescents with ADHD who were resistant to methylphenidate treatment suggested that this agent may have efficacy. In this open trial, reboxetine was initiated and maintained at 4 mg per day. Most common side effects included drowsiness, sedation, and gastrointestinal symptoms. Reboxetine and other new agents in this class await controlled studies to further evaluate their potential efficacy. Table 7–4 lists the FDA-approved medications for ADHD.

TREATMENT OF CNS STIMULANT SIDE EFFECTS. CNS stimulants are generally well tolerated, and the consensus is that once-a-day dosing is preferable with regard to convenience and rebound side effects. A recent study of the long-term tolerability of once-daily mixed amphetamine salts showed mild side effects, most commonly decreased appetite, insomnia, and headache.

Given the predictable side effects of central stimulant medications, strategies have been developed to ameliorate these problems. For example, a variety of strategies have been suggested by experts for a given a child or adolescent with ADHD who responds favorably to methylphenidate (Concerta) but for whom insomnia has become a significant problem. Suggestions for the management of insomnia in such a case include the use of diphenhydramine (25 to 75 mg), a low dose of trazodone (25 to 50 mg), or the addition of an α-adrenergic agent, such as guanfacine. In some cases, insomnia may attenuate on its own after several months of treatment.

Monitoring Pharmacologic Treatment

Stimulants. At baseline, the most recent American Academy of Child and Adolescent Psychiatry (AACAP) practice parameters recommend the following workup before starting use of stimulant medications:

- Physical examination
- Blood pressure
- Pulse
- Weight
- Height

It is recommended that children and adolescents being treated with stimulants have their height, weight, blood pressure, and pulse checked on a quarterly basis and have a physical examination annually.

EVALUATION OF THERAPEUTIC PROGRESS. Monitoring starts with the initiation of medication. Because school performance is most markedly affected, special attention and effort should be given to establishing and maintaining a close collaborative working relationship with a child's school personnel. In most patients, stimulants reduce overactivity, distractibility, impulsiveness, explosiveness, and irritability. No evidence indicates that medications directly improve any existing impairments in learning, although, when the attention deficits diminish, children can learn more effectively. In addition, medication can improve self-esteem when children are no longer constantly reprimanded for their behavior.

Psychosocial Interventions. Medication alone is often not sufficient to satisfy the comprehensive therapeutic needs of children with the disorder and is usually but one facet of a multimodality regimen. Social skills groups, training for parents of children with ADHD, and behavioral interventions at school and at home are often efficacious in the overall management of children with ADHD. Evaluation and treatment of coexisting learning disorders or additional psychiatric disorders is important.

Table 7–4
Food and Drug Administration (FDA)–Approved Medications for the Treatment of Attention-Deficit/Hyperactivity Disorder (ADHD)

Medication	FDA-Approved Dose	Daily Dose Range Used Clinically (mg/kg)	Dose Schedule	Comments
Methylphenidate (MPH)				
Focalin	5–30 mg/day	0.25–1.0	Twice daily or three times daily	Short-acting stimulants may require more frequent dosing; mean daily dose usually 0.75–1.5 mg/kg for D,L-MPH; about half of that for D-MPH
Ritalin	10–60 mg/day (average 20–30 mg/day)	0.5–2.0	Twice daily or three times daily	
MPH		0.5–2.0	Twice daily or three times daily	
Methylin	10–60 mg/day	0.5–2.0	Twice daily or three times daily	
MPH extended duration				
*Focalin	10–20 mg/day	0.25–1.0	Four times daily	Some give 30–40 mg/day
Ritalin SR	10–60 mg/day (average 20–30 mg/day)	0.5–2.0	Four times daily, twice daily, or three times daily	Likely to require immediate-release supplement if given four times daily
Metadate ER	10–60 mg/day (average 20–30 mg/day)	0.5–2.0	Four times daily or twice daily	Likely to require immediate-release supplement if given four times daily
Metadate CD	20 mg/day (max 60 mg/day)	0.5–2.0	Four times daily or twice daily	Likely to require immediate-release supplement if given four times daily
Ritalin LA	20 mg/day (max 60 mg/day)	0.5–2.0	Four times daily or twice daily	Likely to require immediate-release supplement if taken four times daily
Concerta	18–54 mg/day (children); 18–72 mg/day (adolescents)	0.5–2.0	Four times daily	Immediate-release supplement may be used
Daytrana transdermal patch	12.5–37.5 cm^2 (10–30 mg)		Four times daily	Dose determined by wear time (lasts until 3 hrs after removal)
Amphetamine (AMP)				
Dexedrine	2.5–40 mg/day	0.25–1.0	Twice daily or three times daily	
Dextrostat	2.5–40 mg/day	0.25–1.0	Twice daily or three times daily	
Adderall	2.5–40 mg/day	0.25–1.0	Twice daily or three times daily	
Mixed amphetamine salts (generic)	2.5–40 mg/day		Twice daily or three times daily	
Lisdexamfetamine (Vyvanse)	30–70 mg/day		Four times daily	
AMP extended duration				
Dexedrine Spansule	2.5–40 mg/day	0.25–1.0	Four times daily or twice daily	May require immediate-release supplement if given four times daily (especially Dexedrine Spansule)
*Adderall XR	Max 20 mg/day in adults; 30 mg/day in children	0.25–1.0	Four times daily	
Atomoxetine				
*Strattera	Children: target dose is 1.2 mg/kg/day Adults: Start at 40 mg/day, then 80 mg/day (target) and 100 mg/day (max)	Maximum labeled dose 1.4	Four times daily	Nonstimulant; may be given in the morning, evening, or twice daily; may need to start with lower dose and titrate slowly; clinical trials went to the lower of 120 mg or 1.8 mg/kg

Note: Higher-than-approved dosing may be needed to achieve an optimum response.
*FDA-approved for treating adult ADHD.

Children who are prescribed medications should be taught the purpose of the medication and given the opportunity to reveal their feelings about it. Doing so helps dispel misconceptions about medication use (such as "I'm crazy") and makes it clear that the medication helps the child handle situations better than before. When children are helped to structure their environment, their anxiety diminishes. It is often beneficial for parents and teachers to work together to develop a concrete set of expectations for the child and a system of rewards for the child when the expectations are met.

A common goal of therapy is to help parents of children with ADHD recognize and promote the notion that, although the child may not "voluntarily" exhibit symptoms of ADHD, he or she is still capable of being responsible for meeting reasonable expectations. Parents should also be helped to recognize that, despite their child's difficulties, every child faces the normal tasks of maturation, including significant building of self-esteem when he or she develops a sense of mastery. Therefore, children with ADHD do not benefit from being exempted from the requirements, expectations, and planning applicable to other children. Parental training is an integral part of the psychotherapeutic interventions for ADHD. Most parental training is based on helping parents develop usable behavioral interventions with positive reinforcement that target both social and academic behaviors.

Group therapy aimed at both refining social skills and increasing self-esteem and a sense of success may be very useful for children with ADHD, who have great difficulty functioning in group settings, especially in school. A recent year-long group therapy intervention in a clinical setting for boys with the disorder described the goals as helping the boys improve skills in game playing and feeling a sense of mastery with peers. The boys were first asked to do a task that was fun, in pairs, and then were gradually asked to do projects in a group. They were directed in following instructions, waiting, and paying attention and were praised for successful cooperation. This level of highly structured group therapeutic "play" is developmentally appropriate for these children, who benefit from an increased ability to participate in any group activities.

ATTENTION-DEFICIT/HYPERACTIVITY DISORDER NOT OTHERWISE SPECIFIED

The text revision of the fourth edition of the *Diagnostic and Statistical Manual of Mental Disorders* (DSM-IV-TR) includes ADHD not otherwise specified as a residual category for disturbances with prominent symptoms of inattention or hyperactivity that do not meet the criteria for ADHD (Table 7–5).

Table 7–5
DSM-IV-TR Diagnostic Criteria for Attention-Deficit/Hyperactivity Disorder Not Otherwise Specified

This category is for disorders with prominent symptoms of inattention or hyperactivity-impulsivity that do not meet criteria for attention-deficit/hyperactivity disorder. Examples include:

1. Individuals whose symptoms and impairment meet the criteria for attention-deficit/hyperactivity disorder, predominantly inattentive type but whose age at onset is 7 years or after
2. Individuals with clinically significant impairment who present with inattention and whose symptom pattern does not meet the full criteria for the disorder but have a behavioral pattern marked by sluggishness, daydreaming, and hypoactivity

From American Psychiatric Association. *Diagnostic and Statistical Manual of Mental Disorders.* 4th ed. Text rev. Washington, DC: American Psychiatric Association; copyright 2000, with permission.

ADULT MANIFESTATIONS OF ADHD

Attention-deficit/hyperactivity disorder was historically believed to be a childhood condition resulting in delayed development of impulse control that would be outgrown by adolescence. Only in the last few decades have adults with ADHD been identified, diagnosed, and successfully treated. Longitudinal follow-up has shown that up to 40 to 60 percent of children with ADHD have persistent impairment from symptoms into adulthood. Genetic studies, brain imaging, and neurocognitive and pharmacologic studies in adults with ADHD have virtually replicated findings demonstrated in children with ADHD. Increased public awareness and treatment studies within the last decade have led to widespread acceptance of the need for diagnosis and treatment of adults with ADHD.

Epidemiology

Among adults, evidence suggests an approximate 4 percent prevalence of ADHD in the population. ADHD in adulthood is generally diagnosed by self-report, given the lack of school information and observer information available; therefore, it is more difficult to make an accurate diagnosis.

Etiology

ADHD is believed to be largely transmitted genetically, and increasing evidence supports this hypothesis, including the genetic studies, twin studies, and family studies outlined in the child and adolescent ADHD section. Brain imaging studies have obtained data suggesting that adults with ADHD exhibit decreased prefrontal glucose metabolism on PET compared with adults without ADHD. It is unclear whether these data reflect the presence of the disorder or a secondary effect of having ADHD over a period of time. Further studies using single photon emission tomography (SPECT) have revealed increased dopamine transporter (DAT) binding densities in the striatum of the brain in samples of adults with ADHD. This finding may be understood within the context of treatment for ADHD, in that standard stimulant treatment for ADHD, such as methylphenidate, acts to block

DAT activity, possibly leading to a normalization of the striatal brain region in individuals with ADHD.

Factors associated with early childhood emergence of ADHD include premature birth, maternal use of nicotine during the pregnancy, and increased serum lead levels. Factors that protect against emergence of ADHD until later in childhood are not known.

Diagnosis and Clinical Features

The clinical phenomenology of ADHD in children that has evolved over the last few decades has resulted in features of inattention and manifestations of impulsivity prevailing as the core of this disorder. For adults, a leading figure in the development of criteria for adult manifestations of ADHD is Paul Wender of the University of Utah, who began his work on adult ADHD in the 1970s. Wender developed criteria that could be applied to adults (Table 7–6). They included a retrospective diagnosis of ADHD in childhood and evidence of current impairment from ADHD symptoms in adulthood. Furthermore, evidence exists of several additional symptoms that are typical of adult behavior as opposed to childhood behaviors.

In adults, residual signs of the disorder include impulsivity and attention deficit (e.g., difficulty in organizing and completing work, inability to concentrate, increased distractibility, and sudden decision making without thought of the consequences). Many people with the disorder have a secondary depressive disorder associated with low self-esteem related to their impaired performance and which affects both occupational and social functioning.

Table 7–6
Utah Criteria for Adult Attention-Deficit/Hyperactivity Disorder (ADHD)

I. Retrospective childhood ADHD diagnosis
  A. Narrow criterion: met DSM-IV criteria in childhood by parent interview[a]
  B. Broad criterion: both (1) and (2) are met as reported by patient[b]
    1. Childhood hyperactivity
    2. Childhood attention deficits
II. Adult characteristics: five additional symptoms, including ongoing difficulties with inattentiveness and hyperactivity and at least three other symptoms:
  A. Inattentiveness
  B. Hyperactivity
  C. Mood lability
  D. Irritability and hot temper
  E. Impaired stress tolerance
  F. Disorganization
  G. Impulsivity
III. Exclusions: not diagnosed in presence of severe depression, psychosis, or severe personality disorder

[a]Parent report aided with 10-item Parent Rating Scale of Childhood Behavior.
[b]Patient self-report of retrospective childhood symptoms aided by Wender Utah Rating Scale.
DSM-IV, American Psychiatric Association, *Diagnostic and Statistical Manual of Mental Disorders*. 4th ed. Washington, DC: American Psychiatric Association.

A 24-year-old man complained of poor attention span, distractibility, and feelings of restlessness. In childhood, he had persistent problems with academic achievement and behavior. He endorsed a history of seven inattentive and nine hyperactive-impulsive DSM-IV ADHD symptoms during early grade school. He was frequently sent to the principal, and his parents were similarly frustrated at home. Although he was considered a bright student, he made average grades and had no aspirations for college. He worked in construction after graduation, but became dissatisfied with his job prospects. As a result of urging from a friend, he enlisted in the military, and, surprisingly, thrived under military discipline. After receiving an honorable discharge, he enrolled in community college, hoping to become a paralegal.

The ADHD rating scales of childhood behavior confirmed considerable difficulties with inattentive and hyperactive-impulsive symptoms. Ratings of current symptoms were notable for inattention. Clinical review of current DSM symptoms revealed impairment from six inattentive and three hyperactive symptoms. The patient was diagnosed with adult ADHD; no evidence was seen of other coexisting psychopathology.

After receiving education about the nature of ADHD, the patient agreed to a medication trial. Escalating doses of a once-a-day stimulant were titrated over several weeks. At his return visit, the physician reviewed response during the titration and determined an optimal dose. The patient experienced significant reduction of his inattentive symptoms and reported greatly improved academic functioning. He continued to take medication regularly and subsequently transferred to a 4-year university. He married his longtime girlfriend before beginning law school.

Differential Diagnosis

A diagnosis of ADHD is likely when symptoms of inattention and impulsivity are described by adults as a lifelong problem, not as episodic events. The overlap of ADHD and hypomania, bipolar II disorder, and cyclothymia is controversial and difficult to sort out retrospectively. Clear-cut histories of discrete episodes of hypomania and mania, with or without periods of depression, are suggestive of a mood disorder rather than a clinical picture of ADHD; however, ADHD may have predated the emergence of a mood disorder in some individuals. In such a case, ADHD and bipolar disorder can be diagnosed as comorbid disorders. Adults with an early history of chronic school difficulties related to paying attention, activity level, and impulsive behavior are generally diagnosed with ADHD, even when a mood disorder occurs later in life. Anxiety disorders can coexist with ADHD and are less difficult than hypomania to distinguish from it.

Course and Prognosis

The prevalence of ADHD diminishes over time, although at least half of children and adolescents may have the disorder into adulthood. Many children initially diagnosed with ADHD, combined type, exhibit fewer impulsive-hyperactive symptoms as they get older and, by the time they are adults, meet criteria for ADHD, inattentive type. As with children, adults with ADHD demonstrate higher rates of learning disorders, anxiety disorders, mood disorders, and substance use disorder compared with the general population.

Treatment

Treatment of ADHD in adults targets pharmacotherapy similar to that used with children and adolescents with ADHD. Central nervous stimulants, including methylphenidate, amphetamine, and amphetamine salts, are the first line of treatment. Signs of a positive response are an increased attention span, decreased impulsiveness, and improved mood. Psychopharmacologic therapy may be needed indefinitely. Clinicians should use standard ways to monitor drug response and patient compliance.

8

Disruptive Behavior Disorders

Oppositional and aggressive behaviors during childhood are among the most frequent reasons that a given youth is referred for mental health evaluation. Many youth who exhibit negativistic or oppositional behaviors will find other forms of expression as they mature and will no longer demonstrate these behaviors in adulthood. Children who develop enduring patterns of aggressive behaviors that begin in early childhood and violate the basic rights of peers and family members, however, may be destined to an entrenched pattern of conduct-disordered behaviors over time. Controversy has arisen over whether a set of "voluntary" antisocial behaviors can be construed as a psychiatric disorder or can be better accounted for as maladaptive responses to overly harsh or punitive parenting or as strategies that have survival value in chronically threatening environmental situations. Longitudinal studies have demonstrated that, for some youth, early patterns of disruptive behavior may become a lifelong pervasive repertoire culminating in adult antisocial personality disorder. The origin of stable patterns of disruptive behavior is widely accepted as a convergence of multiple contributing factors, including biologic, temperamental, learned, and psychologic conditions.

Disruptive behavior disorders can be divided into two distinct constellations of symptoms categorized as oppositional defiant disorder and conduct disorder, both of which result in impaired social or academic functioning in a child. Some defiance and refusal to comply with adult requests is developmentally appropriate and marks growth in all children, yet children with the following disorders are themselves impaired by the frequency and severity of their disruptive behaviors.

Oppositional defiant disorder is characterized by enduring patterns of negativistic, disobedient, and hostile behavior toward authority figures, as well as an inability to take responsibility for mistakes, leading to placing blame on others. Children with oppositional defiant disorder frequently argue with adults and become easily annoyed by others, leading to a state of anger and resentment. Children with oppositional defiant disorder may have difficulty in the classroom and with peer relationships but generally do not resort to physical aggression or significantly destructive behavior.

In contrast, children with *conduct disorder* engage in severe repeated acts of aggression that can cause physical harm to themselves and others and frequently violate the rights of others. Children with conduct disorder usually have behaviors characterized by aggression to persons or animals, destruction of property, deceitfulness or theft, and multiple violations of rules, such as truancy from school. These behavior patterns cause distinct difficulties in school life as well as in peer relationships. Conduct disorder has been divided into a childhood-onset subtype, in which at least one symptom has emerged repeatedly before age 10 years, and adolescent-onset type, in which no characteristic persistent symptoms were seen until after age 10 years. Although some young children show persistent patterns of behavior consistent with violating the rights of others or destroying property, the diagnosis of conduct disorder in children appears to increase with age.

OPPOSITIONAL DEFIANT DISORDER

In oppositional defiant disorder, a child's temper outbursts, active refusal to comply with rules, and annoying behaviors exceed expectations for these behaviors for children of the same age. The disorder is an enduring pattern of negativistic, hostile, and defiant behaviors in the absence of serious violations of social norms or of the rights of others.

Epidemiology

Oppositional, negativistic behavior, in moderation, is developmentally normal in early childhood and adolescence. Epidemiologic studies of negativistic traits in nonclinical populations found such behavior in 16 to 22 percent of school-age children. According to the text revision of the fourth edition of the *Diagnostic and Statistical Manual of Mental Disorders* (DSM-IV-TR), prevalence rates for this disorder range from 2 to 16 percent. Although oppositional defiant disorder can begin as early as 3 years of age, it typically is noted by 8 years of age and usually not later than adolescence. Oppositional defiant disorder has been reported to occur at rates ranging from 2 to 16 percent. The disorder seems more prevalent in boys than in girls before puberty, and the sex ratio appears to be equal after puberty. One authority suggests that girls are classified as having oppositional disorder more frequently than boys because boys more often receive the diagnosis of conduct disorder. No distinct family patterns have been noted, but many parents of children with the disorder are themselves overly concerned with issues of power, control, and autonomy.

Etiology

The ability of a child to communicate his or her will and oppose the will of others is crucial to normal development as a route toward establishing autonomy, forming an identity, and setting inner standards and controls. The most dramatic example of normal oppositional behavior peaks between 18 and 24 months, the "terrible two's," when toddlers behave negativistically as an expression of growing autonomy. Pathology begins when this developmental phase persists abnormally, authority figures overreact, or oppositional behavior recurs considerably more frequently than in most children of the same mental age.

Children exhibit a range of temperamental predispositions to strong will, strong preferences, or great assertiveness. Parents who model more extreme ways of expressing and enforcing their will may contribute to the development of chronic struggles with their children that are then reenacted with other authority figures. What begins for an infant as an effort to establish self-determination may become transformed into an exaggerated behavioral pattern. In late childhood, environmental trauma, illness, or chronic incapacity, such as mental retardation, can trigger oppositionalism as a defense against helplessness, anxiety, and loss of self-esteem. Another normative oppositional stage occurs in adolescence as an expression of the need to separate from the parents and to establish an autonomous identity.

Classic psychoanalytic theory implicates unresolved conflicts as fueling aggressive behaviors targeting authority figures. Behaviorists have suggested that oppositionality is a reinforced, learned behavior through which a child exerts control over authority figures; for example, by having a temper tantrum when an undesired act is requested, a child coerces the parents to withdraw their request. In addition, increased parental attention—for example, long discussions about the behavior—can reinforce the behavior.

Table 8–1
DSM-IV-TR Diagnostic Criteria for Oppositional Defiant Disorder

A. A pattern of negativistic, hostile, and defiant behavior lasting at least 6 months, during which four (or more) of the following are present:
  (1) often loses temper
  (2) often argues with adults
  (3) often actively defies or refuses to comply with adults' requests or rules
  (4) often deliberately annoys people
  (5) often blames others for his or her mistakes or misbehavior
  (6) is often touchy or easily annoyed by others
  (7) is often angry and resentful
  (8) is often spiteful or vindictive

Note: Consider a criterion met only if the behavior occurs more frequently than is typically observed in individuals of comparable age and developmental level.

B. The disturbance in behavior causes clinically significant impairment in social, academic, or occupational functioning.

C. The behaviors do not occur exclusively during the course of a psychotic or mood disorder.

D. Criteria are not met for conduct disorder, and, if the individual is age 18 years or older, criteria are not met for antisocial personality disorder.

From American Psychiatric Association. *Diagnostic and Statistical Manual of Mental Disorders*. 4th ed. Text rev. Washington, DC: American Psychiatric Association; copyright 2000, with permission.

Diagnosis and Clinical Features

Children with oppositional defiant disorder often argue with adults, lose their temper, and are angry, resentful, and easily annoyed by others. Frequently, they actively defy adults' requests or rules and deliberately annoy other persons. They tend to blame others for their own mistakes and misbehavior. Manifestations of the disorder are almost invariably present in the home, but they may not be present at school or with other adults or peers. In some cases, features of the disorder from the beginning of the disturbance are displayed outside the home; in other cases, the behavior starts in the home but is later displayed outside. Typically, symptoms of the disorder are most evident in interactions with adults or peers whom the child knows well. Thus, a child with the disorder is likely to show little or no sign of the disorder when examined clinically. Usually, these children do not regard themselves as oppositional or defiant, but justify their behavior as a response to unreasonable circumstances. The disorder appears to cause more distress to those around the child than to the child. Diagnostic criteria for oppositional defiant disorder from DSM-IV-TR are given in Table 8–1.

Chronic oppositional defiant disorder almost always interferes with interpersonal relationships and school performance. These children are often friendless and perceive human relationships as unsatisfactory. Despite adequate intelligence, they do poorly or fail in school, as they withhold participation, resist external demands, and insist on solving problems without others' help. Secondary to these difficulties are low self-esteem, poor frustration tolerance, depressed mood, and temper outbursts. Adolescents may abuse alcohol and illegal substances. Often, the disturbance evolves into a conduct disorder or a mood disorder.

Pathology and Laboratory Examination. No specific laboratory tests or pathologic findings help to diagnose oppositional defiant disorder. Because some children with the disorder become physically aggressive and violate the rights of others as they get older, they may share some of the same characteristics under investigation in violent people, such as low serotonin levels in the central nervous system (CNS).

Differential Diagnosis

Because oppositional behavior is both normal and adaptive at specific developmental stages, these periods of negativism must be distinguished from oppositional defiant disorder.

Developmental-stage oppositional behavior, which is of shorter duration than oppositional defiant disorder, is neither considerably more frequent nor more intense than that seen in other children of the same mental age.

Oppositional defiant behavior occurring temporarily in reaction to a stress should be diagnosed as an adjustment disorder. When features of oppositional defiant disorder appear during the course of conduct disorder, schizophrenia, or a mood disorder, the diagnosis of oppositional defiant disorder should not be made. Oppositional and negativistic behaviors can also be present in attention-deficit/hyperactivity disorder (ADHD), cognitive disorders, and mental retardation. Whether a concomitant diagnosis of oppositional defiant disorder should be made depends on the severity, pervasiveness, and duration of such behavior. Some young children who receive a diagnosis of oppositional defiant disorder go on in several years to meet the criteria for conduct disorder. Some investigators believe that the two disorders may be developmental variants of each other, with conduct disorder being the natural progression of oppositional defiant behavior when a child matures. Most children with oppositional defiant disorder, however, do not later meet the criteria for conduct disorder, and up to one fourth of children with oppositional defiant disorder may not meet the diagnosis several years later.

The subtype of oppositional defiant disorder that tends to progress to conduct disorder is one in which aggression is prominent. Most children who have ADHD and conduct disorder develop conduct disorder before the age of 12 years. Most children who develop conduct disorder have a history of oppositional defiant disorder. Overall, the consensus is that two subtypes of oppositional defiant disorder may exist. One type, which is likely to progress to conduct disorder, includes certain symptoms of conduct disorder (e.g., fighting, bullying). The other type, which is characterized by less aggression and fewer antisocial traits, does not progress to conduct disorder.

Jared, age 8 years, was brought to the clinic for evaluation of misbehavior by his mother. She complained that he has frequent tantrums, usually in response to limits on his behavior or not getting his way. She describes the tantrums as consisting of shouting, cursing, crying, slamming doors, and sometimes throwing books or objects on the floor. She states that these outbursts occur almost daily. She feels that sometimes it seems as though he is trying to provoke her. Recently, he was kicking his foot against his mother's chair and she asked him to stop. He looked at her and continued to kick her chair. She says that she has given up on asking him to pick up his room or help with chores, because it inevitably results in an argument. Jared appears sullen and irritable on interview. He says that it was his mother's fault and she is always after him about one thing or another. He interrupts her several times during the joint interview, saying that she was lying or giving his version of events. His grades at school are excellent, and there are no reports of any behavior problems or disobedience at school. His mother says that he does not have many friends, because he has difficulty sharing his things and tends to be bossy. He had a series of ear infections as an infant and occasionally experiences seasonal allergies, but is otherwise in good health, with normal physical development. His mother describes him as being fussy as an infant and difficult to comfort when upset. He is an only child, and his parents separated and divorced when he was 3. He has had no contact with his father since then. His mother was depressed for a year after the divorce until she sought treatment. She has always felt guilty that his father is not in his life and worries that he blames her for not having his father around. She believes his behaviors have become worse since she recently started dating again. (Courtesy of Christopher R. Thomas, M.D.)

Course and Prognosis

The course of oppositional defiant disorder depends largely on the severity of the symptoms and the ability of the child to develop more-adaptive responses to authority. The stability of oppositional defiant disorder varies over time. Persistence of oppositional defiant symptoms poses an increased risk of additional disorders, such as conduct disorder and substance use disorders. Positive outcomes are more likely for intact families who can modify their own expression of demands and give less attention to the child's argumentative behaviors.

About one fourth of all children who receive the diagnosis of oppositional defiant disorder do not continue to meet diagnostic criteria over the next several years. It is not clear in these cases whether the criteria captured children whose behavior was not developmentally abnormal or whether the disorder spontaneously remitted. Patients in whom the diagnosis persists may remain stable or go on to violate the rights of others and, thus, develop conduct disorder. Such patients should receive a guarded prognoses.

An association exists between conduct disorder and later substance use disorders, as well as elevated rates of mood disorders, in children with oppositional defiant disorder, conduct disorder, and ADHD. Parental psychopathology, such as antisocial personality disorder and substance abuse, appears to be more common in families with children who have oppositional defiant disorder than in the general population, which creates additional risks for chaotic and troubled home environments. The prognosis for oppositional defiant disorder in a child depends somewhat on family functioning and the development of comorbid psychopathology.

Treatment

The primary treatment of oppositional defiant disorder is family intervention using both direct training of the parents in child management skills and careful assessment of family interactions. Behavior therapists emphasize teaching parents how to alter their behavior to discourage the child's oppositional behavior and encourage appropriate behavior. Behavior therapy focuses on selectively reinforcing and praising appropriate behavior and ignoring or not reinforcing undesired behavior.

Children with oppositional defiant behavior may also benefit from individual psychotherapy insofar as the child is exposed to a situation with an adult in which to "practice" more-adaptive responses. In the therapeutic relationship, the child can learn new strategies to develop a sense of mastery and success in social situations with peers and families. In the safety of a more "neutral" relationship, children may discover that they are capable of less provocative behavior. Often, self-esteem must be restored before a child with oppositional defiant disorder can make more positive responses to external control. Parent–child conflict strongly predicts conduct problems; patterns of harsh physical and verbal punishment particularly evoke the emergence of aggression and deviance in children. Thus, it is likely that eliminating harsh, punitive parenting and increasing positive parent–child interactions may positively influence the course of oppositional and defiant behaviors.

CONDUCT DISORDER

Children with conduct disorder are likely to demonstrate behaviors in the following four categories: physical aggression or threats of harm to people, destruction of their own property or that of others, theft or acts of deceit, and frequent violation of age-appropriate rules. Conduct disorder is an enduring set of behaviors that evolves over time, usually characterized by aggression and violation of the rights of others. Conduct disorder is associated with many other psychiatric disorders, including ADHD, depression, and learning disorders, and it is also associated with certain psychosocial factors, such as harsh, punitive parenting; family discord; lack of appropriate parental supervision; lack of social competence; and low socioeconomic level. The DSM-IV-TR criteria require 3 specific behaviors of the 15 listed, which include bullying, threatening, or intimidating others and staying out at night despite parental prohibitions, beginning before 13 years of age. DSM-IV-TR also specifies that truancy from school must begin before 13 years of age to be considered a symptom of conduct disorder. The disorder can be diagnosed in a person older than 18 years only if the criteria for antisocial personality disorder are not met. DSM-IV-TR describes a mild level of the disorder as showing few, if any, conduct problems in excess of those needed to make the diagnosis and conduct problems that cause only minor harm to others. According to DSM-IV-TR, the severe level shows many conduct problems in excess of the minimal diagnostic criteria or conduct problems that cause considerable harm to others.

Epidemiology

Occasional rule breaking and rebellious behavior is common during childhood and adolescence, but in youth with conduct disorder, behaviors that violate the rights of others are repetitive and pervasive. Estimated rates of conduct disorder among the general population range from 1 to 10 percent, with a general population rate of approximately 5 percent. The disorder is more common among boys than girls, and the ratio ranges from 4:1 to as much as 12:1. Conduct disorder occurs with greater frequency in the children of parents with antisocial personality disorder and alcohol dependence than in the general population. The prevalence of conduct disorder and antisocial behavior is associated with socioeconomic factors.

Etiology

No single factor can fully account for a child's antisocial behavior and conduct disorder. Instead, many biopsychosocial factors contribute to development of the disorder.

Parental Factors. Harsh, punitive parenting characterized by severe physical and verbal aggression is associated with the development of children's maladaptive aggressive behaviors. Chaotic home conditions are associated with conduct disorder and delinquency. Divorce is considered a risk factor, but the persistence of hostility, resentment, and bitterness between divorced parents may be the more important contributor to maladaptive behavior. Parental psychopathology, child abuse, and negligence often contribute to conduct disorder. Sociopathy, alcohol dependence, and substance abuse in the parents are associated with conduct disorder in their children. Parents may be so negligent that a child's care is shared by relatives or assumed by foster parents. Many such parents were scarred by their own upbringing and tend to be abusive, negligent, or engrossed in getting their own personal needs met.

In the 1980s, particularly in urban areas, cocaine abuse and acquired immunodeficiency syndrome (AIDS) increased family dysfunction. Recent studies suggest that many parents of children with conduct disorder have serious psychopathology, including psychotic disorders. Psychodynamic hypotheses suggest that children with conduct disorder unconsciously act out their parents' antisocial wishes; however, data suggest that children who exhibit a pattern of aggressive behavior have received physically or emotionally harsh parenting.

Sociocultural Factors. Socioeconomically deprived children are at higher risk for the development of conduct disorder, as are children and adolescents who grow up in urban environments. Unemployed parents, lack of a supportive social network, and lack of positive participation in community activities seem to predict conduct disorder. Associated findings that may influence the development of conduct disorder in urban areas are increased rates and prevalence of substance use. A recent survey of alcohol use and mental health in adolescents found that weekly alcohol use among adolescents is associated with increased delinquent and aggressive behavior. Significant interactions between frequent alcohol use and age indicated that those adolescents with weekly alcohol use at younger ages were most likely to exhibit aggressive behaviors and mood disorders. Although drug and alcohol use does not cause conduct disorder, it increases the risks associated with it. Drug intoxication can also aggravate the symptoms. Thus, all factors that increase the likelihood of regular substance use may, in fact, promote and expand the disorder.

Psychologic Factors. Children brought up in chaotic, negligent conditions often express poor modulation of emotions, including anger, frustration, and sadness. Poor modeling of impulse control and the chronic lack of having their needs met leads to a less well-developed sense of empathy.

Neurobiologic Factors. Neurobiologic factors in conduct disorder have been little studied, but research in ADHD yields some important findings, and this disorder often coexists with conduct disorder. In some children with conduct disorder, a low level of plasma dopamine β-hydroxylase, an enzyme that converts dopamine to norepinephrine, has been found. This finding supports a theory of decreased noradrenergic functioning in conduct disorder. Some conduct-disordered juvenile offenders have high serotonin levels in blood. Evidence indicates that blood serotonin levels correlate inversely with levels of the serotonin metabolite 5-hydroxyindoleacetic acid (5-HIAA) in the cerebrospinal fluid (CSF) and that low 5-HIAA levels in CSF correlate with aggression and violence.

Neurologic Factors. A recent Canadian study investigated the relationship between resting frontal brain electrical activity (electroencephalogram [EEG]), emotional intelligence, and aggression and rule breaking in 10-year-old children. Frontal resting brain electrical activity has been hypothesized to reflect the ability to regulate emotionality. Results of this study indicate that children with higher reported externalizing behaviors had significantly greater relative right frontal EEG activity during rest than children with little or no reported aggressive behavior. Boys tended to show lower emotional intelligence and greater aggressive behavior than girls. No relationship, however, was found between emotional intelligence and pattern of frontal EEG activation. This study suggests an association between resting pattern of EEG activation and aggressive behavior.

Child Abuse and Maltreatment. It is widely accepted that children chronically exposed to violence, especially those receiving repeated physical or sexual abuse that starts at a young age, are at high risk for behaving aggressively. Children who are exposed to caregivers who are exposed to violence are also likely to demonstrate disruptive and aggressive behaviors. A recent study of female caregivers' exposed to intimate partner violence revealed a strong association with offspring aggression and mood disturbance. Children who are exposed as witnesses to maternal abuse or who are recipients of abuse themselves may be reticent to verbalize their experiences because of direct threats from the abusive adult and therefore may instead demonstrate their feelings through aggressive and destructive behaviors. Severely abused children and adolescents tend to be hypervigilant; in some cases, they misperceive benign situations as directly threatening and respond with violence. Not all expressed physical behavior in adolescents is synonymous with conduct disorder, but children with a pattern of hypervigilance and violent responses are likely to violate the rights of others.

Comorbid Factors. ADHD, CNS dysfunction or damage, and early extremes of temperament can predispose a child to conduct disorder. Propensity to violence correlates with CNS dysfunction and signs of severe psychopathology, such as delusional tendencies. Longitudinal temperament studies suggest that many behavioral deviations are initially a straightforward response to a poor fit between a child's temperament and emotional needs, on one hand, and parental attitudes and child-rearing practices, on the other.

Diagnosis and Clinical Features

Conduct disorder does not develop overnight; instead, many symptoms evolve over time until a consistent pattern develops that involves violating the rights of others. Very young children are unlikely to meet the criteria for the disorder because they are not developmentally able to exhibit the symptoms typical of older children with conduct disorder. A 3-year-old does not break into someone's home, steal with confrontation, force someone into sexual activity, or deliberately use a weapon that can cause serious harm. School-age children, however, can become bullies, initiate physical fights, destroy property, or set fires. The DSM-IV-TR diagnostic criteria for conduct disorder are given in Table 8–2.

The average age of onset of conduct disorder is younger in boys than in girls. Boys most commonly meet the diagnostic criteria by 10 to 12 years of age, whereas girls often reach 14 to 16 years of age before the criteria are met.

Children who meet the criteria for conduct disorder express their overt aggressive behavior in various forms. Aggressive antisocial behavior can take the form of bullying, physical aggression, and cruel behavior toward peers. Children may be hostile, verbally abusive, impudent, defiant, and negativistic toward adults. Persistent lying, frequent truancy, and vandalism are common. In severe cases, destructiveness, stealing, and physical violence often occur. Some adolescents with conduct disorder make little attempt to conceal their antisocial behavior. Sexual behavior and regular use of tobacco, liquor, or nonprescribed psychoactive substances begin unusually early for such children and adolescents. Suicidal thoughts, gestures, and acts are frequent in children and adolescents with conduct disorder who are in conflict with peers, family members, or the law and are unable to problem solve their difficulties.

Some children with aggressive behavioral patterns have impaired social attachments, as evidenced by their difficulties with peer relationships. Some may befriend a much older or younger person or have superficial relationships with other antisocial youngsters. Many children with conduct problems have poor

Table 8–2
DSM-IV-TR Diagnostic Criteria for Conduct Disorder

A. A repetitive and persistent pattern of behavior in which the basic rights of others or major age-appropriate societal norms or rules are violated, as manifested by the presence of three (or more) of the following criteria in the past 12 months, with at least one criterion present in the past 6 months:

Aggression to people and animals

(1) often bullies, threatens, or intimidates others
(2) often initiates physical fights
(3) has used a weapon that can cause serious physical harm to others (e.g., a bat, brick, broken bottle, knife, gun)
(4) has been physically cruel to people
(5) has been physically cruel to animals
(6) has stolen while confronting a victim (e.g., mugging, purse snatching, extortion, armed robbery)
(7) has forced someone into sexual activity

Destruction of property

(8) has deliberately engaged in fire setting with the intention of causing serious damage
(9) has deliberately destroyed others' property (other than by fire setting)

Deceitfulness or theft

(10) has broken into someone else's house, building, or car
(11) often lies to obtain goods or favors or to avoid obligations (i.e., "cons" others)
(12) has stolen items of nontrivial value without confronting a victim (e.g., shoplifting, but without breaking and entering; forgery)

Serious violations of rules

(13) often stays out at night despite parental prohibitions, beginning before age 13 years
(14) has run away from home overnight at least twice while living in parental or parental surrogate home (or once without returning for a lengthy period)
(15) is often truant from school, beginning before age 13 years

B. The disturbance in behavior causes clinically significant impairment in social, academic, or occupational functioning.

C. If the individual is age 18 years or older, criteria are not met for antisocial personality disorder.

Code based on age at onset:

Conduct disorder, childhood-onset type: onset of at least one criterion characteristic of conduct disorder prior to age 10 years

Conduct disorder, adolescent-onset type: absence of any criteria characteristic of conduct disorder prior to age 10 years

Conduct disorder, unspecified onset: age at onset is not known

Specify severity:

Mild: few if any conduct problems in excess of those required to make the diagnosis and conduct problems cause only minor harm to others

Moderate: number of conduct problems and effect on others intermediate between "mild" and "severe"

Severe: many conduct problems in excess of those required to make the diagnosis or conduct problems cause considerable harm to others

From American Psychiatric Association. *Diagnostic and Statistical Manual of Mental Disorders.* 4th ed. Text rev. Washington, DC: American Psychiatric Association; copyright 2000, with permission.

self-esteem, although they may project an image of toughness. They may lack the skills to communicate in socially acceptable ways and appear to have little regard for the feelings, wishes, and welfare of others. Children and adolescents with conduct disorders often feel guilt or remorse for some of their behaviors but try to blame others to stay out of trouble.

Many children and adolescents with conduct disorder suffer from the deprivation of having few of their dependency needs met and may have had either overly harsh parenting or a lack of appropriate supervision. The deficient socialization of many children and adolescents with conduct disorder can be expressed in physical violation of others and, for some, in sexual violation of others. Severe punishments for behavior in children with conduct disorder almost invariably increases their maladaptive expression of rage and frustration rather than ameliorating the problem.

In evaluation interviews, children with aggressive conduct disorders are typically uncooperative, hostile, and provocative. Some have a superficial charm and compliance until they are urged to talk about their problem behaviors. Then, they often deny any problems. If the interviewer persists, the child may attempt to justify misbehavior or become suspicious and angry about the source of the examiner's information and perhaps bolt from the room. Most often, the child becomes angry with the examiner and expresses resentment of the examination with open belligerence or sullen withdrawal. Their hostility is not limited to adult authority figures but is expressed with equal venom toward their age-mates and younger children. In fact, they often bully those who are smaller and weaker than they are. By boasting, lying, and expressing little interest in a listener's responses, such children reveal their lack of trust in adults to understand their position.

Evaluation of the family situation often reveals severe marital disharmony, which initially may center on disagreements about management of the child. Because of a tendency toward family instability, parent surrogates are often in the picture. Children with conduct disorder are more likely to have been unplanned or unwanted babies. The parents of children with conduct disorder, especially the father, have higher rates of antisocial personality disorder or alcohol dependence. Aggressive children and their family show a stereotyped pattern of impulsive and unpredictable verbal and physical hostility. A child's aggressive behavior rarely seems directed toward any definable goal and offers little pleasure, success, or even sustained advantages with peers or authority figures.

In other cases, conduct disorder includes repeated truancy, vandalism, and serious physical aggression or assault against others by a gang, such as mugging, gang fighting, and beating. Children who become part of a gang usually have the skills for age-appropriate friendships. They are likely to show concern for the welfare of their friends or their own gang members and are unlikely to blame them or inform on them. In most cases, gang members have a history of adequate or even excessive conformity during early childhood that ended when the youngster became a member of the delinquent peer group, usually in preadolescence or during adolescence. Also present in the history is some evidence of early problems, such as marginal or poor school performance, mild behavior problems, anxiety, and depressive symptoms. Some family social or psychologic pathology is usually evident. Patterns of paternal discipline are rarely ideal and can vary from harshness and excessive strictness to inconsistency or relative absence of supervision and control. The mother has often protected the child from the consequences of early mild misbehavior but does not seem to encourage delinquency actively. Delinquency, also called juvenile delinquency, is most often associated with conduct disorder but can also result from other psychologic or neurologic disorders.

Violent Video Games and Violent Behavior. Over the last few decades violent video games have become ubiquitous in Western societies, especially as frequent activities for younger and adolescent males. A recent review of the literature of the effect of violent video games on children and adolescents revealed that violent video game playing is related to aggressive affect, physiologic arousal, and aggressive behaviors. It stands to reason that the degree of exposure to violent games would be related to a greater preoccupation with violent themes.

Pathology and Laboratory Examination

No specific laboratory test or neurologic pathology helps to make the diagnosis of conduct disorder. Some evidence indicates that amounts of certain neurotransmitters, such as serotonin in the CNS, are low in some persons with a history of violent or aggressive behavior toward others or themselves. Whether this association is related to the cause, or is the effect, of violence or is unrelated to the violence is not clear.

Differential Diagnosis

Disturbances of conduct may be part of many childhood psychiatric conditions, ranging from mood disorders to psychotic disorders to learning disorders. Therefore, clinicians must obtain a history of the chronology of the symptoms to determine whether the conduct disturbance is a transient or reactive phenomenon or an enduring pattern. Isolated acts of antisocial behavior do not justify a diagnosis of conduct disorder; an enduring pattern must be present. The relation of conduct disorder to oppositional defiant disorder is under debate. Historically, oppositional defiant disorder has been conceptualized as a mild precursor of conduct disorder, which is likely to be diagnosed in young children at risk for conduct disorder. Children who progress from oppositional defiant disorder to conduct disorder maintain their oppositional characteristics, but some evidence indicates that the two disorders are independent. Many children with oppositional defiant disorder never go on to have conduct disorder, and when conduct disorder first appears in adolescence, it may be unrelated to oppositional defiant disorder. The main distinguishing clinical feature of the two disorders is that in conduct disorder, the basic rights of others are violated, whereas in oppositional defiant disorder, hostility and negativism fall short of seriously violating the rights of others.

Mood disorders are often present in children who exhibit irritability and aggressive behavior. Both major depressive disorder and bipolar disorders must be ruled out, but the full syndrome of conduct disorder can occur and be diagnosed during the onset of a mood disorder. Substantial comorbidity exists of conduct disorder and depressive disorders. A recent report concluded that the high correlation between the two disorders arises from shared risk factors for both disorders rather than a causal relation. Thus, a series of factors, including family conflict, negative life events, early history of conduct disturbance, level of parental involvement, and affiliation with delinquent peers, contributes to the development of affective disorders and conduct disorder. This is not the case with oppositional defiant disorder, which cannot be diagnosed if it occurs exclusively during a mood disorder.

Attention-deficit/hyperactivity disorder and learning disorders are commonly associated with conduct disorder. Usually, the symptoms of these disorders predate the diagnosis of conduct disorder. Substance abuse disorders are also more common in adolescents with conduct disorder than in the general population. Evidence indicates an association between fighting behaviors as a child and substance use as an adolescent. Once a pattern of drug use is formed, this pattern may interfere with the development of positive mediators, such as social skills and problem solving, which could enhance remission of the conduct disorder. Thus, once substance abuse develops, it may promote continuation of the conduct disorder. Obsessive-compulsive disorder also frequently seems to coexist with disruptive behavior disorders. All the disorders described here should be noted when they co-occur. Children with ADHD often exhibit impulsive and aggressive behaviors that may not meet the full criteria for conduct disorder.

John, age 12 years, was referred for outpatient evaluation after being picked up by police for running away from home. He states that he just wanted to get out of the house and visit his friends. His mother says that he has been out of the home overnight on three other occasions in the past year, but usually returns the next morning. She complains that he is constantly in trouble. He has shoplifted on several occasions that she knows of, the first time at age 8 years. She suspects that he also steals from neighbors or school, because there are always items at home that he claims he found. The police have been involved only for his running away from home. He has a quick temper, and she knows he was involved in several fights over the past year in the neighborhood. He is particularly cruel to his younger brother, constantly taunting and teasing him. She stated that he lies constantly, sometimes for no apparent reason. When he was 6 years of age, he was fascinated with fire and set several small fires at home, fortunately with no serious injury or damage. She ended by saying that John is just like his no-good father and that she wished she never had him. John initially refused to answer questions but gradually began to talk. He presented a tough image with an indifferent attitude about the various problems. He denies any abuse at home, saying that he ran off because he was bored. He acknowledged his misbehaviors, but dismissed them as just having fun. He explained the fights as provoked by the others and denied the use of any weapons, although he bragged about breaking the nose of another youth. His record indicates that he was evaluated for symptoms of ADHD when he was in first grade. Methylphenidate (Ritalin) was prescribed; however, the family did not continue with treatment, and he is currently on no medication. He is currently in 6th grade special education classes, having failed and repeated 5th grade. His current grades are failing, and he may have to repeat 6th grade. He admits to truancy on several occasions this year in addition to his problems with completing schoolwork. His previous evaluation indicates that child protective services evaluated the family for possible neglect when he was 5 years of age after he and his brother were found barefoot and unkempt on the street late one evening. Apparently, the family was referred for counseling and never attended, but the case was eventually dismissed. Both of John's parents have a history of drug and alcohol abuse. His birth was unplanned, and his mother used drugs during pregnancy. His parents separated soon after his birth, and his mother returned to live with her parents briefly. He and his mother moved to live with her boyfriend when John was 3 years of age after she became pregnant with his younger brother. This relationship ended within a year, and only John, his mother, and his brother live in their apartment. She has worked several different jobs, and John thinks she still has a drinking problem. (Courtesy of Christopher R. Thomas, M.D.)

Course and Prognosis

In general, the prognosis for children with conduct disorder is most guarded in those who have symptoms at a young age, exhibit the greatest number of symptoms, and express them most frequently. This finding is true partly because those with severe conduct disorder seem to be most vulnerable to comorbid disorders later in life, such as mood disorders and substance use disorders. It stands to reason that the more concurrent mental disorders a person has, the more troublesome life will be. A recent report found that, although assaultive behavior in childhood and parental criminality predict a high risk for incarceration later in life, the diagnosis of conduct disorder per se was not correlated with imprisonment. A good prognosis is predicted for mild conduct disorder in the absence of coexisting psychopathology and the presence of normal intellectual functioning.

Treatment

Multimodality treatment programs that use all of the available family and community resources are likely to bring about the best results in efforts to control conduct-disordered behavior. Multimodal treatments can involve the use of behavioral interventions in which rewards may be earned for prosocial and nonaggressive behaviors, social skills training, family education and therapy, and pharmacologic interventions. Overall, treatment programs have been more successful in decreasing overt symptoms of conduct, such as aggression, than the covert symptoms, such as lying or stealing. Treatment strategies for young children that focus on increasing social behavior and social competence are believed to reduce aggressive behavior. A recent study of 548 third-graders administered a school-based intervention instead of a regular health curriculum in several public schools in North Carolina, called Making Choices: Social Problem Solving Skills For Children (MC), along with supplemental teacher and parent components. Compared with third-graders receiving the routine health curriculum, children exposed to the MC program were rated lower on posttest social and overt aggression and higher on social competence. They further scored higher on an information-processing skills posttest. These findings support the notion that school-based prevention programs have the potential to strengthen social and emotional skills and diminish aggressive behavior among normal populations of school-age children. No treatment is considered curative for the entire spectrum of behaviors that contribute to conduct disorder, but a variety of treatments may be helpful in containing symptoms and promoting prosocial behavior.

An environmental structure that provides support, along with consistent rules and expected consequences, can help to control a variety of problem behaviors. The reduction of violence and aggression in schools is an important setting for interventions. A thoughtful approach to the management of threats of violence includes provision of a functioning security hierarchy, peer-participant programs, threat assessment, and crisis response initiatives. All of these strategies increase the structure necessary to maintain a safe school environment. The structure can be applied to family life in some cases, so that parents become aware of behavioral techniques and grow proficient at using them to foster appropriate behaviors. Families in which psychopathology or environmental stressors prevent parental understanding of the techniques may require parental psychiatric evaluation and treatment before making such an endeavor. When a family is abusive or chaotic, the child may have to be removed from the home to benefit from a consistent and structured environment. School settings can also use behavioral techniques to promote socially acceptable behavior toward peers and to discourage covert antisocial incidents.

Behaviorally based individual psychotherapy targeting problem-solving skills with appropriate rewards can be useful because children with conduct disorder may have a longstanding pattern of maladaptive responses to daily situations. The age at which treatment begins is important because the longer the maladaptive behaviors continue, the more entrenched they become.

Pharmacotherapy. Pharmacologic treatments for aggression have become more accepted adjunctive treatment in the context of conduct disorder. Overt explosive aggression responds to several medications. Early studies of antipsychotics, most notably haloperidol (Haldol), reported decreased aggressive and assaultive behaviors in children with a variety of psychiatric disorders. Currently, the atypical antipsychotics risperidone (Risperdal), olanzapine (Zyprexa), quetiapine (Seroquel), ziprasidone (Geodon), and aripiprazole (Abilify) have replaced the older antipsychotics because of their comparable efficacy and improved side effect profiles. Placebo-controlled, randomized trials have shown risperidone to reduce aggression in children with disruptive behavior disorders, particularly in populations with pervasive developmental disorders and aggression. Growing evidence suggests that atypical antipsychotics are efficacious in contributing to the management of aggression among children and adolescents. Long-term effects of the use of these agents are largely unknown and require further investigation. Side effects include sedation, increased prolactin levels (with risperidone use), and extrapyramidal symptoms, including akathisia. In general, however, the atypical antipsychotics appear to be well tolerated. A preliminary study of clozapine (Clozaril), used mainly in the treatment of refractory schizophrenia, reported decreased aggressive behavior in a sample of treatment-refractory children and adolescents with schizophrenia and aggressive behavior. Lithium (Eskalith) has been reported to have efficacy for some aggressive children with or without comorbid bipolar disorders. Although previous trials suggested that carbamazepine (Tegretol) may help to control aggression, a double-blind, placebo-controlled study did not show superiority of carbamazepine over placebo in decreasing aggression. A recent pilot study found that clonidine (Catapres) may decrease aggression. The selective serotonin reuptake inhibitors (SSRIs), such as fluoxetine (Prozac), sertraline (Zoloft), paroxetine (Paxil), and citalopram (Celexa), have been used in an attempt to diminish impulsivity, irritability, and lability of mood, which often occur with conduct disorder. Conduct disorder frequently coexists with ADHD, learning disorders, and, over time, mood disorders and substance-related disorders; thus, the treatment of any concurrent disorders must also be addressed.

Table 8–3
DSM-IV-TR Diagnostic Criteria for Disruptive Behavior Disorder Not Otherwise Specified

This category is for disorders characterized by conduct or oppositional defiant behaviors that do not meet the criteria for conduct disorder or oppositional defiant disorder. For example, include clinical presentations that do not meet full criteria either for oppositional defiant disorder or conduct disorder, but in which there is clinically significant impairment.

From American Psychiatric Association. *Diagnostic and Statistical Manual of Mental Disorders.* 4th ed. Text rev. Washington, DC: American Psychiatric Association; copyright 2000, with permission.

DISRUPTIVE BEHAVIOR DISORDER NOT OTHERWISE SPECIFIED

According to the DSM-IV-TR, the category of disruptive behavior disorder not otherwise specified can be used for disorders of conduct or oppositional defiant behaviors that do not meet the diagnostic criteria for either conduct disorder or oppositional defiant disorder but in which there is notable impairment (Table 8–3).

9

Feeding and Eating Disorders of Infancy or Early Childhood

Feeding disorders during infancy and early childhood highlight the interactive nature between the infant and caregiver. In broad terms, feeding disorder is characterized by a variety of conditions, including food refusal, food avoidance, active attempts to reject the feeding process, and delay in self-feeding. Feeding disorder has been an underlying process in some children who have been described as picky eaters, poor eaters, or demonstrating feeding resistances. A feeding disorder may or may not be accompanied by physical sequelae of the maladaptive eating patterns, but without well-defined criteria, the term has been used interchangeably with *failure to thrive*, which refers to inadequate weight gain based on standard growth charts. In some cases, failure-to-thrive syndromes are caused by a medical disease process; however, this term is often applied to children without medical illness who have been exposed to parental deprivation or neglect. The text revision of the fourth edition of the *Diagnostic and Statistical Manual of Mental Disorders* (DSM-IV-TR) includes three distinct disorders of feeding and eating in this age group: pica, rumination disorder, and feeding disorder of infancy or early childhood. A high rate of spontaneous recovery from all of these feeding disorders occurs, although a subset of infants refuses to eat and has persistent eating problems throughout childhood. Additional maladaptive feeding patterns that cause impaired nutritional intake that are not included in the DSM-IV-TR include (1) infantile anorexia, (2) feeding disorder of caregiver–infant reciprocity, (3) sensory food aversions, and (4) posttraumatic feeding disorder.

PICA

In the DSM-IV-TR, pica is described as persistent eating of nonnutritive substances for at least 1 month. The behavior must be developmentally inappropriate, not culturally sanctioned, and sufficiently severe to merit clinical attention. Pica is diagnosed even when these symptoms occur in the context of another disorder, such as autistic disorder, schizophrenia, or Kleine-Levin syndrome. Pica appears much more frequently in young children than in adults; it also occurs in persons with mental retardation. Among adults, certain forms of pica, including geophagia (clay eating) and amylophagia (starch eating), have been reported in pregnant women.

Epidemiology

A survey of a large clinic population reported that 75 percent of 12-month-old infants and 15 percent of 2- to 3-year-old toddlers placed nonnutritive substances in their mouth. Pica is more common among children and adolescents with mental retardation. It has been reported in up to 15 percent of persons with severe mental retardation. Pica appears to affect both sexes equally.

Etiology

Pica is most often a transient disorder that typically lasts for several months and then remits. In younger children, it is more frequently seen among children with developmental speech and social developmental delays. Among adolescents with pica, a substantial number exhibit depressive symptoms and use of substances. Several theories have been proposed to explain the phenomenon of pica, but none has been universally accepted. A higher-than-expected incidence of pica seems to occur in the relatives of persons with the symptoms. Nutritional deficiencies have been postulated as causes of pica; in particular circumstances, cravings for nonedible substances have been produced by dietary insufficiencies. For example, cravings for dirt and ice are sometimes associated with iron and zinc deficiencies, which are corrected by their administration. A high incidence of parental neglect and deprivation has been associated with cases of pica. Theories relating children's psychologic deprivation and subsequent ingestion of inedible substances have suggested that pica is a compensatory mechanism to satisfy oral needs.

Diagnosis and Clinical Features

Eating nonedible substances repeatedly after 18 months of age is usually considered abnormal. The onset of pica is usually between ages 12 and 24 months, and the incidence declines with age. The specific substances ingested vary with their accessibility, and they increase with a child's mastery of locomotion and the resultant increased independence and decreased parental supervision. Typically, young children ingest paint, plaster, string, hair, and cloth; older children with pica may ingest dirt, animal feces, stones, and paper. The clinical implications can be benign

Table 9–1
DSM-IV-TR Diagnostic Criteria for Pica

A. Persistent eating of nonnutritive substances for a period of at least 1 month.
B. The eating of nonnutritive substances is inappropriate to the developmental level.
C. The eating behavior is not part of a culturally sanctioned practice.
D. If the eating behavior occurs exclusively during the course of another mental disorder (e.g., mental retardation, pervasive developmental disorder, schizophrenia), it is sufficiently severe to warrant independent clinical attention.

From American Psychiatric Association. *Diagnostic and Statistical Manual of Mental Disorders.* 4th ed. Text rev. Washington, DC: American Psychiatric Association; copyright 2000, with permission.

or life threatening, depending on the objects ingested. Among the most serious complications are lead poisoning (usually from lead-based paint), intestinal parasites after ingestion of soil or feces, anemia and zinc deficiency after ingestion of clay, severe iron deficiency after ingestion of large quantities of starch, and intestinal obstruction from the ingestion of hair balls, stones, or gravel. Except in persons with mental retardation, pica usually remits by adolescence. Pica associated with pregnancy is usually limited to the pregnancy itself. The DSM-IV-TR diagnostic criteria for pica are given in Table 9–1.

Susan was 3 years of age when her mother took her to the pediatrician because of abdominal pain and lack of appetite. The mother complained that Susan put everything in her mouth but did not want to eat regular food. The pediatrician observed that Susan looked pale, thin, and withdrawn. She sucked her thumb and quietly looked down while her mother reported that Susan liked to chew on newspapers and put plaster in her mouth.

The medical examination revealed that Susan was anemic and suffered from lead poisoning. She was admitted to the hospital for treatment, and a psychiatric consultation was obtained.

Further exploration of the history and the observation of mother and child during feeding and play revealed that the mother was overwhelmed with the care of three young children and had little affection for Susan. The mother was unmarried and lived with her three children and five other family members in a three-bedroom apartment in an old housing project. Her 4-year-old son was hyperactive and demanded almost constant supervision. The 18-month-old infant was an engaging and active little girl, whereas Susan would sit quietly, rock herself, suck her thumb, or chew on newspaper.

The treatment plan included the involvement of social services and protective services to remove any lead paint from the walls in the present apartment and to look for better living arrangements for the family. The mother was helped to enroll Susan and her brother in a preschool program that provided them with more structure and stimulation and gave the mother a few hours of relief every day. In addition, Susan was seen with her mother and her younger sister in play therapy to help the mother understand the different temperament of each child and to make her more responsive to Susan's weak attempts to engage her mother. Once the mother felt more supported and less overwhelmed by her situation, she became more empathic and understanding of Susan. When Susan put something in her mouth, the mother was able to engage her in a play activity rather than screaming at her and scolding her for whatever she was doing. Over the period of 1 year, the relationship between Susan and her mother gradually improved, and Susan seemed less in need of putting her thumb or inedible things in her mouth. (Courtesy of Irene Chatoor, M.D.)

Pathology and Laboratory Examination

No single laboratory test confirms or rules out a diagnosis of pica, but several laboratory tests are useful because pica has frequently been associated with abnormal indexes. Levels of iron and zinc in serum should always be determined; in many cases of pica, these levels are low and may contribute to the development of pica. Pica may disappear when oral iron and zinc are administered. A patient's hemoglobin level should be determined; if the level is low, anemia can result. In children with pica, the lead level in serum should be determined; lead poisoning can result from ingesting lead. When a child's lead level is high, this condition must be treated.

Differential Diagnosis

The differential diagnosis of pica includes iron and zinc deficiencies. Pica also can occur in conjunction with failure to thrive and several other mental and medical disorders, including schizophrenia, autistic disorder, anorexia nervosa, and Kleine-Levin syndrome. In psychosocial dwarfism, a dramatic but reversible endocrinologic and behavioral form of failure to thrive, children often show bizarre behaviors, including ingesting toilet water, garbage, and other nonnutritive substances. A recent case report presented an association of pica with hypersomnolence, lead intoxication, and precocious puberty. Precocious puberty implicates the hypothalamus as a site for at least part of the dysfunction. Lead intoxication is known to be associated with pica, as well as several other neuropsychiatric abnormalities in memory and cognitive performance. A few children with autistic disorder and schizophrenia may have pica. For children who exhibit pica along with another medical disorder, both disorders should be coded according to the DSM-IV-TR.

In certain regions of the world and among certain cultures, such as the Australian aborigines, rates of pica in pregnant women are reportedly high. According to the DSM-IV-TR, however, if such practices are culturally accepted, the diagnostic criteria for pica are not met.

Course and Prognosis

The prognosis for pica is usually good because in children of normal intelligence it generally remits spontaneously within several months. In childhood, pica usually resolves with increasing age; in pregnant women, pica is usually limited to the term of the pregnancy. In some adults, however, especially those with mental retardation, pica can continue for years. Follow-up data on these populations are too limited to permit conclusions.

Treatment

The first step in the treatment of pica is determining the cause whenever possible. When pica is associated with situations of neglect or maltreatment, these circumstances naturally need to be altered. Exposure to toxic substances, such as lead, must also be eliminated. No definitive treatment exists for pica; most treatment is aimed at education and behavior modification. Treatments emphasize psychosocial, environmental, behavioral, and family guidance approaches. An effort should be made to ameliorate any significant psychosocial stressors. When lead is present in the surroundings, it must be eliminated or rendered inaccessible or the child must be moved to new surroundings.

Several behavioral techniques have been used with some effect. The most rapidly successful technique seems to be mild aversion therapy or negative reinforcement (e.g., a mild electric shock, an unpleasant noise, or an emetic drug). Positive reinforcement, modeling, behavioral shaping, and overcorrection treatment have also been used. Increasing parental attention, stimulation, and emotional nurturance may yield positive results. One study found that pica was negatively correlated with involvement with play materials and occurred most frequently in impoverished environments. In some patients, correcting an iron or zinc deficiency eliminated pica. Medical complications (e.g., lead poisoning) that develop secondarily to the pica must also be treated.

RUMINATION DISORDER

Rumination can be observed in developmentally normal infants who put their thumb or hand in the mouth, suck their tongue rhythmically, and arch their back to initiate regurgitation. This behavior pattern is not infrequently observed in infants who receive inadequate emotional interaction and have learned to soothe and stimulate themselves through rumination. The onset of the disorder generally occurs after 3 months of age; once the regurgitation occurs, the food may be swallowed or spit out. Infants who ruminate are observed to strain to bring the food back into their mouths and appear to find the experience pleasurable. Infants who are "experienced" ruminators are able to bring up the food through tongue movements and may not spit out the food at all, but hold it in their mouths and reswallow it. The disorder is rare in older children, adolescents, and adults. It varies in severity and is sometimes associated with medical conditions, such as hiatal hernia, that result in esophageal reflux. In its most severe form, the disorder can be fatal.

The diagnosis of rumination disorder can be made whether or not an infant has attained a normal weight for his or her age. Failure to thrive, therefore, is not a necessary criterion of this disorder, but it is sometimes a sequela. According to the DSM-IV-TR, the disorder must be present for at least 1 month after a period of normal functioning, and it is not associated with gastrointestinal illness or other general medical conditions.

Rumination has been recognized for hundreds of years. An awareness of the disorder is important so that it is correctly diagnosed and unnecessary surgical procedures and inappropriate treatment are avoided. *Rumination* is derived from the Latin word *ruminare*, meaning "to chew the cud." The Greek equivalent is *merycism*, the act of regurgitating food from the stomach into the mouth, rechewing the food, and reswallowing it.

Epidemiology

Rumination is a rare disorder. It seems to be more common among male infants, and emerges between 3 months and 1 year of age. It persists more frequently among children and adults with mental retardation. Adults with rumination usually maintain a normal weight. No reliable figures on predisposing factors or familial patterns are available.

Etiology

Rumination and gastroesophageal reflux often coexist, leading to a spectrum of variable contributions from organic and psychologic factors for the emergence of the disorder. In some cases, vomiting secondary to gastroesophageal reflux or an acute illness precedes a pattern of rumination that lasts for several months. It appears, for some infants, that the rumination behavior is self-soothing or produces a sense of relief, leading to a continuation of behaviors to bring it about. In those with mental retardation, the disorder may be attributed to self-stimulatory behavior. Psychodynamic theories hypothesize various disturbances in the mother–child relationship as a contributing factor in the development of rumination disorder. The mothers of infants with the disorder have been characterized as immature, exposing the infant to increased levels of marital conflict, leading to understimulation and inadequate emotional attention to the baby. These factors are hypothesized to result in insufficient emotional gratification and stimulation for the infant who seeks to self-stimulate. The rumination is interpreted as the infant's attempt to recreate the feeding process and to provide gratification that the mother does not.

Overstimulation and tension have also been suggested as causes of rumination. A dysfunctional autonomic nervous system may be implicated. As sophisticated and accurate investigative techniques have been refined, a substantial number of children classified as ruminators have been shown to have gastroesophageal reflux or hiatal hernia.

Table 9–2
DSM-IV-TR Diagnostic Criteria for Rumination Disorder

A. Repeated regurgitation and rechewing of food for a period of at least 1 month following a period of normal functioning.
B. The behavior is not due to an associated gastrointestinal or other general medical condition (e.g., esophageal reflux).
C. The behavior does not occur exclusively during the course of anorexia nervosa or bulimia nervosa. If the symptoms occur exclusively during the course of mental retardation or a pervasive developmental disorder, they are sufficiently severe to warrant independent clinical attention.

From American Psychiatric Association. *Diagnostic and Statistical Manual of Mental Disorders.* 4th ed. Text rev. Washington, DC: American Psychiatric Association; copyright 2000, with permission.

Behaviorists attribute rumination to the positive reinforcement of pleasurable self-stimulation and to the attention the baby receives from others as a consequence of the disorder.

Diagnosis and Clinical Features

The DSM-IV-TR diagnostic criteria for rumination disorder are given in Table 9–2. The DSM-IV-TR notes that the essential feature of the disorder is repeated regurgitation and rechewing of food for a period of at least 1 month after a period of normal functioning. Partially digested food is brought up into the mouth without nausea, retching, disgust, or associated gastrointestinal disorder. This activity can be distinguished from vomiting by the clear, purposeful movements the infant makes to induce it. The food is then ejected from the mouth or reswallowed. A characteristic position of straining and arching of the back, with the head held back, is observed. The infant makes sucking movements with the tongue and gives the impression of gaining considerable satisfaction from the activity. Usually, the infant is irritable and hungry between episodes of rumination.

Initially, rumination may be difficult to distinguish from the regurgitation that frequently occurs in normal infants. In fully developed cases, however, the diagnosis is obvious. Food or milk is regurgitated without nausea, retching, or disgust and is subjected to what appears to be innumerable pleasurable sucking and chewing movements. The food is then reswallowed or ejected from the mouth.

Although spontaneous remissions are common, severe secondary complications can develop, such as progressive malnutrition, dehydration, and lowered resistance to disease. Failure to thrive, with absence of growth and developmental delays in all areas, can occur. A mortality rate as high as 25 percent has been reported in severe cases. An additional complication is that the mother or caretaker is often discouraged by failure to feed the infant successfully and can become alienated if this is not already the case. Further alienation often occurs as the noxious odor of the regurgitated material leads to avoidance of the infant.

Justin was 9 months old when he was referred by a gastroenterologist for a psychiatric evaluation because of concerns that he continued to vomit because of rumination. Justin was born full-term and had developed nicely until he was approximately 6 weeks old, when he began to vomit increasing amounts of milk during and after feedings. He was diagnosed with gastroesophageal reflux, which was treated with thickened feedings and medication. Justin responded well to the treatment; he stopped vomiting almost completely and gained weight adequately. Because Justin was doing so well, his mother decided to go back to work when Justin was 8 months old. She transitioned his care to a young woman who would come to the house during the mother's working hours. Justin started to vomit soon after his mother left the house. The vomiting seemed to increase from day to day in frequency and in intensity, and, after 2 weeks of the mother's return to work, Justin vomited several times daily and was losing weight. He was seen by a gastroenterologist, and during the barium swallow, it was noticed that Justin put his hand in his mouth, which seemed to trigger vomiting. Justin was put back on medication for gastroesophageal reflux, but he continued to vomit with increasing frequency, which led to the psychiatric consultation.

Observation of mother and infant during feeding revealed that, as soon as Justin finished feeding, he put his hand in his mouth and vomited. When his mother restricted his hand, Justin moved his tongue back and forth in a rhythmic manner until he vomited again. This happened repeatedly, and Justin continued the rhythmic tongue movements even when he could not bring up any more milk.

Because of his poor nutritional state and moderate dehydration, Justin was admitted to the hospital, and a nasojejunal tube was inserted for feedings. When Justin was awake, a special nurse or the parents played with him and tried to distract him whenever he attempted to put his hand in his mouth or thrust his tongue rhythmically. Justin became increasingly engaged, and his ruminatory activity decreased accordingly. After 1 week in the hospital, small feedings were started; however, Justin tried to ruminate again, and the oral feedings had to be stopped. At this point, the mother decided to stop working and take Justin home to continue the treatment at home. The mother started small feedings, played with Justin after feedings, and was able to keep him from ruminating. After 4 weeks of slow increments in his feedings, Justin was able to take all his feedings by mouth without ruminating, and the nasojejunal tube could be removed. (Courtesy of Irene Chatoor, M.D.)

Pathology and Laboratory Examination

No specific laboratory examination is pathognomonic of rumination disorder. Clinicians must rule out physical causes of vomiting, such as pyloric stenosis and hiatal hernia, before making the diagnosis of rumination disorder. Rumination disorder can be associated with failure to thrive and varying degrees of starvation. Thus, laboratory measures of endocrinologic function (thyroid function tests, dexamethasone-suppression test), serum electrolytes, and a hematologic workup help to determine the severity of the effects of rumination disorder.

Differential Diagnosis

To make the diagnosis of rumination disorder, clinicians must rule out gastrointestinal congenital anomalies, infections, and other medical illnesses. Pyloric stenosis is usually associated with projectile vomiting and is generally evident before 3 months of age, when rumination has its onset. Rumination has been associated with various mental retardation syndromes in which other stereotypic behaviors and eating disturbances, such as pica, are present. Rumination disorder can occur in patients with other eating disorders, such as bulimia nervosa.

Course and Prognosis

Rumination disorder is believed to have a high rate of spontaneous remission. Indeed, many cases of rumination disorder may develop and remit without ever being diagnosed. Only limited data are available about the prognosis of rumination disorder in adults.

Treatment

The treatment of rumination disorder is often a combination of education and behavioral techniques. Sometimes, an evaluation of the mother–child relationship reveals deficits that can be influenced by offering guidance to the mother. Behavioral interventions, such as squirting lemon juice into the infant's mouth whenever rumination occurs, can be effective in diminishing the behavior. This practice appears to be the most rapidly effective treatment, with rumination reportedly eliminated in 3 to 5 days. In the aversive-conditioning reports on rumination disorder, infants were doing well at 9- or 12-month follow-up, with no recurrence of the rumination and with weight gains, increased activity levels, and increased responsiveness to persons. Rumination may be decreased by the technique of withdrawing attention from the child whenever this behavior occurs. The effectiveness of treatments is difficult to evaluate. Most reported are single-case studies; patients are not randomly assigned to controlled studies.

Treatments include improvement of the child's psychosocial environment, increased tender loving care from the mother or caretakers, and psychotherapy for the mother or both parents. When anatomic abnormalities, such as hiatal hernia, are present, surgical repair may be necessary. If an infant is malnourished and continues to lose most nutrition through rumination, a jejunal tube may need to be inserted before other treatments can be used.

Medications are not a standard part of the treatment of rumination. Case reports, however, cite a variety of medications that have been tried, including metoclopramide (Reglan) and cimetidine (Tagamet), and antipsychotics such as haloperidol (Haldol) and thioridazine (Mellaril) have been cited to be helpful according to anecdotal reports. One study showed that when infants were allowed to eat as much as they wanted, the rate of rumination decreased.

The treatment of adolescents with rumination disorder is often complex and includes a multidisciplinary approach consisting of individual psychotherapy, nutritional intervention, and pharmacologic treatment for the frequent comorbid anxiety and depressive symptoms.

FEEDING DISORDER OF INFANCY OR EARLY CHILDHOOD

Feeding disorder of infancy, a broadly defined maladaptive pattern of eating behaviors in infants, features the interactive process between caregiver and infant. This disorder has variable components that range from food refusal, food selectivity, eating too little, and food avoidance to delayed self-feeding. According to the DSM-IV-TR, feeding disorder of infancy or early childhood is a persistent failure to eat adequately, reflected in significant failure to gain weight or in significant weight loss over 1 month. The symptoms are not better accounted for by a medical condition or by another mental disorder and are not caused by lack of food (Table 9–3). The disorder has its onset before the age of 6 years.

Children with feeding disorders display less affectionate touch, more negative touch, and more rejection of mother's touch than children without feeding problems. In addition, more rejecting maternal responses to the child's touch have been observed, and children with feeding disorders are more often positioned out of reach of their mothers' arms. Children with feeding disorders are often withdrawn, and touch is diminished during the entire feeding process compared with other children. It is likely that patterns of proximity and touch between mothers and infants during feeding may serve as an index of risk for future feeding difficulties and potential growth failure.

Table 9–3
DSM-IV-TR Diagnostic Criteria for Feeding Disorder of Infancy or Early Childhood

A. Feeding disturbance as manifested by persistent failure to eat adequately with significant failure to gain weight or significant loss of weight over at least 1 month.
B. The disturbance is not due to an associated gastrointestinal or other general medical condition (e.g., esophageal reflux).
C. The disturbance is not better accounted for by another mental disorder (e.g., rumination disorder) or by lack of available food.
D. The onset is before age 6 years.

From American Psychiatric Association. *Diagnostic and Statistical Manual of Mental Disorders.* 4th ed. Text rev. Washington, DC: American Psychiatric Association; copyright 2000, with permission.

Epidemiology

It is estimated that between 15 and 35 percent of infants and young children have transient feeding difficulties. A recent survey of feeding problems in nursery school children revealed a prevalence of 4.8 percent with equal gender distribution. Children with feeding problems exhibited more somatic complaints, and mothers of affected infants exhibited increased risk of anxiety symptoms. Data from community samples estimate a prevalence of failure-to-thrive syndromes in approximately 3 percent of infants, with approximately half of those infants exhibiting feeding disorders.

Differential Diagnosis

Feeding disorder of infancy must be differentiated from structural problems with the infants' gastrointestinal tract that may be contributing to discomfort during the feeding process. Because feeding disorders and organic causes of swallowing difficulties often coexist, it is important to rule out medical reasons for feeding difficulties. A recent study of videofluoroscopic evaluation of children with feeding and swallowing problems revealed that clinical evaluation was 92 percent accurate in identifying those children at increased risk of aspiration. This type of evaluation is necessary before psychotherapeutic interventions in cases in which a medical contribution to feeding problems is suspected.

Course and Prognosis

Most infants with feeding disorders exhibit symptoms within the first year of life and, with appropriate recognition and intervention, do not go on to develop failure to thrive. When feeding disorders have their onset later, in children 2 to 3 years of age, growth and development can be affected when the disorder lasts for several months. It is estimated that about 70 percent of infants who persistently refuse food in the first year of life continue to have some feeding problems during childhood.

Thomas was 3 months old when he was referred for a psychiatric evaluation because of his feeding difficulties and poor weight gain since birth. His parents were college-educated, and both had pursued their professional careers until Thomas was born. Although Thomas was full-term and weighed 7 pounds at birth, he had difficulty drinking from the breast. When he was 4 weeks old, his mother had reluctantly switched him to bottle feedings because he was losing weight. Although his intake improved somewhat on bottle feedings, he gained weight very slowly and was still less than 8 pounds at 3 months of age. His mother appeared tired and described how Thomas would drink only 1, 2, or 3 ounces at a time; wiggle and cry; and refuse to continue with the feeding. But after a few hours, he might cry again as if he were hungry. However, she could not settle him to feed and he would continue to cry inconsolably. The mother described that she would attempt to feed him on an average of 10 to 15 times in a 24-hour period, that Thomas would cry a lot during the day and at night, and that everybody in the family was getting very little sleep.

The observation of mother–infant interactions during feeding and play revealed that Thomas was a very alert and wiggly baby who had difficulty settling in his mother's arms. While drinking from the bottle he would kick his feet and move around with his arms, and soon the nipple of the bottle would slip out of his mouth. This upset him, and he started crying. His mother appeared anxious and tried to restart him by changing his position in various ways, but this only agitated him more. After repeated unsuccessful attempts to continue the feeding, mother and baby appeared exhausted, and the mother gave up.

The assessment revealed that Thomas was a very active and excitable baby who had difficulty keeping calm during feedings. After reviewing the videotape with the mother, the therapist explored ways in which the mother could better facilitate calming during feedings. Using a quiet corner in the house, swaddling Thomas in a blanket, and singing to him before starting the feeding were the most useful suggestions. Thomas stayed calm during feedings, was able to drink larger amounts of milk, and waited longer between feedings. This, in turn, relieved the mother's anxiety and helped both to have calmer interactions. (Courtesy of Irene Chatoor, M.D.)

Treatment

Treatments for feeding disorders need to be individualized and include interventions aimed at the infant and the mother, most often targeting the interactions between the infant and mother or caregiver.

If an infant tires before ingesting an adequate amount of nutrition, it may be necessary to begin treatment with the placement of a nasogastric tube for supplemental oral feedings. On the other hand, if the mother or caregiver is unable to participate in the intervention, it may be necessary to include additional caregivers to contribute to feeding the infant. In rare cases, an infant may require hospitalization until adequate nutrition on a daily basis is accomplished.

Most interventions for feeding disorders are aimed at optimizing the interaction between the mother and infant during feedings and identifying any factors that can be changed to promote greater ingestion. The mother is helped to become more aware of the infant's stamina for length of individual feedings, the infant's biologic regulation patterns, and when the infant is fatigued, with a goal of increasing the level of engagement between mother and infant during feeding.

A transactional model of intervention has been proposed by Irene Chatoor, M.D., a leading expert in the field, for infants who exhibit the "difficult" temperamental traits of emotional intensity, stubbornness, lack of hunger cues, irregular eating and sleeping patterns and strong will in refusing to eat a sufficient amount and who are intensely interested in noneating exploration of their environment. The treatment includes education for the parents regarding the temperamental traits of the infant, exploration of the parents' anxieties about the infant's nutrition, and training for the parents regarding changing their behaviors to promote internal regulation of eating in the infant. Parents are encouraged to feed the infant on a regular basis at 3- to 4-hour intervals and offer only water between meals. The parents are trained to deliver praise to the infant for any self-feeding efforts, regardless of the amount of food ingested. Furthermore, parents are guided to limit any distracting stimulation during meals and give attention and praise to positive eating behaviors rather than intense negative attention to inappropriate behavior during meals. It is recommended that this training process for parents be done in an intense manner within a short period of time. Many parents are able to facilitate improved eating patterns in the infant in a short period of time.

For older children with severe feeding disorders resulting in failure-to-thrive syndromes, hospitalization and nutritional supplementation is necessary before optimal psychotherapeutic interventions. Medication is not a standard component of treatment for feeding disorders, although several anecdotal reports have suggested benefit with adjunctive pharmacologic agents. One recent case report indicated that in several preadolescents with failure-to-thrive and feeding disorders who received enteral nutritional interventions and were comorbid for anxiety and mood symptoms, the addition of risperidone (Risperdal) was associated with an increase in oral intake and accelerated weight gain.

10

Tic Disorders

Tic disorders are distinguished by the type of tic symptoms, their frequency, and the pattern in which they emerge over time. Tics are abnormal movements or vocalizations that most commonly affect the muscles of the face and neck, such as eye blinking, head jerking, mouth grimacing, or head shaking. Typical vocal tics include throat clearing, grunting, snorting, and coughing. Tics are defined as rapid and repetitive muscle contractions resulting in movements or vocalizations that are experienced as involuntary. Children and adolescents may exhibit tic behaviors that occur after a stimulus or in response to an internal urge. Tic disorders—a group of neuropsychiatric disorders—generally begin in childhood or adolescence, with a stable or fluctuating course in childhood that generally wanes by adolescence. Although tics are not volitional, in some individuals they may be suppressed for periods.

The most widely known and most severe tic disorder is Gilles de la Tourette syndrome, also known as Tourette's disorder. The text revision of the fourth edition of the *Diagnostic and Statistical Manual of Mental Disorders* (DSM-IV-TR) includes several other tic disorders, such as chronic motor or vocal tic disorder, transient tic disorder, and tic disorder not otherwise specified. Although tics have no particular purpose, they often consist of motions that are used in volitional movements. One half to two thirds of children with Tourette's disorder exhibit a reduction or complete remission of tic symptoms during adolescence. Obsessive-compulsive symptoms or disorder (OCD) has been found to coexist in one third to two thirds of children and adolescents with Tourette's disorder, and about one third of adults with Tourette's disorder have persistent OCD into adulthood. The obsessive-compulsive symptoms most likely to occur in those individuals with Tourette's disorder are characteristically related to ordering, symmetry, counting, and repetitive touching, whereas OCD disorders in the absence of tic disorders are characterized by symptoms more often associated with fears of contamination and fears of harming others. A recent study found that the risk of developing OCD symptoms in children with Tourette's disorder by early adulthood was significantly higher in children with higher intellectual quotients (IQs), that is, above 120, compared with those with an average of 100.

Motor and vocal tics are divided into simple and complex types. *Simple motor tics* are those composed of repetitive, rapid contractions of functionally similar muscle groups—for example, eye blinking, neck jerking, shoulder shrugging, and facial grimacing. Common *simple vocal tics* include coughing, throat clearing, grunting, sniffing, snorting, and barking. *Complex motor tics* appear to be more purposeful and ritualistic than simple tics. Common *complex motor tics* include grooming behaviors, the smelling of objects, jumping, touching behaviors, echopraxia (imitation of observed behavior), and copropraxia (display of obscene gestures). *Complex vocal tics* include repeating words or phrases out of context, coprolalia (use of obscene words or phrases), palilalia (a person's repeating his or her words), and echolalia (repetition of the last-heard words of others).

Some persons with tic disorders can suppress the tics for minutes or hours, but others, especially young children, either are not cognizant of their tics or experience their tics as irresistible. Tics may be attenuated by sleep, relaxation, or absorption in an activity. Tics often, but not always, disappear during sleep.

TOURETTE'S DISORDER

According to the DSM-IV-TR, tics in Tourette's disorder are multiple motor tics and one or more vocal tics. The tics occur many times a day for more than 1 year. Tourette's disorder causes distress or significant impairment in important areas of functioning. The disorder has an onset before the age of 18 years, and it is not caused by a substance or by a general medical condition.

Georges Gilles de la Tourette (1857–1904) first described a patient with what was later known as Tourette's disorder in 1885 while he was studying with Jean-Martin Charcot in France. De la Tourette noted a syndrome in several patients that included multiple motor tics, coprolalia, and echolalia.

Epidemiology

The lifetime prevalence of Tourette's disorder is estimated to be 4 to 5 per 10,000. More children exhibit this disorder than adults, such that 5 to 30 of 10,000 children are affected, but by adulthood, only 1 to 2 of 10,000 meet diagnostic criteria. The onset of the motor component of the disorder generally occurs by the age of 7 years; vocal tics emerge on average by the age of 11 years. Tourette's disorder occurs about three times more often in boys than in girls.

Etiology

Genetic Factors. Twin studies, adoption studies, and segregation analysis studies all support a genetic cause for Tourette's disorder. Twin studies indicate that concordance for the disorder in monozygotic twins is significantly greater than that in dizygotic twins. That Tourette's disorder and chronic motor or vocal tic disorder are likely to occur in the same families lends support to the view that the disorders are part of a genetically determined spectrum. The sons of mothers with Tourette's disorder seem to be at the highest risk for the disorder. Evidence in some families indicates that Tourette's disorder is transmitted in an autosomal dominant fashion. Recent studies of a long family pedigree suggest that Tourette's disorder may be transmitted in a bilinear mode; that is, Tourette's disorder appears to be inherited through an autosomal pattern in some families, intermediate between dominant and recessive. A recent study of 174 unrelated probands with Tourette's disorder identified a greater-than-chance occurrence of a rare sequence variant in *SLITRK1* believed to be a candidate gene on chromosome 13q31.

A relation is found between Tourette's disorder and attention-deficit/hyperactivity disorder (ADHD); up to half of all patients with Tourette's disorder also have ADHD. A relation also appears between Tourette's disorder and OCD; up to 40 percent of all those with Tourette's disorder also have OCD. In addition, first-degree relatives of persons with Tourette's disorder are at high risk for the development of the disorder, chronic motor or vocal tic disorder, and OCD. The presence of symptoms of ADHD in more than half of persons with Tourette's disorder raises questions about a genetic relation between these two disorders.

Neurochemical and Neuroanatomic Factors. Compelling but indirect evidence of dopamine system involvement in tic disorders includes the observations that pharmacologic agents that antagonize dopamine (haloperidol [Haldol], pimozide [Orap], and fluphenazine [Prolixin]) suppress tics and that agents that increase central dopaminergic activity (methylphenidate [Ritalin], amphetamines, pemoline [Cylert], and cocaine) tend to exacerbate tics. The relation of tics to neurotransmitter systems is complex and not well understood; for example, in some cases, antipsychotic medications, such as haloperidol, are not effective in reducing tics, and the effect of stimulants on tic disorders reportedly varies. In some cases, Tourette's disorder has emerged during treatment with antipsychotic medications.

More direct analyses of the neurochemistry of Tourette's disorder have been possible using brain proton magnetic resonance spectroscopy, a method only recently used to investigate this disorder. A recent investigation examining the cellular neurochemistry of patients with Tourette's disorder using magnetic resonance spectroscopy of the frontal cortex, caudate nucleus, putamen, and thalamus demonstrated that these patients had a reduced amount of choline and *N*-acetylaspartate in the left putamen along with reduced levels of bilaterally in the putamen. In the frontal cortex, patients with Tourette's disorder were found to have lower concentrations of *N*-acetylaspartate bilaterally, lower levels of creatine on the right side, and reduced myoinositol on the left side. These results imply that deficits in the density of neuronal and nonneuronal cells are present in patients with Tourette's disorder.

Endogenous opioids may be involved in tic disorders and OCD. Some evidence indicates that pharmacologic agents that antagonize endogenous opiates—for example, naltrexone (ReVia)—reduce tics and attention deficits in patients with Tourette's disorder. Abnormalities in the noradrenergic system have been implicated in some cases by the reduction of tics with clonidine (Catapres). This adrenergic agonist reduces the release of norepinephrine in the central nervous system and thus may reduce activity in the dopaminergic system. Abnormalities in the basal ganglia result in various movement disorders, such as Huntington's disease, and are implicated as possible sites of disturbance in Tourette's disorder, OCD, and ADHD.

Immunologic Factors and Postinfection. An autoimmune process that is secondary to streptococcal infections is a potential mechanism for Tourette's disorder. Such a process could act synergistically with a genetic vulnerability for this disorder. Poststreptococcal syndromes have also been associated with one potential causative factor in the development of OCD in children.

Diagnosis and Clinical Features

To make a diagnosis of Tourette's disorder, clinicians must obtain a history of multiple motor tics and the emergence of at least one vocal tic at some point in the disorder. According to the DSM-IV-TR, the tics must occur many times a day nearly every day or intermittently for more than 1 year. The average age of onset of tics is 7 years, but tics can occur as early as age 2 years. The onset must occur before the age of 18 years (Table 10–1).

In Tourette's disorder, the initial tics are in the face and neck. Over time, the tics tend to occur in a downward progression. The most commonly described tics are those affecting the face and head, the arms and hands, the body and lower extremities, and the respiratory and alimentary systems. In these areas, the tics take the form of grimacing; forehead puckering; eyebrow raising; eyelid blinking; winking; nose wrinkling; nostril trembling; mouth twitching; displaying the teeth; biting the lips and other parts; tongue extruding; protracting the lower jaw; nodding, jerking, or shaking the head; twisting the neck; looking sideways; head rolling; hand jerking; arm jerking; plucking fingers; writhing fingers; fist clenching; shoulder shrugging; foot, knee, or toe shaking; walking peculiarly; body writhing; jumping; hiccupping; sighing; yawning; snuffing; blowing through the nostrils; whistling; belching; sucking or smacking sounds; and clearing the throat. Several assessment instruments are available that are useful in making diagnoses of tic disorders,

Table 10–1
DSM-IV-TR Diagnostic Criteria for Tourette's Disorder

A. Both multiple motor and one or more vocal tics have been present at some time during the illness, although not necessarily concurrently. (A tic is a sudden, rapid, recurrent, nonrhythmic, stereotyped motor movement or vocalization.)
B. The tics occur many times a day (usually in bouts) nearly every day or intermittently throughout a period of more than 1 year, and during this period there was never a tic-free period of more than 3 consecutive months.
C. The onset is before age 18 years.
D. The disturbance is not due to the direct physiologic effects of a substance (e.g., stimulants) or a general medical condition (e.g., Huntington's disease or postviral encephalitis).

From American Psychiatric Association. *Diagnostic and Statistical Manual of Mental Disorders.* 4th ed. Text rev. Washington, DC: American Psychiatric Association; copyright 2000, with permission.

including comprehensive self-report assessment tools, such as the Tic Symptom Self Report and the Yale Global Tic Severity Scale, administered by a clinician (Table 10–2).

Typically, prodromal behavioral symptoms (e.g., irritability, attention difficulties, and poor frustration tolerance) are evident before, or coincide with the onset of, tics. More than 25 percent of persons in some studies received stimulants for a diagnosis of ADHD before receiving a diagnosis of Tourette's disorder. The most frequent initial symptom is an eye-blink tic, followed by a head tic or a facial grimace. Most complex motor and vocal symptoms emerge several years after the initial symptoms. Coprolalia usually begins in early adolescence and occurs in about one third of all patients. Mental coprolalia—in which a patient thinks a sudden, intrusive, socially unacceptable thought or obscene word—can also occur. In some severe cases, physical injuries, including retinal detachment and orthopedic problems, have resulted from severe tics.

Obsessions, compulsions, attention difficulties, impulsivity, and personality problems have been associated with Tourette's disorder. Attention difficulties often precede the onset of tics, whereas obsessive-compulsive symptoms often occur after their onset. Whether these problems usually develop secondarily to a patient's tics or are caused primarily by the same underlying pathologic condition is being debated. Many tics have an aggressive or sexual component that may result in serious social consequences for the patient. Phenomenologically, tics resemble a failure of censorship, both conscious and unconscious, with increased impulsivity and inability to inhibit a thought from being put into action.

Todd, age 8 years, came to the Tourette Syndrome Clinic for an evaluation of tics, hyperactivity, and impulsive behavior. He is a third-grade student in a regular class at the local public school. Before the consultation, parent and teacher ratings, including the Child Behavior Checklist (CBCL), Swanson, Nolan, and Pelham-IV (SNAP-IV), Conners' Parent and Teacher Questionnaires, Tic Symptom Self-Report (TSSR), and medical history survey, were sent to his family (Table 10–2). His mother and the classroom teacher rated him well above the norm for hyperactivity, inattention, and impulsiveness. He was failing in school, often argued with adults, was occasionally aggressive, and had few friends. His tics were rated as mild.

Todd's mother recalls difficulties with overactivity and reckless behavior since preschool. At age 5, his kindergarten teacher encouraged the family to obtain consultation for his behavior. The family's pediatrician made a diagnosis of ADHD and recommended a trial of methylphenidate (Ritalin), which eventually occurred in the first grade. Within 2 weeks of starting medication, his behavior showed a dramatic improvement. He was able to stay in his seat and complete his work and was more able to wait his turn on the playground. The next several months went well. After a dosage increase in the spring of his first-grade year, however, he began showing motor and phonic tics consisting of head jerking, facial

Table 10–2
Clinical Assessment Tools in Tic Disorders

Domain	Type	Reliability and Validity	Sensitive to Change
Tics			
Tic Symptom Self-Report	Parent/self	Good	Yes
Yale Global Tic Severity Scale	Clinician	Excellent	Yes
Attention-deficit/hyperactivity disorder			
Swanson, Nolan, and Pelham-IV	Parent/teacher	Excellent	Yes
Abbreviated Conners' Questionnaire	Parent/teacher	Excellent	Yes
Obsessive-compulsive disorder			
Yale-Brown Obsessive Compulsive Scale and Children's Yale-Brown Obsessive Compulsive Scale	Clinician	Excellent	Yes
National Institute of Mental Health Global	Clinician	Excellent	Yes
General			
Child Behavior Checklist	Parent/teacher	Excellent	No

movements, coughing, and grunting. The medication was immediately stopped and, although the tics subsided, they did not go away. In hindsight, Todd's mother recalled that he had shown blinking and throat clearing before starting methylphenidate, but she had dismissed these tics as unimportant.

Off medication, the second grade did not go well, and Todd was placed in special education class. At his mother's insistence, Todd returned to the regular class for third grade. However, his adjustment to the third-grade classroom was poor. The family went back to the pediatrician, who made the referral to the Tourette Syndrome Clinic.

Todd is healthy with no history of serious illness or injuries. The pregnancy, labor, and delivery were uncomplicated, and his developmental milestones were achieved at appropriate times. Intelligence testing completed by the school psychologist revealed average intellectual ability. His appetite is good. His mother notes that Todd has long-standing trouble falling asleep but sleeps through the night. Although he is described as argumentative and easily frustrated with frequent outbursts of temper, his mood is generally upbeat.

BEHAVIORAL OBSERVATIONS

Todd is of average height and weight with no dysmorphic features. His speech is rapid in tempo but normal in tone and volume. His discourse is coherent and developmentally appropriate, and no evidence is seen of thought disorder. He does not appear depressed and denies worries about everyday issues such as friends and school performance, although he recognizes that school is not going so well. He also denies recurring worries about contamination or harm coming to him or family members, or fears of acting on unwanted impulses. Other than mild touching habits involving the need to touch objects with each hand three times or in combinations of three, he denies repetitive rituals. Several tics were observed during the evaluation session, including blinking, facial grimacing, head jerking, and grunting. He was restless and easily distracted throughout the session and often needed assistance with entertaining himself when not directly involved in conversation.

IMPRESSION

Given the history of enduring motor and phonic tics, which are confirmed by direct observation, Todd meets criteria for Tourette's syndrome. Based on history, he also meets criteria for ADHD, combined type.

TREATMENT PLAN

Although recent studies have shown that children with a tic disorder can tolerate stimulant medication without inducing an exacerbation in tics, some children show an increase in tics on exposure to stimulants. Thus, guanfacine (Systemic), 0.5 mg, is recommended with planned increases of 0.5 mg every 4 to 5 days as tolerated to a maximum of 3 mg per day in three divided doses. Blood pressure, pulse, sleep, appetite, energy level, and tics will be monitored every 2 weeks during the dose adjustment phase. Parent and teacher ratings will be obtained at 4 and 8 weeks to assess response.

Parents will be given educational materials about Tourette's syndrome and ADHD and referred for parent training. The parent training will focus on distinguishing between tics and oppositional behavior, how to modify disruptive behavior, and how to cultivate positive behavior. With the parents' permission, the school will be informed of the diagnosis, and a special education classification in the "other health impaired" category is likely. Although Todd may remain in the regular classroom, he may benefit from a teacher's aide to monitor his behavior and help him organize his school work. (Courtesy of L. Scahill M.S.N., Ph.D., and J.F. Leckman, M.D.)

Pathology and Laboratory Examination

No specific laboratory diagnostic test exists for Tourette's disorder, but many patients with Tourette's disorder have nonspecific abnormal electroencephalographic findings. Computed tomography (CT) and magnetic resonance imaging (MRI) scans have revealed no specific structural lesions, although about 10 percent of all patients with Tourette's disorder show some nonspecific abnormality on CT scans.

Differential Diagnosis

Tics must be differentiated from other disordered movements (e.g., dystonic, choreiform, athetoid, myoclonic, and hemiballismic movements) and the neurologic diseases that they characterize (e.g., Huntington's disease, Parkinsonism, Sydenham's chorea, and Wilson's disease), as listed in Table 10–3. Tremors, mannerisms, and stereotypic movement disorder (e.g., head banging or body rocking) must also be distinguished from tic disorders. Stereotypic movement disorders, including movements such as rocking, hand gazing, and other self-stimulatory behaviors, seem to be voluntary and often produce a sense of comfort, in contrast to tic disorders. Although tics in children and adolescents may or may not feel controllable, they rarely produce a sense of well-being. Compulsions are sometimes difficult to distinguish from complex tics and may be on the same continuum biologically. Tic disorders also occur comorbidly with multiple behavioral and mood disturbances. In a recent survey, the greater the severity of tics, the higher is the probability of both aggressive and depressive symptoms in children. Even in a given child with Tourette's disorder, it has been reported that when there is exacerbation of tic symptoms, behavior and mood also seem to deteriorate. This phenomenon occurs with children who have Tourette's disorder and ADHD and also with those who have depression or oppositional-defiant disorders. In children with Tourette's disorder and ADHD, even when the tic disorder had always been mild, a high frequency of disruptive behavior problems and mood disorder exists. Both autistic children and

Table 10–3
Differential Diagnosis of Tic Disorders

Disease or Syndrome	Age at Onset	Associated Features	Course	Predominant Type of Movement
Hallervorden-Spatz	Childhood–adolescence	May be associated with optic atrophy, club feet, retinitis pigmentosa, dysarthria, dementia, ataxia, emotional lability, spasticity, autosomal recessive inheritance	Progressive to death in 5–20 years	Choreic, athetoid, myoclonic
Dystonia musculorum deformans	Childhood–adolescence	Autosomal recessive inheritance commonly, primarily among Ashkenazi Jews; a more benign autosomal dominant form also occurs	Variable course, often progressive but with rare remissions	Dystonia
Sydenham's chorea	Childhood, usually 5–15 yrs	More common in females, usually associated with rheumatic fever (carditis elevated ASLO titers)	Usually self-limited	Choreiform
Huntington's disease	Usually 30–50 yrs, but childhood forms are known	Autosomal dominant inheritance, dementia, caudate atrophy on CT scan	Progressive to death in 10–15 years after onset	Choreiform
Wilson's disease (hepatolenticular degeneration)	Usually 10–25 yrs	Kayser-Fleischer rings, liver dysfunction, inborn error of copper metabolism; autosomal recessive inheritance	Progressive to death without chelating therapy	Wing-beating tremor, dystonia
Hyperreflexias (including latah, myriachit, jumper disease of Maine)	Generally in childhood (dominant inheritance)	Familial; may have generalized rigidity and autosomal inheritance	Nonprogressive	Excessive startle response; may have echolalia, coprolalia, and forced obedience
Myoclonic disorders	Any age	Numerous causes, some familial, usually no vocalizations	Variable, depending on cause	Myoclonus
Myoclonic dystonia	5–47 yrs	Nonfamilial, no vocalizations	Nonprogressive	Torsion dystonia with myoclonic jerks
Paroxysmal myoclonic dystonia with vocalization	Childhood	Attention, hyperactive, and learning disorders; movements interfere with ongoing activity	Nonprogressive	Bursts of regular, repetitive clonic (less tonic) movements and vocalizations
Tardive Tourette's disorder syndromes	Variable (after antipsychotic medication use)	Reported to be precipitated by discontinuation or reduction of medication	May terminate after increase or decrease of dose	Orofacial dyskinesias, choreoathetosis, tics, vocalization
Neuroacanthocytosis	Third or fourth decade	Acanthocytosis, muscle wasting, Parkinsonism, autosomal recessive inheritance	Variable	Orofacial dyskinesia and limb chorea, tics, vocalization
Encephalitis lethargica	Variable	Shouting fits, bizarre behavior, psychosis, Parkinson's disease	Variable	Simple and complex motor and vocal tics, coprolalia, echolalia, echopraxia, palilalia
Gasoline inhalation	Variable	Abnormal EEG; symmetrical theta and theta bursts frontocentrally	Variable	Simple motor and vocal tics
Postangiographic complications	Variable	Emotional lability, amnestic syndrome	Variable	Simple motor and complex vocal tics, palilalia
Postinfectious	Variable	EEG: occasional asymmetrical theta bursts before movements, elevated ASLO titers	Variable	Simple motor and vocal tics, echopraxia

(*continued*)

Table 10–3 (Continued)

Disease or Syndrome	Age at Onset	Associated Features	Course	Predominant Type of Movement
Posttraumatic	Variable	Asymmetrical tic distribution	Variable	Complex motor tics
Carbon monoxide poisoning	Variable	Inappropriate sexual behavior	Variable	Simple and complex motor and vocal tics, coprolalia, echolalia, palilalia
XYY genetic disorder	Infancy	Aggressive behavior	Static	Simple motor and vocal tics
XXY and 9p mosaicism	Infancy	Multiple physical anomalies, mental retardation	Static	Simple motor and vocal tics
Duchenne's muscular dystrophy (X-linked recessive)	Childhood	Mild mental retardation	Progressive	Motor and vocal tics
Fragile X syndrome	Childhood	Mental retardation, facial dysmorphism, seizures, autistic features	Static	Simple motor and vocal tics, coprolalia
Developmental and perinatal disorders	Infancy, childhood	Seizures, EEG and CT abnormalities, psychosis, aggressivity, hyperactivity, Ganser's syndrome, compulsivity, torticollis	Variable	Motor and vocal tics, echolalia

ASLO, anti–streptolysin O serum; CT, computed tomography; EEG, electroencephalogram.

children with mental retardation may exhibit symptoms similar to those seen in tic disorders, including Tourette's disorder. A greater-than-expected occurrence of Tourette's disorder, autistic disorder, and bipolar disorder also is present.

Before instituting treatment with an antipsychotic medication, clinicians must make a baseline evaluation of preexisting abnormal movements; such medication can mask abnormal movements, and, if the movements occur later, they can be mistaken for tardive dyskinesia. Stimulant medications (e.g., methylphenidate, amphetamines, and pemoline) have reportedly exacerbated preexisting tics in some cases. These effects have been reported primarily in some children and adolescents being treated for ADHD. In most but not all cases, after the drug was discontinued, the tics remitted or returned to premedication levels. Most experts suggest that children and adolescents who experience tics while receiving stimulants are probably genetically predisposed and would have experienced tics regardless of their treatment with stimulants. Until the situation is clarified, clinicians should use great caution and should frequently monitor children at risk for tics who are given stimulants.

Course and Prognosis

Tourette's disorder is a childhood-onset neuropsychiatric disorder that includes both motor and vocal tics with a natural history leading to reduction or complete resolution of tics symptoms in most cases by adolescence. During childhood, individual tic symptoms may decrease, persist, or increase, and old symptoms may be replaced by new ones. Severely afflicted persons may have serious emotional problems, including major depressive disorder. Impairment may also be associated with the motor and vocal tic symptoms of Tourette's disorder; however, in many cases, interference in function is exacerbated by comorbid ADHD and OCD, both of which frequently coexist with the disorder. When the aforementioned three disorders are comorbid, severe social, academic, and occupational problems may ensue. Although most children with Tourette's disorder experience a decline in the frequency and severity of tic symptoms during adolescence, no clinical measures exist to predict which children may have persistent symptoms into adulthood. Imaging studies provided cross-sectional data showing that Tourette's disorder is associated with reduced caudate nucleus volume. A recent prospective investigation measuring clinical symptom severity and basal ganglia volumes in 43 children over an average length of 7.5 years found that the smaller the volume of the caudate nucleus, as measured by high-resolution MRI, the more likely were tic symptoms and OCD to persist into early adulthood. Thus, caudate volumes in children with Tourette's disorder were predictive of severity and persistence of symptoms over time. Caudate volumes were not correlated, however, with the severity of symptoms in childhood when the initial magnetic resonance scans were done. Thus, the severity of childhood tics does not always predict persistence or severity of symptoms in adulthood.

Children with mild forms of Tourette's disorder often have satisfactory peer relationships, function well in school, and develop adequate self-esteem and may not require treatment.

Treatment

Consideration of a child's or adolescent's overall functioning is the first step in determining the most appropriate treatments for tic disorders. Families, teachers, and peers sometimes misinterpret tics as purposeful behaviors, and a child may be treated as if he or she has a "behavior" problem when the tics are actually experienced as involuntary. Treatment should begin with comprehensive education for families so that children are not unwittingly punished for their tic behaviors. Families must also understand the waxing and waning nature of many tic disorders. In mild cases, children with tic disorders who are functioning well socially and academically may not require treatment. In more severe cases, children with tic disorders may be ostracized by peers and have academic work compromised by the disruptive nature of tics, and a variety of treatments must be considered.

Pharmacologic interventions have some efficacy in tic suppression, and behavioral interventions such as "habit reversal" techniques are being used to help children and adolescents become more aware of their tics and initiate voluntary movements that can "counter" tics. Older children, adolescents, and adults often report tics to be preceded by an unpleasant sensation denoted as a "premonitory urge." Premonitory urge phenomena may play an important role in behavioral interventions, in that a patient's ability to recognize and respond to a premonitory urge can become the basis of replacing the tic behavior with a desired behavior before it emerges. A scale for premonitory urge called the Premonitory Urge for Tics Scale (PUTS) was recently devised and examined psychometrically and was found to be internally consistent and correlated with overall tic severity in youths older than 10 years of age.

Other behavioral techniques were reviewed by Stanley A. Hobbs, including massed (negative) practice, self-monitoring, incompatible response training, presentation and removal of positive reinforcement, and habit reversal treatment. He reported that tic frequency was reduced in many cases, particularly with habit reversal treatment; additional studies are under way to replicate the efficacy of these techniques. Behavioral techniques, including relaxation, may reduce the stress that often exacerbates Tourette's disorder. It is hypothesized that behavioral techniques and pharmacotherapy together have a synergistic effect.

Pharmacotherapy. Haloperidol (Haldol) and pimozide (Orap) are the two best-investigated antipsychotic agents in the treatment of Tourette's disorder, although atypical antipsychotics such as risperidone (Risperdal) and olanzapine (Zyprexa) are often chosen as first-line agents due to their safer side-effect profiles. High-potency dopamine receptor antagonists (typical antipsychotics), such as haloperidol, trifluoperazine (Stelazine), and pimozide, have been shown to reduce tics significantly. Up to 80 percent of patients have some favorable response; their symptoms decrease by as much as 70 to 90 percent of baseline frequency. Follow-up studies, however, indicate that only 20 to 30 percent of these patients continue to take long-term maintenance therapy. Discontinuation is often based on the drug's adverse effects, including extrapyramidal effects and dysphoria. The initial daily haloperidol dose for adolescents is usually between 0.25 and 0.5 mg. Haloperidol is not approved for use in children younger than 3 years of age. For children between 3 and 12 years of age, the recommended total daily dose is between 0.05 and 0.075 mg per kg, administered in divided doses either two or three times a day.

The initial daily dose of pimozide is usually 1 to 2 mg in divided doses; the dose may be increased every other day. Most patients are maintained on a daily dose of less than 0.2 mg per kg or 10 mg, whichever is less. A daily dose of 0.3 mg per kg or 20 mg should never be exceeded because of cardiotoxic adverse effects. Pimozide appears to be relatively safe at recommended doses, with cardiotoxicity limited to prolonged QT-wave intervals. Electrocardiography is needed at baseline and periodically during treatment. Little experience is reported in administering pimozide to children less than 12 years of age.

Clinicians must warn patients and families of the possibility of acute dystonic reactions and Parkinsonian symptoms when use of a conventional or atypical antipsychotic medication is to be initiated. Atypical antipsychotics (serotonin-dopamine antagonists), including risperidone and olanzapine (Zyprexa), can be initiated as a treatment option instead of the conventional antipsychotics in the hope that adverse effects will be less pervasive. Risperidone has been used in the treatment of Tourette's disorder in doses ranging from 1 to 6 mg per day with some success. Adverse effects include weight gain, sedation, and extrapyramidal adverse effects. Risperidone and pimozide were found to be of equal efficacy in one study of 50 children, adolescents, and adults with Tourette's disorder. Olanzapine is generally well tolerated, although weight gain and reports of cognitive dulling have limited its use. Even with the serotonin-dopamine antagonists, diphenhydramine (Benadryl) or benztropine (Cogentin) may be required to control extrapyramidal adverse effects.

Although not presently approved by the U.S. Food and Drug Administration (FDA) for use in Tourette's disorder, several studies reported that clonidine, an α_2-adrenergic agonist, was efficacious; 40 to 70 percent of patients benefited from the medication. In addition to the reduction in tic symptoms, patients may experience less tension and improved attention span. Another α_2-adrenergic agonist, guanfacine (Tenex), has also been used in the treatment of tic disorders. Clonidine has generally been used in doses ranging from 0.05 mg orally thrice daily to 0.1 mg four times daily, and guanfacine is usually used in doses ranging from 1 to 4 mg per day. When used in these dose ranges, adverse effects of the α-adrenergic agents include drowsiness, headache, irritability, and occasional hypotension.

In view of the frequent comorbidity of tic behaviors and obsessive-compulsive symptoms or disorders, the selective serotonin reuptake inhibitors (SSRIs) have been used alone or in combination with antipsychotics in the treatment of Tourette's disorder. Some data suggest that SSRIs, such as fluoxetine (Prozac), may be helpful.

Although clinicians must weigh the risks and benefits of using stimulants in cases of severe hyperactivity and comorbid tics, a recent study reported that methylphenidate does not increase the rate or intensity of motor or vocal tics in most children with hyperactivity and tic disorders. A recent study of atomoxetine (Strattera) at doses ranging from 0.5 to 1.5 mg per kg in the treatment of children and adolescents with ADHD and tic disorders revealed that the atomoxetine did not exacerbate tics and may be associated with some tic reduction. One case report on the use of bupropion (Wellbutrin), an antidepressant of the aminoketone class, indicated increased tic behavior in several children being treated for Tourette's disorder and ADHD. Other antidepressants, such as imipramine (Tofranil) and desipramine (Norpramin, Pertofrane), may decrease disruptive behavior in children with Tourette's disorder but are no longer widely used because of their potentially serious cardiac adverse effects.

CHRONIC MOTOR OR VOCAL TIC DISORDER

In the DSM-IV-TR, chronic motor or vocal tic disorder is defined as the presence of either motor tics or vocal tics but not both. The other features are the same as those of Tourette's disorder, but chronic motor or vocal tic disorder cannot be diagnosed if the criteria for Tourette's disorder have ever been met. According to DSM-IV-TR criteria, the disorder must have its onset before the age of 18 years.

Epidemiology

The rate of chronic motor or vocal tic disorder has been estimated to be from 100 to 1,000 times greater than that of Tourette's disorder. School-age boys are at highest risk, but the incidence is unknown. Although the disorder was once believed to be rare, current estimates of the prevalence of chronic motor or vocal tic disorder range from 1 to 2 percent.

Etiology

Tourette's disorder and chronic motor or vocal tic disorder aggregate in the same families. Twin studies have found a high concordance for either Tourette's disorder or chronic motor tics in monozygotic twins. This finding supports the importance of hereditary factors in the transmission of at least some tic disorders.

Diagnosis and Clinical Features

The onset of chronic motor or vocal tic disorder appears to be in early childhood. The types of tics and their locations are similar to those in transient tic disorder. Chronic vocal tics are considerably rarer than chronic motor tics. The chronic vocal tics are usually much less conspicuous than those in Tourette's disorder. The vocal tics are usually not loud or intense and are not primarily produced by the vocal cords; they consist of grunts or other noises caused by thoracic, abdominal, or diaphragmatic contractions. The DSM-IV-TR diagnostic criteria are given in Table 10–4.

Table 10–4
DSM-IV-TR Diagnostic Criteria for Chronic Motor or Vocal Tic Disorder

A. Single or multiple motor or vocal tics (i.e., sudden, rapid, recurrent, nonrhythmic, stereotyped motor movements or vocalizations), but not both, have been present at some time during the illness.
B. The tics occur many times a day nearly every day or intermittently throughout a period of more than 1 year, and during this period there was never a tic-free period of more than 3 consecutive months.
C. The onset is before age 18 years.
D. The disturbance is not due to the direct physiologic effects of a substance (e.g., stimulants) or a general medical condition (e.g., Huntington's disease or postviral encephalitis).
E. Criteria have never been met for Tourette's disorder.

From American Psychiatric Association. *Diagnostic and Statistical Manual of Mental Disorders*. 4th ed. Text rev. Washington, DC: American Psychiatric Association; copyright 2000, with permission.

Differential Diagnosis

Chronic motor tics must be differentiated from a variety of other motor movements, including choreiform movements, myoclonus, restless legs syndrome, akathisia, and dystonias. Involuntary vocal utterances can occur in certain neurologic disorders, such as Huntington's disease and Parkinson's disease.

Course and Prognosis

Children whose tics start between the ages of 6 and 8 years seem to have the best outcomes. Symptoms usually last for 4 to 6 years and stop in early adolescence. Children whose tics involve the limbs or trunk tend to do less well than those with only facial tics.

Treatment

The treatment of chronic motor or vocal tic disorder depends on the severity and frequency of the tics; the patient's subjective distress; the effects of the tics on school or work, job performance, and socialization; and the presence of any other concomitant mental disorder. Psychotherapy may be indicated to minimize the secondary social difficulties caused by severe tics. Several studies found that behavioral techniques, particularly habit reversal treatments, were effective in treating chronic motor or vocal tic disorder. Antianxiety agents have been unsuccessful. Haloperidol has been helpful in some cases, but the risks must be weighed against the possible clinical benefits because of

Table 10–5
DSM-IV-TR Diagnostic Criteria for Transient Tic Disorder

A. Single or multiple motor and/or vocal tics (i.e., sudden, rapid, recurrent, nonrhythmic, stereotyped motor movements or vocalizations)
B. The tics occur many times a day, nearly every day for at least 4 weeks, but for no longer than 12 consecutive months.
C. The onset is before age 18 years.
D. The disturbance is not due to the direct physiologic effects of a substance (e.g., stimulants) or a general medical condition (e.g., Huntington's disease or postviral encephalitis).
E. Criteria have never been met for Tourette's Disorder or Chronic Motor or Vocal Tic Disorder.

Specify if:
Single episode or **Recurrent**

the drug's adverse effects, including the development of tardive dyskinesia.

TRANSIENT TIC DISORDER

In the DSM-IV-TR, transient tic disorder is defined as the presence of a single tic or multiple motor or vocal tics or both. The tics occur many times a day for at least 4 weeks but no longer than 12 months. The other features are the same as those for Tourette's disorder, but transient tic disorder cannot be diagnosed if the criteria for Tourette's disorder or chronic motor or vocal tic disorder have ever been met. According to the DSM-IV-TR, the disorder must have its onset before the age of 18 years.

Epidemiology

Transient tic-like movements and nervous muscular twitches are common in children. From 5 to 24 percent of all school-age children have a history of tics. The prevalence of tics as defined here is unknown.

Etiology

Transient tic disorder probably has organic origins, with some tics combining psychogenic contributions as well. Early onset of tics, which are probably most likely to progress to Tourette's disorder, occur with greater frequency in children with an increased family history of tics. Tics that progress to chronic motor or vocal tic disorder are most likely to have components of both organic and psychogenic origin. Tics of all sorts are *exacerbated* by stress and anxiety, but no evidence indicates that tics are *caused* by stress or anxiety.

Table 10–6
DSM-IV-TR Diagnostic Criteria for Tic Disorder Not Otherwise Specified

This category is for disorders characterized by tics that do not meet criteria for a specific tic disorder. Examples include tics lasting less than 4 weeks or tics with an onset after age 18 years.

Diagnosis and Clinical Features

The DSM-IV-TR criteria for establishing the diagnosis of transient tic disorder are as follows: The tics are single or multiple, motor or vocal. They occur many times a day nearly every day for at least 4 weeks but no longer than 12 consecutive months. The patient has no history of Tourette's disorder or chronic motor or vocal tic disorder. The onset is before age 18 years. The tics do not occur exclusively during substance intoxication, and they are not caused by a general medical condition. The diagnosis should specify whether a single episode or recurrent episodes are present (Table 10–5). Transient tic disorder can be distinguished from chronic motor or vocal tic disorder and Tourette's disorder only by observing symptom progression over time.

Course and Prognosis

Motor tics are frequent among young children and, in general, are not associated with severe impairment. Over time, tics either disappear permanently or recur during periods of special stress. Only a small percentage of those with tics develop chronic motor or vocal tic disorder or Tourette's disorder.

Treatment

Whether the tics will disappear spontaneously, progress, or become chronic is unclear at the beginning of treatment. Focusing much attention on mild or infrequent tics may serve to cause undue stress for a child, but if tics are sufficiently severe to cause impairment in social, academic, or emotional function, psychiatric and pediatric neurologic examinations are recommended. Psychopharmacology is recommended when symptoms are severe and disabling. Several studies found that behavioral techniques, particularly habit reversal treatment, are effective in treating transient tics.

TIC DISORDER NOT OTHERWISE SPECIFIED

According to the DSM-IV-TR, tic disorder not otherwise specified refers to disorders characterized by tics but not otherwise meeting the criteria for a specific tic disorder (Table 10–6).

11 Elimination Disorders

The developmental milestones of mastering control over bowel and bladder function are complex processes that occur over a period of months for the typical toddler. Infants generally void small volumes of urine approximately every hour, commonly stimulated by feeding, and may have incomplete emptying of the bladder. As the infant matures to be a toddler, bladder capacity increases, and between 1 and 3 years of age, cortical inhibitory pathways develop allowing the child to have voluntary control over reflexes that control the bladder muscles. The ability to have muscular control over the bowel occurs even before bladder control for most toddlers, and the assessment of fecal soiling includes determining whether the clinical presentation occurs with or without chronic constipation and overflow soiling. The normal sequence of developing control over bowel and bladder functions is the development of nocturnal fecal continence, diurnal fecal continence, diurnal bladder control, and nocturnal bladder control. Bowel and bladder control develops gradually over time. Toilet training is affected by many factors, such as a child's intellectual capacity and social maturity, cultural determinants, and the psychologic interactions between child and parents.

Enuresis and encopresis are the two elimination disorders described in the text revision of the fourth edition of the *Diagnostic and Statistical Manual of Mental Disorders* (DSM-IV-TR). These disorders are considered after age 4 years for encopresis and after age 5 years for enuresis, when a child is chronologically, developmentally, and physiologically expected to be able to master these skills. Normal development encompasses a range of time in which a given child is able to devote the attention, motivation, and physiologic skills to exhibit competency in elimination processes. Encopresis is defined as a pattern of passing feces in inappropriate places, such as in clothing or other places, at least once per month for 3 consecutive months, whether the passage is involuntary or intentional. The child with encopresis typically exhibits dysregulated bowel function—for example, with infrequent bowel movements, constipation, or recurrent abdominal pain and sometimes pain on defecations. Encopresis is a nonorganic condition in a child who is chronologically at least 4 years old. Enuresis is the repeated voiding of urine into clothes or bed, whether the voiding is involuntary or intentional. The behavior must occur twice weekly for at least 3 months or must cause clinically significant distress or impairment socially or academically. The child's chronologic or developmental age must be at least 5 years.

ENCOPRESIS

Epidemiology

Incidence rates for encopretic behavior decrease drastically with increasing age. Although the diagnosis is not made until after age 4 years, encopretic behavior is present in 8.1 percent of 3-year-olds, 2.2 percent of 5-year-olds, and 0.75 percent of 10-to-12 year olds. In Western cultures, bowel control is established in more than 95 percent of children by their fourth birthday and in 99 percent by the fifth birthday. Encopresis is virtually absent in youth with normal intellectual function by the age of 16 years. Males are found to be about six times more likely to have encopresis than females. A significant relation exists between encopresis and enuresis.

Etiology

Encopresis involves an often complicated interplay between physiologic and psychologic factors. Although encopresis is considered a nonorganic disorder, a typical child with encopresis may show evidence of chronic constipation, leading to infrequent defecation, withholding of bowel movements, and avoidance of defecation. Children may avoid the pain of having a bowel movement by holding in the bowel movement, which then leads to impaction and eventual overflow soiling. This pattern is observed in more than 75 percent of children with encopretic behavior. This common set of circumstances in most children with encopresis supports a behavioral intervention with a focus on ameliorating constipation while increasing appropriate toileting behavior. Inadequate training or the lack of appropriate toilet training may delay a child's attainment of continence.

Evidence indicates that some encopretic children have lifelong inefficient and ineffective sphincter control. Other children may soil involuntarily because of either the inability to control the sphincter adequately or the presence of excessive fluid caused by a retentive overflow.

Encopresis has been demonstrated to occur with significantly greater frequency among children with known sexual abuse than among a sample of normal children, and it occurs with greater frequency among children with a variety of psychiatric disturbances than among controls. Encopresis, however, is not a specific indicator of sexual abuse because it also occurs with increased frequency in nonabused children with other behavioral problems. Some evidence indicates that encopresis in children is associated with measures of maternal hostility and harsh and punitive parenting. A recent study evaluating the frequency of encopresis and enuresis in children with prepubertal and early adolescent bipolar I disorder found a greater prevalence of encopresis among children with bipolar disorder than among healthy controls; in most cases, however, the encopresis predated the onset of the affective illness.

It is evident that once a given child has developed a pattern of withholding bowel movements with resulting pain with attempts to defecate, a child's fear and resistance to changing the pattern can lead to a power struggle between child and parent over effective toileting behavior. Perpetual battles often aggravate the disorder and frequently cause secondary behavioral difficulties. Many children with encopresis who are not reported to have early behavioral problems end up being socially ostracized and rejected because of the encopresis. The social consequences of soiling can further lead to the development of psychiatric problems. On the other hand, children with encopresis who clearly can control their bowel function adequately but chronically deposit feces of relatively normal consistency in abnormal places are more likely to have a preexisting neurodevelopmental problems, easy distractibility, short attention span, low frustration tolerance, hyperactivity, or poor coordination. Occasionally, a child has a specific fear of using the toilet, leading to a phobia.

In some children, encopresis can be considered secondary, that is, emerging after a period of normal bowel habits in conjunction with a disruptive life event, such as the birth of a sibling or a move to a new home. When encopresis manifests after a long period of fecal continence, it may reflect a response indicative of a developmental regressive behavior—for example, based on a severe stressor, such as a parental separation, loss of a best friend, or an unexpected academic failure.

Psychogenic Megacolon. Most children with encopresis retain feces and become constipated, either voluntarily or secondarily to painful defecation. In some cases a subclinical preexisting anorectal dysfunction exists that contributes to the constipation. In either case, resulting chronic rectal distention from large, hard fecal masses can cause loss of tone in the rectal wall and desensitization to pressure. Thus, children in this situation become even less aware of the need to defecate, and overflow encopresis occurs, usually with relatively small amounts of liquid or soft stool leaking out.

Anecdotal reports indicate that children whose parenting has been harsh and punitive and who have been severely punished for "accidents" during toilet training are at greater risk of developing encopresis.

Table 11–1
DSM-IV-TR Diagnostic Criteria for Encopresis

A. Repeated passage of feces into inappropriate places (e.g., clothing or floor) whether involuntary or intentional.
B. At least one such event a month for at least 3 months.
C. Chronologic age is at least 4 years (or equivalent developmental level).
D. The behavior is not due exclusively to the direct physiologic effects of a substance (e.g., laxatives) or a general medical condition except through a mechanism involving constipation.

Code as follows:
With constipation and overflow incontinence
Without constipation and overflow incontinence

From American Psychiatric Association. *Diagnostic and Statistical Manual of Mental Disorders.* 4th ed. Text rev. Washington, DC: American Psychiatric Association; copyright 2000, with permission.

Diagnosis and Clinical Features

According to the DSM-IV-TR, encopresis is diagnosed when feces are passed into inappropriate places on a regular basis (at least once a month) for 3 months (Table 11–1). Encopresis may be present in children who have bowel control and intentionally deposit feces in their clothes or other places for a variety of emotional reasons. Anecdotal reports have suggested that occasionally encopresis is attributable to an expression of anger or rage in a child whose parents have been punitive or of hostility at a parent. In such a case, once a child develops this inappropriate repetitive behavior eliciting negative attention, it is difficult to break the cycle of continuous negative attention. In other children, sporadic episodes of encopresis can occur during times of stress—for example, proximal to the birth of a new sibling—but in such cases, the behavior is usually transient and does not fulfill the diagnostic criteria for the disorder.

Encopresis can also be present on an involuntary basis in the absence of physiologic abnormalities. In these cases, a child may not exhibit adequate control over the sphincter muscles because either the child is absorbed in another activity or he or she is unaware of the process. The feces may be of normal, near-normal, or liquid consistency. Some involuntary soiling occurs from chronic retaining of stool, which results in liquid overflow. In rare cases, the involuntary overflow of stool results from psychologic causes of diarrhea or anxiety disorder symptoms.

The DSM-IV-TR breaks down the types of encopresis into encopresis *with* constipation and overflow incontinence and encopresis *without* constipation and overflow incontinence. To receive a diagnosis of encopresis, a child must have a developmental or chronologic level of at least 4 years. If the fecal incontinence is directly related to a medical condition, encopresis is not diagnosed.

Studies have indicated that children with encopresis who do not have gastrointestinal illnesses have high rates of abnormal anal sphincter contractions. This finding is particularly prevalent among children with encopresis with constipation and overflow incontinence who have difficulty relaxing their anal sphincter muscles when trying to defecate. Children with constipation who have difficulties with sphincter relaxation are not likely to respond well to laxatives in the treatment of their encopresis. Children with encopresis without abnormal sphincter tone are likely to improve over a short period.

Jack was a 9-year-old boy with daily encopresis, enuresis, and a history of hoarding behaviors, along with hiding the feces around the house. He resided with his adoptive parents, having been removed from his biological parents at age 3 years because of neglect, and physical and sexual abuse. He was reported to be cocaine addicted at birth, but was otherwise healthy. His mother was a known drug and alcohol user, and his father had spent time in jail for drug sales. Jack has always been enuretic at night, and when he was younger he had a history of daytime enuresis as well. Jack had a short attention span, was highly impulsive, and had great difficulty staying in his seat at school and remaining on task. He had reading difficulties and was placed in a contained special education classroom because of his disruptive behavior as well as his academic difficulties. Jack also qualified for a diagnosis of oppositional-defiant disorder. Despite experiencing physical and sexual abuse, he has not experienced flashbacks or other symptoms indicating the presence of post-traumatic stress disorder. Jack is being treated for attention-deficit/hyperactivity disorder (ADHD) and is responding to methylphenidate (Concerta 36 mg per day).

Jack's adoptive family resided in an urban area that had access to a university hospital with an outpatient program that had expertise in the behavioral treatment of encopresis. This program coupled the bowel training method with a psychoeducational component and psychotherapy. It was determined that Jack's encopresis was not of the retentive-overflow type, and the feces were always well formed. Much to the surprise of the psychiatric consultant, several-week outpatient bowel training course coupled with the psychoeducational component and psychotherapy resulted in significant improvement in the frequency of the encopresis. Jack was proud and gave his therapist a diagram of the functioning of the digestive system that was part of the psychoeducational program. In retrospect, it appeared that although there were symbolic aspects to Jack's encopretic behavior, the soiling was ego-dystonic, and he was motivated to change the behavior. (Courtesy of Edwin J. Mikkelsen, M.D., and Caroly Pataki, M.D.)

Pathology and Laboratory Examination

Although no specific test indicates a diagnosis of encopresis, clinicians must rule out medical illnesses, such as Hirschsprung's disease, before making a diagnosis. If it is unclear whether fecal retention is responsible for encopresis with constipation and overflow incontinence, a physical examination of the abdomen is indicated, and an abdominal X-ray can help to determine the degree of constipation present. Sophisticated tests to determine whether sphincter tone is abnormal are generally not conducted in simple cases of encopresis.

Differential Diagnosis

In encopresis with constipation and overflow incontinence, constipation can begin as early as the child's first year and can peak between the second and fourth years. Soiling usually begins at age 4 years. Frequent liquid stools and hard fecal masses are found in the colon and the rectum on abdominal palpation and rectal examination. Complications include impaction, megacolon, and anal fissures.

Encopresis with constipation and overflow incontinence can be caused by faulty nutrition; structural disease of the anus, rectum, and colon; medicinal adverse effects; or nongastrointestinal medical (endocrine or neurologic) disorders. The chief differential problem is aganglionic megacolon or Hirschsprung's disease, in which a patient may have an empty rectum and no desire to defecate, but may still have an overflow of feces. The disorder occurs in 1 in 5,000 children; signs appear shortly after birth.

Given the frequency of comorbid psychiatric disorders and increased incidence of encopresis among children who have been sexually abused, it is imperative to investigate the possibility of sexual and physical abuse during the evaluation of encopresis.

Course and Prognosis

The outcome of encopresis depends on the cause, the chronicity of the symptoms, and coexisting behavioral problems. In many cases, encopresis is self-limiting, and it rarely continues beyond middle adolescence. Encopresis in children who have contributing physiologic factors, such as poor gastric motility and an inability to relax the anal sphincter muscles, is more difficult to treat than that in those with constipation but normal sphincter tone.

Encopresis is a particularly repugnant disorder to most persons, including family members; thus, family tension is often high. The child's peers are also sensitive to the developmentally inappropriate behavior and often ostracize the child. A child with encopresis is often scapegoated by peers and shunned by adults. Many of these children have abysmally low self-esteem and are aware of their constant rejection. Psychologically, the child may appear blunted toward the symptoms or may be entrenched in a pattern of encopresis as a mode of expressing anger. The outcome of cases of encopresis is affected by the family's willingness and ability to participate in treatment without being overly punitive and by the child's awareness of when the passage of feces is about to occur.

Treatment

The treatment plan for encopresis cannot be established until a medical assessment of bowel function is completed together with a full psychiatric assessment. A typical treatment plan for a child with encopresis includes an initial medical plan to address constipation, in most cases, as well as an ongoing behavioral intervention to enhance appropriate bowel behavior and diminish anxiety related to bowel movement. By the time a child is brought for treatment, considerable family discord and distress are common. Family tensions about the symptom must be reduced and a nonpunitive atmosphere established. Similar efforts should be made to reduce the child's embarrassment at school. Many changes of underwear with a minimum of fuss should be arranged. Education of the family and correction of misperceptions that a family may have about soiling must occur before treatment. A useful physiologic approach involves a combination of daily laxatives or mineral oil along with a behavioral intervention in which the child sits on the toilet for timed intervals daily and is rewarded for successful defecation. Laxatives are not necessary for children who are not constipated and do have good bowel control, but regular, timed intervals on the toilet may be useful with these children as well.

A recent report confirms the success of an interactive parent–child family guidance intervention for young children with encopresis based on psychologic and behavioral interventions for children younger than the age of 9 years.

Supportive psychotherapy and relaxation techniques may be useful in treating the anxieties and other sequelae of children with encopresis, such as low self-esteem and social isolation. Family interventions can be helpful for children who have bowel control but continue to deposit their feces in inappropriate locations. A good outcome occurs when a child feels in control of life events. Coexisting behavior problems predict a poorer outcome. In all cases, proper bowel habits may need to be taught. In some cases, biofeedback techniques have been of benefit.

ENURESIS

Epidemiology

The prevalence of enuresis decreases with increasing age. The diagnosis of enuresis is not made until the chronologic and developmental age of 5 years, but enuretic behavior nocturnally and during the daytime is common, with reported prevalence from 2 to 5 percent among school-aged children. Enuretic behavior is considered developmentally appropriate among young toddlers, precluding diagnoses of enuresis; however, enuretic behavior occurs in 82 percent of 2-year-olds, 49 percent of 3-year-olds, 26 percent of 4-year-olds, and 7 percent of 5-year-olds on a regular basis. Prevalence rates vary, however, on the basis of the population studied and the tolerance for the symptoms in various cultures and socioeconomic groups.

The Isle of Wight study reported that 15.2 percent of 7-year-old boys were enuretic occasionally and that 6.7 percent of them were enuretic at least once a week. The study reported that 3.3 percent of girls at the age of 7 years were enuretic at least once a week. By age 10, the overall prevalence of enuresis was reported to be 3 percent. The rate drops drastically for teenagers; a prevalence of 1.5 percent has been reported for 14-year-olds. Enuresis affects about 1 percent of adults.

Although most children with enuresis do not have a comorbid psychiatric disorder, children with enuresis are at higher risk for the development of a variety of developmental and behavioral disturbances than children without enuresis.

Nocturnal enuresis is about 50 percent more common in boys and accounts for about 80 percent of children with enuresis. Diurnal enuresis is also more often seen in boys, who often delay voiding until it is too late. The rate of spontaneous resolution of nocturnal enuresis is about 15 percent per year. Nocturnal enuresis consists of a normal volume of voided urine, whereas, when small volumes of urine are voided at night, other medical causes may be present.

Etiology

Most children with nocturnal enuresis do not exhibit neurologic conditions that account for the symptoms. Voiding dysfunction in the absence of a specific neurogenic cause is believed to originate from behavioral factors that affect normal voiding habits and inhibit the maturation of normal voluntary control.

The most severe form of dysfunctional voiding is called Hinman's syndrome and is thought of as a nonneurogenic neurogenic bladder resulting from habitual, voluntary tightening of the external sphincter during urges to urinate. The pattern may be set in a young child who may start out with a normal or overactive detrusor muscle in the bladder but, in any case, repeatedly attempts to prevent leaking or urination when there is an urge to void. Over time, the sensation of the urge to urinate is diminished and the bladder does not empty regularly, leading to enuresis at night when the bladder is relaxed and can empty without resistance. This immature pattern of urinating can account for some cases of enuresis, especially when the pattern has been in place since early childhood. Most children are not enuretic by intention or even with awareness until after they are wet. Physiologic factors often play a role in the development of enuresis, and behavioral patterns are likely to maintain the maladaptive urination. Normal bladder control, which is acquired gradually, is influenced by neuromuscular and cognitive development, socioemotional factors, toilet training, and genetic factors. Difficulties in one or more of these areas can delay urinary continence.

Genetic factors are believed to play a role in the expression of enuresis, given that the emergence of enuresis has been found to be significantly greater in first-degree relatives. A longitudinal study of child development found that children with enuresis were about twice as likely to have concomitant developmental delays as those who did not have enuresis. About 75 percent of children with enuresis have a first-degree relative who has or has had enuresis. A child's risk for enuresis has been found to be more than seven times greater if the father was enuretic. The concordance rate is higher in monozygotic twins than in dizygotic twins. A strong genetic component is suggested, and much can be accounted for by tolerance for enuresis in some families and by other psychosocial factors.

Studies indicated that children with enuresis with a normal anatomic bladder capacity report urge to void with less urine in the bladder than do children without enuresis. Other studies reported that nocturnal enuresis occurs when the bladder is full because of lower-than-expected levels of nighttime antidiuretic hormone. This could lead to a higher-than-usual urine output. Enuresis does not appear to be related to a specific stage of sleep or time of night; rather, bed-wetting appears randomly. In most cases, the quality of sleep is normal. Little evidence indicates that children with enuresis sleep more soundly than other children.

Psychosocial stressors appear to precipitate enuresis in a subgroup of children with the disorder. In young children, the disorder has been particularly associated with the birth of a sibling, hospitalization between the ages of 2 and 4 years, the start of school, the breakup of a family because of divorce or death, and a move to a new home.

Table 11–2
DSM-IV-TR Diagnostic Criteria for Enuresis

A. Repeated voiding of urine into bed or clothes (whether involuntary or intentional).
B. The behavior is clinically significant as manifested by either a frequency of twice a week for at least 3 consecutive months or the presence of clinically significant distress or impairment in social, academic (occupational), or other important areas of functioning.
C. Chronologic age is at least 5 years (or equivalent developmental level).
D. The behavior is not due exclusively to the direct physiologic effect of a substance (e.g., a diuretic) or a general medical condition (e.g., diabetes, spina bifida, a seizure disorder).

Specify type:
Nocturnal only
Diurnal only
Nocturnal and diurnal

From American Psychiatric Association. *Diagnostic and Statistical Manual of Mental Disorders.* 4th ed. Text rev. Washington, DC: American Psychiatric Association; copyright 2000, with permission.

Diagnosis and Clinical Features

Enuresis is the repeated voiding of urine into a child's clothes or bed; the voiding may be involuntary or intentional. For the diagnosis to be made, a child must exhibit a developmental or chronologic age of at least 5 years. According to the DSM-IV-TR, the behavior must occur twice weekly for a period of at least 3 months or must cause distress and impairment in functioning to meet the diagnostic criteria. Enuresis is diagnosed only if the behavior is not caused by a medical condition. Children with enuresis are at higher risk for ADHD than the general population. They are also more likely to have comorbid encopresis. The DSM-IV-TR and the 10th revision of the *International Statistical Classification of Diseases and Related Health Problems* (ICD-10) break down the disorder into three types: nocturnal only, diurnal only, and nocturnal and diurnal (Table 11–2).

Pathology and Laboratory Examination

No single laboratory finding is pathognomonic of enuresis, but clinicians must rule out organic factors, such as the presence of urinary tract infections, that may predispose a child to enuresis. Structural obstructive abnormalities may be present in up to 3 percent of children with apparent enuresis. Sophisticated radiographic studies are usually deferred in simple cases of enuresis with no signs of repeated infections or other medical problems.

Differential Diagnosis

To make the diagnosis of enuresis, organic causes of bladder dysfunction must be investigated and ruled out. Organic syndromes, such as urinary tract infections, obstructions, or anatomic conditions, are found most often in children who experience both nocturnal and diurnal enuresis combined with urinary frequency and urgency. The organic features include genitourinary pathology—structural, neurologic, and infectious—such as obstructive uropathy, spina bifida occulta, and cystitis; other organic disorders that can cause polyuria and enuresis, such as diabetes mellitus and diabetes insipidus; disturbances of consciousness and sleep, such as seizures, intoxication, and sleepwalking disorder, during which a child urinates; and adverse effects from treatment with antipsychotics (e.g., thioridazine [Mellaril]).

Course and Prognosis

Enuresis is often self-limited, and a child with enuresis may have a spontaneous remission without psychologic sequelae. Most such children find their symptoms ego-dystonic and enjoy enhanced self-esteem and improved social confidence when they become continent. About 80 percent of affected children have never achieved a year-long period of dryness. Enuresis after at least one dry year usually begins between the ages of 5 and 8 years; if it occurs much later, especially during adulthood, organic causes must be investigated. Some evidence indicates that late onset of enuresis in children is more frequently associated with a concomitant psychiatric difficulty than is enuresis without at least one dry year. Relapses occur in children with enuresis who are becoming dry spontaneously and in those who are being treated. The significant emotional and social difficulties of these children usually include poor self-image, decreased self-esteem, social embarrassment and restriction, and intrafamilial conflict. The course of children with enuresis may be influenced by whether they receive appropriate evaluation and treatment for common comorbid disorders such as ADHD.

Treatment

A treatment plan for typical enuresis can be developed after organic causes of urinary dysfunction have been ruled out.

Modalities that have been used successfully for enuresis include both behavioral and pharmacologic interventions. A relatively high rate of spontaneous remission over long periods also occurs. The first step in any treatment plan is to review appropriate toilet training. If toilet training was not attempted, the parents and the patient should be guided in this undertaking. Record keeping is helpful in determining a baseline and following the child's progress and may itself be a reinforcer. A star chart may be particularly helpful. Other useful techniques include restricting fluids before bed and night lifting to toilet train the child. Another basic intervention for children with enuresis and bowel dysfunction is to assess whether chronic constipation is contributing to urinary dysfunction and consider increasing dietary fiber to diminish constipation.

Behavioral Therapy. Classic conditioning with the bell (or buzzer) and pad apparatus is generally the most effective treatment for enuresis, with dryness resulting in more than 50 percent of cases. The treatment is equally effective in children with and without concomitant mental disorders, and no evidence suggests symptom substitution. Difficulties may include child and family noncompliance, improper use of the apparatus, and relapse. Bladder training—encouragement or reward for delaying micturition for increasing times during waking hours—has also been used. Although sometimes effective, this method is decidedly inferior to the bell and pad.

Pharmacotherapy. Medication is considered when enuresis is causing impairment in social, family, and school function and behavioral, dietary, and fluid restriction have not been efficacious. When the problem interferes significantly with a child's functioning, several medications can be considered, although the problem often recurs as soon as medications are withdrawn.

Imipramine (Tofranil) is efficacious and has been approved for use in treating childhood enuresis, primarily on a short-term basis. Initially, up to 30 percent of patients with enuresis stay dry, and up to 85 percent wet less frequently than before treatment. The success often does not last, however, and tolerance can develop after 6 weeks of therapy. Once the drug is discontinued, relapse and enuresis at former frequencies usually occur within a few months. The drug's adverse effects, which include cardiotoxicity, are also a serious problem.

The tricyclic drugs are not used frequently for enuresis because of their risks and reports of sudden death in several children with ADHD who were taking desipramine (Norpramin, Pertofrane). Desmopressin (DDAVP), an antidiuretic compound that is available as an intranasal spray, has shown some initial success in reducing enuresis. Reduction of enuresis has varied from 10 to 90 percent with the use of desmopressin. In most studies, enuresis recurred shortly after discontinuation of this medication. Adverse effects that can occur with desmopressin include headache, nasal congestion, epistaxis, and stomachache. The most serious adverse effect reported with the use of desmopressin to treat enuresis was a hyponatremic seizure experienced by a child.

Reboxetine (Edronax, Vestra), a norepinephrine reuptake inhibitor with a noncardiotoxic side effect profile, has recently been investigated as a safer alternative to imipramine in the treatment of childhood enuresis. A trial in which 22 children with socially handicapping enuresis who had not responded to an enuresis alarm, desmopressin, or anticholinergics were administered 4 to 8 mg of reboxetine at bedtime. Of the 22 children, 13 (59 percent) in this open trial achieved complete dryness with reboxetine alone or in combination with desmopressin. Side effects were minimal and did not lead to discontinuation of the medication in this trial. Future placebo-controlled trials are indicated to determine the efficacy of this promising medication in the treatment of enuresis.

Psychotherapy. Psychotherapy may be useful in dealing with the coexisting psychiatric problems and the emotional and family difficulties that arise secondary to chronic enuresis. Although many psychologic and psychoanalytic theories regarding enuresis have been advanced, controlled studies have found that psychotherapy alone is not effective in the short-term treatment of enuresis.

12

Reactive Attachment Disorder of Infancy or Early Childhood

Reactive attachment disorder (RAD) is a clinical disorder characterized by aberrant social behaviors in a young child reflecting an environment of maltreatment that interfered with the development of normal attachment behavior. Unlike most disorders in the text revision of the fourth edition of the *Diagnostic and Statistical Manual of Mental Disorders* (DSM-IV-TR), a diagnosis of RAD is based on the presumption that the etiology is directly linked to environmental deprivation experienced by the child. The diagnosis of RAD is a relatively recent entity, added to the third edition of the DSM (DSM-III) in 1980. The formation of this diagnosis is largely based on the building blocks of attachment theory, which describes the quality of a child's generalized affective relationship with primary caregivers, usually parents. This basic relationship is the product of a young child's need for protection, nurturance, and comfort and the interaction of the parents and child in fulfilling these needs.

Based on observations of a young child and parents during a brief separation and reunion, designated the "strange situation procedure" pioneered by Mary Ainsworth and colleagues, researchers have designated a child's basic pattern of attachment to be characterized as secure, insecure, or disorganized. Children who exhibit secure attachment behavior are believed to experience their caregivers as emotionally available and appear to be more exploratory and well adjusted than children who exhibit insecure or disorganized attachment behavior. Insecure attachment is believed to result from a young child's perception that the caregiver is not consistently available, whereas a child with disorganized attachment behavior is believed to be experiencing the need for proximity to the caregiver with apprehension in approaching the caregiver. These early patterns of attachment are believed to influence a child's future complex capacities for affect regulation, self-soothing, and relationship building. According to the DSM-IV-TR, RAD of infancy or early childhood is marked by an inappropriate social relatedness that occurs in most contexts. The disorder appears before the age of 5 years and is associated with "grossly pathologic care." It is not accounted for solely by a developmental delay and does not meet the criteria for pervasive developmental disorder. The pattern of care may exhibit lasting disregard for a child's emotional or physical needs or repeated changes of caregivers, as when a child is frequently relocated during foster care. The pathologic care pattern is believed to cause the disturbance in social relatedness.

The disorder has two subtypes: the *inhibited* type, in which the disturbance takes the form of constantly failing to initiate and respond to most social interactions in a developmentally normal way; and the *disinhibited* type, in which the disturbance takes the form of undifferentiated, unselective social relatedness. These developmentally inappropriate behaviors are presumed to be caused mostly by pathogenic caregiving, but less severe disturbances in parenting may also be associated with infants who exhibit the disorder.

The disorder may result in a picture of failure to thrive, in which an infant shows physical signs of malnourishment and does not exhibit the expected developmental motor and verbal milestones. When this is the case, the failure to thrive is coded on Axis III.

EPIDEMIOLOGY

Few data exist on the prevalence, sex ratio, or familial pattern of RAD. It has been estimated to occur in less than 1 percent of the population. Studies have used selected high-risk populations. In a retrospective report of children in one county of the United States who were removed from their homes because of neglect or abuse before the age of 4 years, 38 percent exhibited signs of emotionally withdrawn or indiscriminate RAD. A study in 2004 established the reliability of the diagnosis by reviewing videotaped assessments of children at risk interacting with caregivers along with a structured interview with caregivers. Given that pathogenic care, including maltreatment, occurs more frequently in the presence of general psychosocial risk factors, such as poverty, disrupted families, and mental illness among caregivers, these circumstances are likely to increase the risk of RAD. In unusual circumstances, however, a caregiver may be fully satisfactory for one child, whereas another child in the same household may be maltreated and develops RAD.

ETIOLOGY

The essence of RAD is the malformation of normal attachment behaviors. The inability of a young child to develop normative social interactions that culminate in aberrant attachment behaviors in RAD is inherent in the disorder's definition. RAD is linked to maltreatment, including emotional neglect, physical abuse, or both as well. Grossly pathogenic care of an infant or young child by the caregiver presumably causes the markedly disturbed social relatedness that is usually evident. The emphasis is on the unidirectional cause; that is, the caregiver does something inimical or neglects to do something essential for the infant or child. In evaluating a patient for whom such a diagnosis is appropriate, however, clinicians should consider the contributions of each member of the caregiver–child dyad and their interactions. Clinicians should weigh such things as infant or child temperament, deficient or defective bonding, a developmentally disabled or sensorially impaired child, and a particular caregiver–child mismatch. The likelihood of neglect increases with parental mental retardation; lack of parenting skills because of personal upbringing, social isolation, or deprivation and lack of opportunities to learn about caregiving behavior; and premature parenthood (during early and middle adolescence), in which parents are unable to respond to, and care for, an infant's needs and in which the parents' needs take precedence over their infant's or child's needs. Frequent changes of the primary caregiver—as may occur in institutionalization, repeated lengthy hospitalizations, and multiple foster care placements—may also cause a reactive attachment disorder of infancy or early childhood.

Table 12–1
DSM-IV-TR Diagnostic Criteria for Reactive Attachment Disorder of Infancy or Early Childhood

A. Markedly disturbed and developmentally inappropriate social relatedness in most contexts, beginning before age 5 years, as evidenced by either (1) or (2):
   (1) persistent failure to initiate or respond in a developmentally appropriate fashion to most social interactions, as manifest by excessively inhibited, hypervigilant, or highly ambivalent and contradictory responses (e.g., the child may respond to caregivers with a mixture of approach, avoidance, and resistance to comforting, or may exhibit frozen watchfulness)
   (2) diffuse attachments as manifest by indiscriminate sociability with marked inability to exhibit appropriate selective attachments (e.g., excessive familiarity with relative strangers or lack of selectivity in choice of attachment figures)

B. The disturbance in Criterion A is not accounted for solely by developmental delay (as in mental retardation) and does not meet criteria for a pervasive developmental disorder.

C. Pathogenic care as evidenced by at least one of the following:
   (1) persistent disregard of the child's basic emotional needs for comfort, stimulation, and affection
   (2) persistent disregard of the child's basic physical needs
   (3) repeated changes of primary caregiver that prevent formation of stable attachments (e.g., frequent changes in foster care)

D. There is a presumption that the care in Criterion C is responsible for the disturbed behavior in Criterion A (e.g., the disturbances in Criterion A began following the pathogenic care in Criterion C).

Specify type:

Inhibited type: if Criterion A1 predominates in the clinical presentation

Disinhibited type: if Criterion A2 predominates in the clinical presentation

From American Psychiatric Association. *Diagnostic and Statistical Manual of Mental Disorders.* 4th ed. Text rev. Washington, DC: American Psychiatric Association; copyright 2000, with permission.

DIAGNOSIS AND CLINICAL FEATURES

Children with RAD may initially be identified by a preschool teacher or by a pediatrician based on direct observation of the child's inappropriate social responses. The diagnosis of RAD is based on documenting evidence of pervasive disturbance of attachment leading to inappropriate social behaviors present before the age of 5 years. The clinical picture varies greatly, depending on a child's chronologic and mental ages, but expected social interaction and liveliness are not present. Often, the child is not progressing developmentally or is frankly malnourished. Perhaps the most typical clinical picture of an infant with one form of RAD is the nonorganic failure to thrive. Such infants usually exhibit hypokinesis, dullness, listlessness, and apathy with a poverty of spontaneous activity. Infants look sad, joyless, and miserable. Some infants also appear frightened and watchful, with a radar-like gaze. Nevertheless, they may exhibit delayed responsiveness to a stimulus that would elicit fright or withdrawal from a normal infant (Table 12–1). Infants with failure to thrive and RAD appear significantly malnourished, and many have protruding abdomens. Occasionally, foul-smelling, celiac-like stools are reported. In unusually severe cases, a clinical picture of marasmus appears.

The infant's weight is often below the third percentile and markedly below the appropriate weight for his or her height. If serial weights are available, the weight percentiles may have decreased progressively because of an actual weight loss or a failure to gain weight as height increases. Head circumference is usually normal for the infant's age. Muscle tone may be poor. The skin may be colder and paler or more mottled than the skin of a normal child. Laboratory findings are usually within normal limits, except for abnormal findings coincident with any malnutrition, dehydration, or concurrent illness. Bone age is usually retarded. Growth hormone levels are usually normal or elevated, a finding suggesting that growth failure in these children is secondary to caloric deprivation and malnutrition. The children improve physically and gain weight rapidly after they are hospitalized.

Socially, the infants usually show little spontaneous activity and a marked diminution of both initiative toward others and reciprocity in response to the caregiving adult or examiner. Both mother and infant may be indifferent to separation on hospitalization or to termination of subsequent hospital visits. The infants frequently show none of the normal upset, fretting, or protest about hospitalization. Older infants usually show little interest in their environment. They may not play with toys, even if encouraged; however, they rapidly or gradually take an interest in, and relate to, their caregivers in the hospital.

Classic psychosocial dwarfism or psychosocially determined short stature is a syndrome that usually is first manifest in children 2 to 3 years of age. The children are typically unusually short and have frequent growth hormone abnormalities and severe behavioral disturbances. All of these symptoms result from an inimical caregiver–child relationship. The affectionless character may appear when there is a failure, or lack of opportunity, to form attachments before the age of 2 to 3 years. Children cannot form lasting relationships, and their inability is sometimes accompanied by a lack of guilt, an inability to obey rules, and a need for attention and affection. Some children are indiscriminately friendly.

A 6-year-old boy was referred by his adoptive parents because of hyperactivity and disruptive behavior at school. He had been adopted at 5 years of age, after living most of his life in a Romanian orphanage in which he received care from a rotating shift of caregivers. Although he had been below the 5th percentile for height and weight on arrival, he quickly approached the 10th percentile in his new home. However, both of his adoptive parents were frustrated by their inability to "reach him." They had initially worried about a hearing disturbance, although testing and his capacity to engage many adults and children verbally suggested otherwise. He showed interest in anyone and would often follow strangers willingly. He showed little empathy when others were hurt and blandly resisted redirection in school. He was frequently injured because of seemingly reckless behavior, although he had an extremely high tolerance for pain. Intensive intervention focused on problem behaviors at home decreased his self-endangering behavior, although he remained oddly overfriendly and nonempathic at home and in school. The boy was diagnosed with reactive attachment disorder, disinhibited type. (Courtesy of Neil W. Boris, M.D., and Charles H. Zeanah, Jr., M.D.)

PATHOLOGY AND LABORATORY EXAMINATION

Although no single specific laboratory test is used to make a diagnosis, many children with RAD have disturbances of growth and development. Thus, establishing a growth curve and examining the progression of developmental milestones may be helpful in determining whether associated phenomena, such as failure to thrive, are present.

DIFFERENTIAL DIAGNOSIS

The differential diagnosis of RAD must consider other psychiatric disorders that are more likely to arise in conjunction with conditions of maltreatment, including posttraumatic stress disorders, developmental language disorders, and mental retardation syndromes. Metabolic disorders, pervasive developmental disorders, mental retardation, various neurologic abnormalities, and psychosocial dwarfism are also considerations in the differential diagnosis. Children with autistic disorder are typically well nourished and of age-appropriate size and weight; they are generally alert and active, despite their impairments in reciprocal social interactions. Moderate, severe, or profound mental retardation is present in about 50 percent of children with autistic disorder, whereas when mental retardation is comorbid with RAD, it is generally in milder forms. Unlike most children with RAD, children with autistic disorder do not improve rapidly if they are removed from their homes and placed in a hospital or other favorable environment. Children with mental retardation may show delays in all social skills. Such children, unlike children with RAD, are usually adequately nourished, their social relatedness is appropriate to their mental age, and they show a sequence of development similar to that seen in normal children.

COURSE AND PROGNOSIS

Most of the data on the natural course of children with RAD come from follow-up studies of institutionalized children with histories of serious neglect. Findings from these studies suggest that in children with the inhibited patterns of RAD who are adopted into more normative caring environments, the quality of attachment behaviors tends to become more normalized over time. Children with the indiscriminate sociability and disinhibited forms of RAD appear to persist in their behavioral patterns for years even when they appear to be attached to new caregivers. Children with indiscriminate social behavior tend to exhibit poor peer relationships over time. The prognosis for children with reactive attachment disorders is influenced by the duration and severity of the neglectful and pathogenic parenting and associated complications, such as failure to thrive. Constitutional and nutritional factors interact in children, who may either respond resiliently to treatment or continue to fail to thrive. Outcomes range from the extremes of death to the developmentally healthy child. In general, the longer a child remains in the adverse environment without adequate intervention, the greater is the physical and emotional damage and the worse is the prognosis. After the pathologic environmental situation has been recognized, the amount of treatment and rehabilitation that the family receives affects the child who returns to this family. Children who have multiple problems stemming from pathogenic caregiving may recover physically faster and more completely than they do emotionally.

TREATMENT

Recommendations in the management of RAD must begin with a comprehensive assessment of the current level of safety and adequate caregiving. Thus, the first consideration in treating the disorder is the child's safety. With suspicion of maltreatment persisting in the home, the first decision is often whether to hospitalize the child or to attempt treatment while the child remains in the home. If neglect or emotional, physical, or sexual abuse is suspected, then legally such must be reported to the appropriate law enforcement and child protective services in the area. The child's physical and emotional state and the level of pathologic caregiving determine the therapeutic strategy. A determination must be made regarding the nutritional status of the child and the presence of ongoing physical abuse or threat. Hospitalization is necessary for children with malnourishment. Along with an assessment of the child's physical well-being, an evaluation of the child's emotional condition is important. Immediate intervention must address the parents' awareness and capacity to participate in altering the injurious patterns that have ensued. The treatment team must begin to alter the unsatisfactory relationship between the caregiver and child, which usually requires extensive and intensive intervention and education with the mother or with both parents when possible.

The caregiver–child relationship is the basis of the assessment of RAD symptoms and the substrate from which to modify attachment behaviors. Structured observations allow a clinician to determine the range of attachment behaviors established with various family members. The clinician's first task in the treatment of RAD is to advocate for providing the child with a caregiver who is emotionally available and committed to developing a positive attachment to the child. This may necessitate placement in a foster care situation when no relatives are available to fill this role. The clinician may work closely with the caregiver and the child to facilitate greater sensitivity in their interactions. Three basic psychotherapeutic modalities are helpful in promoting positive bonds between children and caregiver. First, a clinician can target the caregiver to promote positive interaction with a child who does not yet have the repertoire to respond positively. Second, a clinician can work with the child and the caregiver together as a dyad to advocate for practicing appropriate positive reinforcement for each other, and through the use of videotapes, the interactions can then be viewed and modifications can be suggested to increase the positive engagement. The third modality for clinical intervention is through individual work with the child. Working with the child and caregiver together is often more effective in producing more emotionally meaningful exchanges.

Psychosocial interventions for families in which a child has RAD include (1) psychosocial support services, including hiring a homemaker, improving the physical condition of the apartment, or obtaining more adequate housing; improving the family's financial status; and decreasing the family's isolation; (2) psychotherapeutic interventions, including individual psychotherapy, psychotropic medications, and family or marital therapy; (3) educational counseling services, including mother–infant or mother–toddler groups, and counseling to increase awareness and understanding of the child's needs and to increase parenting skills; and (4) provisions for close monitoring of the progression of the patient's emotional and physical well-being. Sometimes, separating a child from the stressful home environment temporarily, as in hospitalization, allows the child to break out of the accustomed pattern. A neutral setting, such as the hospital, is the best place to start with families who are genuinely available emotionally and physically for intervention. If interventions are unfeasible or inadequate or if they fail, placement with relatives or in foster care, adoption, or a group home or residential treatment facility must be considered.

Pharamacotherapy

Pharmacotherapy is not indicated in this disorder unless there is a comorbid condition (i.e., anxiety or depression) that is a contributing factor to the disorder or results as a reaction to it.

13

Stereotypic Movement Disorder and Disorder of Infancy, Childhood, or Adolescence Not Otherwise Specified

STEREOTYPIC MOVEMENT DISORDER

Stereotypic movements are repetitive, voluntary, often rhythmic movements that occur in normal children and with increased frequency in children who have received a diagnosis of pervasive developmental disorder and mental retardation syndromes. These movements appear to be purposeless, but in some cases, such as body rocking, head rocking, or hand flapping, they may be either self-soothing or self-stimulating. In other cases, stereotypic movements such as head banging, face slapping, eye poking, or hand biting can cause significant self-harm. Nail biting, thumb sucking, and nose picking are generally not included as symptoms of stereotypic movement disorder because they rarely cause impairment.

According to the text revision of the fourth edition of the *Diagnostic and Statistical Manual of Mental Disorders* (DSM-IV-TR), stereotypic movement disorder is repetitive, nonfunctional motor behavior that seems to be compulsive. The behavior significantly interferes with normal activities or produces self-inflicted bodily injuries sufficiently severe to require medical care unless the child is protected. For children with mental retardation, the injurious behavior is sufficiently dangerous to become the focus of treatment.

Epidemiology

The incidence of transient stereotypic habits is reported to be about 7 percent in the normal pediatric population, with a prevalence of about 15 to 20 percent in children under the age of 6 years. After age 6 years, the rates of stereotypic movements in the normal population are unknown but believed to be negligible. The prevalence of self-injurious behaviors, however, has been estimated to be in the range of 2 to 3 percent among children and adolescents with mental retardation.

Behaviors such as nail biting are common and affect as many as one half of all school-age children; behaviors such as thumb sucking and rocking are normal in young children but are often maladaptive in older children and adolescents. These behaviors usually do not constitute a stereotypic movement disorder; most children who bite their nails function in daily activities without impairment or self-injury. In one pediatric clinic, as many as 20 percent of children had a history of rocking, head banging, or swaying in one form or another.

Deciding which cases are sufficiently severe to confirm a diagnosis of stereotypic movement disorder may be difficult. The diagnosis is a compilation of many symptoms, and various behaviors must be studied separately to obtain data about prevalence, sex ratio, and familial patterns. It is clear, however, that stereotypic movement disorder is more prevalent in boys than in girls. Stereotypic behaviors are common among children with mental retardation; 10 to 20 percent are affected. Self-injurious behaviors occur in some genetic syndromes, such as Lesch-Nyhan syndrome, and also in some patients with Tourette's disorder. Self-injurious stereotypic behaviors are increasingly common in persons with severe mental retardation. Stereotypic behaviors are also common in children with sensory impairments, such as blindness and deafness.

Etiology

The causes of stereotypic movement disorder can be considered from the standpoint of behavioral factors, developmental factors, and functional and neurobiologic perspectives. Some stereotypic behaviors in young children can be associated with normal development; for example, up to 80 percent of all normal children show rhythmic activities that phase out by 4 years of age. These rhythmic patterns seem to be purposeful, to provide sensorimotor stimulation and tension release, and to be satisfying and pleasurable to the children. The movements may increase at times of frustration, boredom, and tension.

The progression from early expressions of stereotyped behavior in toddlers to stereotypic movement disorder in older children often reflects disordered development, as in mental retardation or a pervasive developmental disorder. Genetic factors likely play a role in some stereotypic movements, such as the X-linked recessive deficiency of enzymes leading to Lesch-Nyhan syndrome, which has predictable features including mental retardation, hyperuricemia, spasticity, and self-injurious behaviors. Other stereotypic movements (e.g., nail biting), although they often cause minimal or no impairment, seem to run in families. Some stereotypic behaviors seem to emerge or become exaggerated in situations of neglect or deprivation; such behaviors as head banging have been associated with psychosocial deprivation.

Stereotypic movements seem to be associated with dopamine activity. Neurobiologic factors may contribute to the development of stereotypic movement disorders. Dopamine agonists induce or increase stereotypic behaviors, whereas dopamine antagonists decrease them. In one report, four children with attention-deficit/hyperactivity disorder (ADHD) who were treated with a stimulant medication began to bite their nails and fingertips. The nail biting ceased when the medication was eliminated. Endogenous opioids also have been implicated in producing self-injurious behaviors.

Diagnosis and Clinical Features

The presence of multiple repetitive stereotyped symptoms tends to occur among those most severely afflicted with mental retardation or a pervasive developmental disorder. Patients with multiple stereotyped movements frequently have other significant mental disorders, including disruptive behavior disorders. In extreme cases, severe mutilation and life-threatening injuries can result, and secondary infection and septicemia may follow self-inflicted trauma. The DSM-IV-TR diagnostic criteria for stereotypic movement disorder are listed in Table 13–1.

Head Banging. Head banging exemplifies a stereotypic movement disorder that can result in functional impairment. According to the DSM-IV-TR, the male-to-female ratio is 3:1. Typically, head banging begins during infancy, between 6 and 12 months of age. Infants strike their heads with a definite rhythmic and monotonous continuity against the crib or another hard surface. They seem to be absorbed in the activity, which can persist until they become exhausted and fall asleep. The head banging is often transitory, but sometimes persists into middle childhood. Head banging that is a component of temper tantrums differs from stereotypic head banging and ceases after the tantrums and their secondary gains have been controlled.

Nail Biting. Nail biting begins as early as 1 year of age and increases in incidence until age 12 years. All nails are usually bitten. Most cases are not sufficiently severe to meet the DSM-IV-TR diagnostic criteria. In other cases, children cause physical damage to the fingers, usually by associated biting of the cuticles, which leads to secondary infections of the fingers and nail beds.

Table 13–1
DSM-IV-TR Diagnostic Criteria for Stereotypic Movement Disorder

A. Repetitive, seemingly driven, and nonfunctional motor behavior (e.g., hand shaking or waving, body rocking, head banging, mouthing of objects, self-biting, picking at skin or bodily orifices, hitting own body).
B. The behavior markedly interferes with normal activities or results in self-inflicted bodily injury that requires medical treatment (or would result in an injury if preventive measures were not used).
C. If mental retardation is present, the stereotypic or self-injurious behavior is of sufficient severity to become a focus of treatment.
D. The behavior is not better accounted for by a compulsion (as in obsessive-compulsive disorder), a tic (as in tic disorder), a stereotypy that is part of a pervasive developmental disorder, or hair pulling (as in trichotillomania).
E. The behavior is not due to the direct physiologic effects of a substance or a general medical condition.
F. The behavior persists for 4 weeks or longer.

Specify if:

With self-injurious behavior: if the behavior results in bodily damage that requires specific treatment (or that would result in bodily damage if protective measures were not used)

From American Psychiatric Association. *Diagnostic and Statistical Manual of Mental Disorders.* 4th ed. Text rev. Washington, DC: American Psychiatric Association; copyright 2000, with permission.

Nail biting seems to occur or increase in intensity when a person is either anxious or bored. Some of the most severe nail biting occurs in those with severe and profound mental retardation and some patients with paranoid schizophrenia; however, some nail biters have no obvious emotional disturbance.

Pathology and Laboratory Examination

No specific laboratory measures are helpful in the diagnosis of stereotypic movement disorder.

Victor, a legally blind 14-year-old boy with severe mental retardation, was evaluated when he transferred to a new residential school for children with multiple disabilities. Observed in his classroom, he was noted to be a small boy who appeared younger than his age. He held his hands in his pockets and spun around in place. Periodically, he approached his teacher, kissed her, positioned himself to receive a return kiss, and clearly enjoyed the contact with her. When offered a toy (which had to be held close to his eyes), he took it and manipulated it for a while. When he was prompted to engage in various tasks that required that he take his hands out of his pockets, he began hitting his head with his hands. If his hands were held by the teacher, he hit his head with his knees. He was adept in contorting himself, so that he could hit or kick himself in almost any position, even while walking. Soon, his face and forehead were covered with black-and-blue marks.

Only sketchy personal history was available. He was a premature baby, with birthweight of 2 pounds. Retinopathy of prematurity and severe mental retardation were diagnosed early in life. His development was delayed in all spheres, and he never developed language. Comprehensive studies did not disclose the etiology of Victor's developmental disabilities other than prematurity. He lived at home and attended a special educational program. His self-injurious behaviors developed early in life, and, when his parents tried to stop him, he became aggressive. Gradually, he became too difficult for them to manage, and, at 3 years of age, he was placed in a special school. The self-abusive and self-restraining (i.e., holding his hands in his pockets) behavior was present throughout his stay there, and, virtually all of the time, he was on one antipsychotic medication or another. He carried a diagnosis of cerebral dysfunction. Although the psychiatrist's notes mentioned improvement in his self-injurious behavior, other notes described it as continuing and fluctuating. He was transferred to the new school because of lack of progress and difficulties in managing him as he became bigger and stronger. His intellectual functioning was within the 34 to 40 intelligence quotient (IQ) range. His adaptive skills were poor. He required full assistance in self-care, could not provide even for his own simple needs, and required constant supervision for his safety.

In a few months, Victor settled into the routine in his new school. His self-injurious behavior fluctuated. It was reduced or even absent when he restrained himself by holding his hands in his pockets or inside his shirt or even by manipulating some object with his hands. If left to himself, he could contort himself, while holding his hands inside his shirt, to such a degree that he was nicknamed Pretzel. Because the stereotypic self-injurious and self-restraining behavior interfered with his daily activities and education, it became a primary focus of a behavior modification program. For a few months, he did well, especially when he developed a good relationship with a new teacher, who was firm, consistent, and nurturing. With him, Victor could engage in some school tasks. When the teacher left, Victor regressed. To prevent injuries, the staff started blocking his self-hitting with a pillow. He was offered activities that he liked and in which he could engage without resorting to self-injury. After several months, his antipsychotic medication was slowly discontinued, over a period of 11 months, without any behavioral deterioration. (Courtesy of Bhavik Shah, M.D.)

Differential Diagnosis

The differential diagnosis of stereotypic movement disorder includes obsessive-compulsive disorder (OCD) and tic disorders, both of which are exclusionary criteria in the DSM-IV-TR. Although stereotypic movements are voluntary and not spasmodic, it is difficult to differentiate these features from tics in all cases. A recent study of stereotyped movements compared with tics found that stereotyped movements tended to be longer in duration and displayed more rhythmic qualities than tics. Tics seemed to occur more when a child was in an "alone" condition than when the child was in a play condition, whereas stereotypic movements occurred with the same frequency in these two different conditions. Stereotypic movements are likely to be self-soothing, whereas tics are often associated with distress. In OCD, the compulsions must be ego-dystonic, although this, too, is difficult to discern in young children.

Differentiating dyskinetic movements from stereotypic movements can be difficult. Because antipsychotic medications can suppress stereotypic movements, clinicians must note any stereotypic movements before initiating treatment with an antipsychotic agent. Stereotypic movement disorder may be diagnosed concurrently with substance-related disorders (e.g., amphetamine use disorders), severe sensory impairments, central nervous system and degenerative disorders (e.g., Lesch-Nyhan syndrome), and severe schizophrenia.

Course and Prognosis

The duration and course of stereotypic movement disorder vary, and the symptoms may wax and wane. As many as 80 percent of normal children show rhythmic activities that seem purposeful and comforting and tend to disappear by 4 years of age. When stereotypic movements are present or emerge more severely later in childhood or in a noncomforting manner, they range from brief episodes occurring under stress to an ongoing pattern in the context of a chronic condition, such as mental retardation or a pervasive developmental disorder. Even in chronic conditions, stereotypic behaviors may come and go. In some cases, stereotypic movements are prominent in early childhood and diminish as a child gets older.

The severity of the dysfunction caused by stereotypic movements also varies with the associated frequency, amount, and degree of self-injury. Children who exhibit frequent, severe, self-injurious stereotypic behaviors have the poorest prognosis. Repetitive episodes of head banging, self-biting, and eye poking can be difficult to control without physical restraints. Most nail biting is benign and often does not meet the diagnostic criteria for stereotypic movement disorder. In severe cases in which the nail beds are repetitively damaged, bacterial and fungal infections can occur. Although chronic stereotypic movement disorders can severely impair daily functioning, several treatments help control the symptoms.

Treatment

Treatment modalities yielding the most promising effects include behavioral techniques, such as habit reversal and differential reinforcement of other behavior, as well as pharmacologic interventions. A recent report on using both habit reversal (in which the child is trained to replace the undesired repetitive behavior with a more acceptable behavior) and reinforcement for reducing the unwanted behavior indicated that these treatments had efficacy among 12 nonautistic children between 6 and 14 years of age.

Pharmacologic interventions have been used in clinical practice to minimize self-injury in children whose stereotyped movements caused significant harm to their bodies. In the past, typical antipsychotics were used; more recently, however, atypical antipsychotics have been favored. Small open-label studies have reported benefit of atypical antipsychotics, and case reports have indicated the use of serotonin reuptake inhibitor agents in the management of self-injurious stereotypies. Valproic acid has been used clinically, although no current controlled trial supports its use.

The dopamine antagonists have been the commonly used medications for treating stereotypic movements and self-injurious behavior. Phenothiazines have been the most frequently used drugs. Opiate antagonists have reduced self-injurious behaviors in some patients without exposing them to tardive dyskinesia or impaired cognition. Additional pharmacologic agents that have been tried in the treatment of stereotypic movement disorder include fenfluramine (Pondimin), clomipramine (Anafranil), and fluoxetine (Prozac). In some reports, fenfluramine diminished stereotypic behaviors in children with autistic disorder; in other studies, the results were less encouraging. Open trials indicate that both clomipramine and fluoxetine may decrease self-injurious behaviors and other stereotypic movements in some patients. Trazodone (Desyrel) and buspirone (BuSpar) have also been tried, with unclear results.

Pharmacotherapy. Pharmacotherapy is not indicated in this disorder unless there is a comorbid condition (i.e., anxiety or depression) that is a contributing factor to the disorder or results from it.

DISORDER OF INFANCY, CHILDHOOD, OR ADOLESCENCE NOT OTHERWISE SPECIFIED

The DSM-IV-TR describes disorder of infancy, childhood, or adolescence not otherwise specified as a category that includes disorders with onset in infancy, childhood, or adolescence that do not meet the criteria for any specific disorder. The DSM-IV-TR diagnostic criteria are shown in Table 13–2. The following two case histories exemplify children who have disorder of regulation and attachment, respectively, that cause impairment but do not fit neatly into any of the other developmental disorders of infancy.

Table 13–2
DSM-IV-TR Diagnostic Criteria for Disorder of Infancy, Childhood, or Adolescence Not Otherwise Specified

This category is a residual category for disorders with onset in infancy, childhood, or adolescence that do not meet criteria for any specific disorder in the classification.

From American Psychiatric Association. *Diagnostic and Statistical Manual of Mental Disorders.* 4th ed. Text rev. Washington, DC: American Psychiatric Association; copyright 2000, with permission.

A 3-year, 2-month-old boy was brought to the infant and preschool clinic by his mother, who was concerned about his extreme and chronic irritability, fussiness, and difficulty adapting to any environmental change. He was described as a difficult infant, the product of an uncomplicated full-term pregnancy, who was slow to develop a stable eating and sleeping cycle and was difficult to soothe. His mother was finding it increasingly difficult to leave him with alternate caretakers (i.e., babysitters) owing to the severe and extended tantrums that would result, and she was becoming anxious about his ability to transition into preschool. On further interview, it was revealed that the child was extremely rigid in a number of areas with which the family had unwittingly complied (and therefore barely recognized as symptoms on interview). The child had a small repertoire of food that he would eat that appeared to be largely limited by texture and temperature. He refused to eat anything that was too warm or too cold: All foods had to be room temperature, and his mother had taken significant care to ensure that this was the case at each meal.

Similarly, the child was extremely sensitive to tactile stimuli as well, tolerating only cotton fabrics and preferring not to wear clothing at all. He had the inclination to take off his clothes while at home, independent of the season. He routinely comforted himself by stroking a soft lambskin blanket, which he found soothing. Strikingly, he was drawn to articles of clothing with a restricted range of colors. Family vacations were nearly impossible, because the child would become extremely irritable and would have a tantrum when faced with the need to sleep in an unfamiliar bed. In particular, he was highly sensitive to the smell and texture of unfamiliar sheets and pillows. He openly expressed his discomfort with the unusual smell of the new setting of the hotel room and was unable to enjoy himself, appearing distressed and whining throughout the trip. The child's verbal skills were within normal limits for his chronologic age, and no core impairment in interpersonal relatedness was present. He was interested in same-age peers and expressed a desire to play with them but insisted on doing this at his own home. After a four-session dyadic evaluation, the diagnosis of a regulatory disorder was made, and the conclusion was that his behavioral dysregulation (e.g., tantrums) was precipitated by his extreme hypersensitivity. Previous clinicians had suggested the diagnosis of pervasive developmental disorder not otherwise specified (NOS); however, his parents felt strongly that he was simply a child with an extremely difficult temperament. (Courtesy of Joan Luby, M.D.)

K.S. was a 3-year-old Romanian girl who was adopted by her parents and brought to the United States from a Romanian orphanage at 8 months of age. No details of her biological family history or perinatal development were known. However, it was clear that conditions in the orphanage were not optimal and that K.S. had spent significant amounts of time in a crib in a room without windows and with little social stimulation. Although she displayed language and motor delays (some growth retardation) at the time of adoption, she made rapid developmental gains during the first 12 months in her new home. Although she appeared to be functioning well in her preschool overall, her parents had become concerned about her lack of spontaneous eye contact, extreme sensitivity, and hypervigilance to potentially frightening noises or events (e.g., sirens and thunderstorms), and the concern that she was not engaging in peer relationships in an age-appropriate manner. Both parents reported that she understood their roles as special caregivers; however, she was unusually friendly to strangers and would become highly engaging with every unfamiliar service person who came to the home.

During two play observations with each parent, it was noted that the child had a tendency to play alone and failed to engage spontaneously either parent in play, although she was responsive to parental overtures. Although she did seem open to, and was not avoidant of, physical contact (or displays of physical affection) with each parent, she did not spontaneously seek physical proximity. She demonstrated no apparent anxiety in engaging with the unfamiliar examiner and was no more inclined to engage a parent in play or to request assistance from a parent than from the examiner. Despite her adequate functioning in the preschool setting, her lack of significant social withdrawal, and the lack of extreme disinhibition (which prevent her from meeting criteria for a DSM-IV-TR reactive attachment disorder), it was determined that she had a clinically significant (but relatively less severe) form of an attachment disorder that was classified using the NOS category, which did require formal psychotherapeutic intervention. (Courtesy of Joan Luby, M.D.)

14

Mood Disorders and Suicide

▲ 14.1 Depressive Disorders and Suicide

Depressive disorders occur in children of all ages but are much more prevalent with increasing age. Children and adolescents with depressive disorders often display irritability, withdrawal from family and peers, and deterioration in academic investment, leading to devastating social isolation. The core features of major depressive disorder have striking similarities in children, adolescents, and adults, although developmental factors influence its clinical presentation.

Although suicidal thoughts and behaviors can occur in the context of a depressive disorder, most youth who contemplate, attempt, or complete suicide are not in the midst of a major depression. Most children and adolescents with depressive disorders do not exhibit suicidal behaviors. Thus, it is not clear that optimal treatments for depression mitigate the risks of suicidality among youth in general.

Mood disorders among children and adolescents have been increasingly recognized over the last three decades, and evidence suggests that combined treatment modalities, including medication and cognitive-behavioral strategies, may have the greatest efficacy. Although clinicians and parents have readily acknowledged transient sadness and despair among youth, it has become clear that the full criteria of persistent disorders of mood can occur even in prepubertal children. Two criteria for mood disorders in childhood and adolescence are a disturbance of mood, such as depression or elation, and irritability.

Although diagnostic criteria for mood disorders in the text revision of the fourth edition of the *Diagnostic and Statistical Manual of Mental Disorders* (DSM-IV-TR) are almost identical across all age groups, the expression of disturbed mood varies in children according to their age. Young, depressed children commonly show symptoms that appear less often as they grow older, including mood-congruent auditory hallucinations, somatic complaints, withdrawn and sad appearance, and poor self-esteem. Symptoms that are more common among depressed youngsters in late adolescence than in young childhood are pervasive anhedonia, severe psychomotor retardation, delusions, and a sense of hopelessness. Symptoms that appear with the same frequency, regardless of age and developmental status, include suicidal ideation, depressed or irritable mood, insomnia, and diminished ability to concentrate.

Developmental issues, however, influence the expression of all symptoms. For example, unhappy young children who exhibit recurrent suicidal ideation are rarely able to propose a realistic suicide plan or to carry out such a plan. Children's moods are especially vulnerable to the influences of severe social stressors, such as chronic family discord, abuse and neglect, and academic failure. Most young children with major depressive disorder have histories of abuse or neglect. Children with depressive disorders in the midst of toxic environments may have remission of some or many depressive symptoms when the stressors diminish or when the children are removed from the stressful environment. Bereavement often becomes a focus of psychiatric treatment when children have lost a loved one, even when a depressive disorder is not present.

Depressive disorders are generally episodic, although their onset may be insidious and remain unidentified until impairment in peer relationships, deterioration in academic function, or withdrawal from sports activities emerges. Attention-deficit/hyperactivity disorder (ADHD), oppositional defiant disorder, and conduct disorder can occur among children who later experience depression. In some cases, conduct disturbances or disorders occur in the context of a major depressive episode and resolve with the resolution of the depressive episode. Clinicians must clarify the chronology of the symptoms to determine whether a given behavior (e.g., poor concentration, defiance, or temper tantrums) was present before the depressive episode and is unrelated to it or whether the behavior is occurring for the first time and is related to the depressive episode.

EPIDEMIOLOGY

Depressive disorders increase in frequency with increasing age in the general population. Mood disorders among preschool-age children are extremely rare; the rate of major depressive disorder in preschoolers is estimated to be about 0.3 percent in the community and 0.9 percent in a clinic setting. Among prepubertal school-age children in the community, the point prevalence is approximately 1 percent. In referred samples of school-age children, depression is about the same in boys as in girls, with some surveys indicating a slightly increased rate among boys.

Among adolescents, reported rates of major depression range from 1 percent to about 6 percent in community samples, and the rate of depression among female adolescents is double the rate in male adolescents. Estimates of cumulative prevalence of depression among older adolescents range between 14 and 25 percent. Reported rates of dysthymic disorder are generally lower than those of major depressive disorder, with rates of 5 of 100,000 in prepubertal children, compared with 1 percent for major depressive disorder. School-age children with dysthymic disorder have a high likelihood of developing major depressive disorder at some point after 1 year of the dysthymic disorder. In adolescents, as in adults, dysthymic disorder is reported to occur in about 5 of 1,000 adolescents, compared with about 5 percent for major depressive disorder.

Among hospitalized children and adolescents, the rates of major depressive disorder are much higher than in the general community; of these, as many as 20 percent of children and 40 percent of adolescents are depressed.

ETIOLOGY

Considerable evidence indicates that the mood disorders in childhood are the same fundamental diseases experienced by adults.

Molecular Genetic Studies

Two genes have been identified as incurring vulnerability for depressive disorder. The first one, the MAOA gene, is responsible for the functioning of monoamine oxidase, and the second is the serotonin transporter gene (5-HTT). The serotonin transporter gene, which is involved in the process of making serotonin available, is present in homozygous long alleles; a heterozygous, one-long- and one-short-allele pair; and homozygous short alleles. A large longitudinal study in New Zealand found a relationship of early environmental stress and subsequent depression in children with one or two short alleles, but not in those children in the sample with two long alleles. Because the short alleles are less efficient in transcription, this finding suggests that the availability of the transporter gene may provide a marker for vulnerability to depression. Thus, a stress-diathesis model for the emergence of depression may best fit with the foregoing data.

Familiality. Mood disorders in children, adolescents, and adult patients tend to cluster in the same families. An increased incidence of mood disorders is generally found among children of parents with mood disorders and relatives of children with mood disorders; having one depressed parent probably doubles the risk for offspring. Having two depressed parents probably quadruples the risk of a child having a mood disorder before age 18 years compared with the risk for children with two unaffected parents. Some evidence indicates that the number of recurrences of parental depression increases the likelihood that the children will be affected, but this increase may be only partly related to the affective loading of the parent's own family tree. Similarly, children with the largest number of severe episodes have shown much evidence of dense and deep familial aggregation for major depressive disorder.

Biological Factors. Studies of prepubertal major depressive disorder and adolescent mood disorder have revealed a variety of biological abnormalities. For example, prepubertal children in an episode of depressive disorder secrete significantly more growth hormone during sleep than do normal children and those with nondepressed mental disorders. These children also secrete significantly less growth hormone in response to insulin-induced hypoglycemia than do nondepressed patients. Both abnormalities persist for at least 4 months of full, sustained clinical response, with the last month in a drug-free state. In contrast, the data conflict regarding cortisol hypersecretion during major depressive disorder; some workers report hypersecretion, whereas others report normal secretion.

Sleep studies are inconclusive in depressed children and adolescents. Polysomnography shows either no change or changes characteristic of adults with major depressive disorder: reduced rapid eye movement (REM) latency and an increased number of REM periods.

Magnetic Resonance Imaging. Magnetic resonance imaging (MRI) scans in more than 100 psychiatrically hospitalized children with mood disturbances report a low frontal lobe volume and a high ventricular volume. These results are consistent with MRI findings in adults with major depression insofar as postmortem studies of depressed adults have demonstrated selective loss of frontal lobe cells and frontal lobe serotonin. Damage to the frontal lobes has also been associated with depressive symptoms in patients after stroke. The frontal lobes seem to have multiple connections with the basal ganglia and the limbic system and are also believed to be involved in the neuropathology of depressive symptomatology.

Endocrine Studies. Thyroid hormone studies have found lower free total thyroxine (FT4) levels in depressed adolescents than in a matched control group. These values were associated with normal thyroid-stimulating hormone (TSH). This finding suggests that, although values of thyroid function remain in the normative range, FT4 levels have been shifted downward. These downward shifts in thyroid hormone possibly contribute to the clinical manifestations of depression. Some data suggest that the addition of exogenous thyroid hormone can potentiate the effects of antidepressant medication in adults with depression. Impairment in mood and cognitive function in adults with subclinical hypothyroidism has been found to be corrected with exogenous thyroid hormone.

Social Factors

The finding that identical twins do not have 100 percent concordance suggests a role for nongenetic factors in the emergence of major depressive disorder. Despite a lack of definitive evidence, given the stress-diathesis hypotheses of depression, genetic vulnerability in combination with a variety of social factors, including level of family conflict, abuse or neglect, family socioeconomic status, and parental separation or divorce, may play a significant role in the emergence of depressive disorders in children. Evidence indicates that boys whose fathers died before they were 13 years of age are at greater risk than controls to develop depression.

The psychosocial impairment that characterizes depressed children lingers far after recovery from the index episode of depression. These deficits can be compounded by the relatively long duration of at least 1 year for a dysthymic episode and an average of 9 months to 1 year for a depressive episode in a child or adolescent. For an adolescent, a major depressive episode significantly interferes with social and academic skills, which are poorly accomplished or unaccomplished during the episode. Among preschoolers with depressive clinical presentations, the role of environmental influences is likely to have a significant impact on the course and recovery of the young child.

DIAGNOSIS AND CLINICAL FEATURES

Major Depressive Disorder

Major depressive disorder in children is diagnosed most easily when it is acute and occurs in a child without previous psychiatric symptoms. Often, however, the onset is insidious, and the disorder occurs in a child who has had several years of difficulties with hyperactivity, separation anxiety disorder, or intermittent depressive symptoms.

According to the DSM-IV-TR diagnostic criteria for major depressive episode, at least five symptoms must be present for a period of 2 weeks, and there must be a change from previous functioning. Among the necessary symptoms is either a depressed or irritable mood or a loss of interest or pleasure. Other symptoms from which the other four diagnostic criteria are drawn include a child's failure to make expected weight gains, daily insomnia or hypersomnia, psychomotor agitation or retardation, daily fatigue or loss of energy, feelings of worthlessness or inappropriate guilt, diminished ability to think or concentrate, and recurrent thoughts of death. These symptoms must produce social or academic impairment. To meet the diagnostic criteria for major depressive disorder, the symptoms cannot be the direct effects of a substance (e.g., alcohol) or a general medical condition. A diagnosis of major depressive disorder is not made within 2 months of the loss of a loved one, except when marked functional impairment, morbid preoccupation with worthlessness, suicidal ideation, psychotic symptoms, or psychomotor retardation is present.

A major depressive episode in a prepubertal child is likely to be manifest by somatic complaints, psychomotor agitation, and mood-congruent hallucinations. Anhedonia is also frequent, but anhedonia, as well as hopelessness, psychomotor retardation, and delusions, are more common in adolescent and adult major depressive episodes than in those of young children. Adults have more problems with sleep and appetite than depressed children and adolescents. In adolescence, negativistic or frankly antisocial behavior and the use of alcohol or illicit substances can occur and may justify the additional diagnoses of oppositional defiant disorder, conduct disorder, and substance abuse or dependence. Feelings of restlessness, grouchiness, aggression, and sulkiness, reluctance to cooperate in family ventures, withdrawal from social activities, and a desire to leave home are all common in adolescent depression. School difficulties are likely. Adolescents may be inattentive to personal appearance and show increased emotionality, with particular sensitivity to rejection in love relationships.

Children can be reliable reporters about their own behavior, emotions, relationships, and difficulties in psychosocial functions. They may, however, refer to their feelings by many names. Clinicians, therefore, must ask children about feeling sad, empty, low, down, blue, or very unhappy; about feeling like crying or about having a bad feeling that is present most of the time. Depressed children usually identify one or more of these terms as their persistent feeling. Clinicians should assess the duration and periodicity of the depressive mood to differentiate relatively universal, short-lived, and sometimes frequent periods of sadness, usually after a frustrating event, from a true, persistent depressive mood. The younger the child, the more imprecise his or her time estimates are likely to be.

Mood disorders tend to be chronic if they begin early. Childhood onset may be the most severe form of mood disorder and tends to appear in families with a high incidence of mood disorders and alcohol abuse. The children are likely to have such secondary complications as conduct disorder, alcohol and other substance abuse, and antisocial behavior. Functional impairment associated with a depressive disorder in childhood extends to practically all areas of a child's psychosocial world; school performance and behavior, peer relationships, and family relationships all suffer. Only highly intelligent and academically oriented children with no more than a moderate depression can compensate for their difficulties in learning by substantially increasing their time and effort. Otherwise, school performance is invariably affected by a combination of difficulty concentrating, slowed thinking, lack of interest and motivation, fatigue, sleepiness, depressive ruminations, and preoccupations. Depression in a child may be misdiagnosed as a learning disorder. Learning problems secondary to depression, even when longstanding, are corrected rapidly after a child's recovery from the depressive episode.

Children and adolescents with major depressive disorder may have hallucinations and delusions. Usually, these psychotic symptoms are thematically consistent with the depressed mood, occur with the depressive episode (usually at its worst), and do not include certain types of hallucinations (such as conversing voices and a commenting voice, which are specific to schizophrenia). Depressive hallucinations usually consist of a single voice speaking to the person from outside his or her head, with derogatory or suicidal content. Depressive delusions center on themes of guilt, physical disease, death, nihilism, deserved punishment, personal inadequacy, and (sometimes) persecution. These delusions are rare in prepuberty, probably because of cognitive immaturity, but are present in about one half of psychotically depressed adolescents.

Adolescent onset of a mood disorder can be difficult to diagnose when first seen if the adolescent has attempted self-medication with alcohol or other illicit substances. In a recent study, 17 percent of young persons with a mood disorder first received medical attention because of substance abuse. Only after detoxification could the psychiatric symptoms be assessed properly and the mood disorder diagnosed correctly.

Dysthymic Disorder

Dysthymic disorder in children and adolescents consists of a depressed or irritable mood for most of the day, for more days than not, over a period of at least 1 year. DSM-IV-TR notes that in children and adolescents, irritable mood can replace the depressed mood criterion for adults, and that the duration criterion is not 2 years but 1 year for children and adolescents. According to the DSM-IV-TR diagnostic criteria, at least three of the following symptoms must accompany the depressed or irritable mood: poor self-esteem, pessimism or hopelessness, loss of interest, social withdrawal, chronic fatigue, feelings of guilt or brooding about the past, irritability or excessive anger, decreased activity or productivity, and poor concentration or memory. During the year of the disturbance, these symptoms do not resolve for more than 2 months at a time. In addition, the diagnostic criteria for dysthymic disorder specify that during the first year, no major depressive episode emerges. To meet the DSM-IV-TR diagnostic criteria for dysthymic disorder, a child must not have a history of a manic or hypomanic episode. Dysthymic disorder is also not diagnosed if the symptoms occur exclusively during a chronic psychotic disorder or if they are the direct effects of a substance or a general medical condition. The DSM-IV-TR provides for specification of early onset (before 21 years of age) or late onset (after 21 years of age).

A child or adolescent with dysthymic disorder may have had a major depressive episode before developing a dysthymic disorder, but it is much more common for a child with dysthymic disorder for more than 1 year to have a major depressive episode. In this case, both depressive diagnoses are given (double depression). Dysthymic disorder in children is known to have an average age of onset that is several years earlier than the age of onset of major depressive disorder. Controversy exists among clinicians and researchers about whether dysthymic disorder is best categorized as a chronic, insidious version of major depressive disorder or represents a separate disorder. Occasionally, young persons fulfill the criteria for dysthymic disorder, except that their episodes last only 2 weeks to several months, with symptom-free intervals lasting for 2 to 3 months. These minor mood presentations in children are likely to indicate severe mood disorder episodes in the future. Current knowledge suggests that the longer, the more recurrent, the more frequent, and perhaps the less related to social stress these episodes are, the greater is the likelihood of a severe mood disorder in the future. When minor depressive episodes follow a significant stressful life event by less than 3 months, it is often part of an adjustment disorder.

Cyclothymic Disorder

The only difference in the DSM-IV-TR diagnostic criteria for child or adolescent cyclothymic disorder is that a period of 1 year of numerous mood swings is necessary instead of the adult criterion of 2 years. Some adolescents with cyclothymic disorder probably experience bipolar I disorder.

Schizoaffective Disorder

The criteria for schizoaffective disorder in children and adolescents are identical to those in adults. Although some adolescents and probably some children fit the criteria for schizoaffective disorder, little is known about the natural course of their illness, family history, psychobiology, and treatment. In DSM-IV-TR, schizoaffective disorder in children is classified as a psychotic disorder.

Bereavement

Bereavement is a state of grief related to the death of a loved one, which can occur with symptoms characteristic of a major depressive episode. Typical depressive symptoms associated with bereavement include feelings of sadness, insomnia, diminished appetite, and, in some cases, weight loss. Grieving children may become withdrawn and appear sad, and they are not easily drawn into even favorite activities.

In the DSM-IV-TR, bereavement is not a mental disorder but is in the category of additional conditions that may be a focus of clinical attention. Children in the midst of a typical bereavement period may also meet the criteria for major depressive disorder when the symptoms persist longer than 2 months after the loss. In some instances, severe depressive symptoms within 2 months of the loss are considered to be beyond the scope of normal grieving, and a diagnosis of major depressive disorder is warranted. Symptoms indicating major depressive disorder exceeding usual bereavement include guilt related to issues beyond those surrounding the death of the loved one, preoccupation with death other than thoughts about being dead to be with the deceased person, morbid preoccupation with worthlessness, marked psychomotor retardation, prolonged serious functional impairment, and hallucinations other than transient perceptions of the voice of the deceased person.

The duration of a normal period of bereavement varies; in children, the duration may depend partly on the support system in place. For example, a child who must be removed from home because of the death of the only parent in the home may feel devastated and abandoned for a long time. Children who lose loved ones may feel that the death occurred because they were bad or did not perform as expected. The reaction to the loss of a loved one can be partly influenced by the child's being prepared for the death because of the person's chronic illness.

PATHOLOGY AND LABORATORY EXAMINATION

No single laboratory test is useful in making a diagnosis of a mood disorder. A screening test for thyroid function can rule out the possibility of an endocrinologic contribution to a mood disorder. Dexamethasone-suppression tests may be performed serially in cases of major depressive disorder to document whether an initial nonsuppressor becomes a suppressor with treatment or with resolution of the symptoms.

DIFFERENTIAL DIAGNOSIS

Substance-induced mood disorder can sometimes be differentiated from other mood disorders only after detoxification. Anxiety symptoms and conduct-disordered behavior can coexist with depressive disorders and frequently can pose problems in differentiating those disorders from nondepressed emotional and conduct disorders.

Of particular importance is the distinction between agitated depressive or manic episodes and ADHD, in which the persistent excessive activity and restlessness can cause confusion. Prepubertal children do not show classic forms of agitated depression, such as hand wringing and pacing. Instead, an inability to sit still and frequent temper tantrums are the most common symptoms. Sometimes, the correct diagnosis becomes evident only after remission of the depressive episode. If a child has no difficulty concentrating, is not hyperactive when recovered from a depressive episode, and is in a drug-free state, ADHD probably is not present.

COURSE AND PROGNOSIS

The course and prognosis of mood disorders in children and adolescents depend on the age of onset, episode severity, and presence of comorbid disorders. In most cases, younger age of onset, recurrent episodes, and comorbid disorders predict a poorer prognosis. The mean length of an episode of major depression in children and adolescents is about 9 months; the cumulative probability of recurrence is 40 percent by 2 years and 70 percent by 5 years. Reportedly, depressed children who live in families with high levels of chronic conflict are more likely to have relapses. Follow-up studies have found that in 20 to 40 percent of adolescents who have a major depression, bipolar I disorder will develop in a period of 5 years after the index depression. Clinical characteristics of the depressive episode that suggest the highest risk of developing bipolar I disorder include delusionality and psychomotor retardation in addition to a family history of bipolar illness. Depressive disorders are associated with short-term and long-term peer relationship difficulties and complications, poor academic achievement, and persistently poor self-esteem. Dysthymic disorder has an even more protracted recovery than major depression; the mean episode length is about 4 years. Early-onset dysthymic disorder is associated with significant risks of comorbidity with major depression (70 percent), bipolar disorder (13 percent), and eventual substance abuse (15 percent). The risk of suicide, which represents 12 percent of mortalities in the adolescent age range, is significant among adolescents with depressive disorders.

TREATMENT

Hospitalization

Safety is the most immediate consideration in evaluating a child or adolescent with major depression, and determining whether hospitalization is indicated to keep the child or adolescent safe becomes the first decision point. Children and adolescents who are depressed and express suicidal thoughts or behaviors need an extended evaluation in the hospital to provide maximal protection against the patient's self-destructive impulses and behavior. Hospitalization also may be needed when a child or adolescent has coexisting substance abuse or dependence.

Evidence-Based Treatments

The literature reflects evidence of efficacy of various treatments for childhood and adolescent depression based on randomized, placebo-controlled trials (RCTs) with various pharmacologic agents, RCTs comparing cognitive-behavioral therapy (CBT) with other psychosocial interventions, and one large multicenter trial that assessed the efficacy of combined CBT and a serotonin reuptake inhibitor with each of the aforementioned treatment strategies alone. This recent investigation, by the Treatment for Adolescents with Depression Study (TADS) Team (2004), divided 439 adolescents between the ages of 12 and 17 years into three treatment groups of 12 weeks: fluoxetine (Prozac) alone (10 to 40 mg per day), fluoxetine with the same dose range in combination with CBT, or CBT alone. Based on ratings of the Children's Depression Rating Scale-Revised (CDRS-R) and clinical global ratings, the group of depressed adolescents receiving the combination treatment had significantly superior response rates compared with either treatment alone. Based on clinical global improvement, rates of much or very much improvement were 71 percent for the group that received the combined treatment, 61 percent for the group that received fluoxetine, and 43 percent for the CBT alone. The placebo group had a 35 percent response rate. Thus, based on this large study, combination treatment appears to be the optimal strategy in the treatment of depression among youth.

Psychotherapy

Cognitive-behavioral therapy is widely recognized as an efficacious intervention for the treatment of moderately severe depression in children and adolescents. Cognitive-behavioral therapy aims to challenge maladaptive beliefs and enhance problem-solving abilities and social competence. A recent review of controlled cognitive-behavioral studies in children and adolescents revealed that, as with adults, both children and adolescents showed consistent improvement with these methods. Other "active" treatments, including relaxation techniques, were also shown to be helpful as adjunctive treatment for mild to moderate depression. Findings from one large controlled study comparing cognitive-behavioral interventions with nondirective supportive psychotherapy and systemic behavioral family therapy showed that 70 percent of adolescents had some improvement with each of the interventions; cognitive-behavioral intervention had the most rapid effect. Another controlled study comparing a brief course of CBT with relaxation therapy favored the cognitive-behavioral intervention. At a 3- to 6-month follow-up, however, no significant differences existed between the two treatment groups. This effect resulted from relapse in the cognitive-behavioral group, along with continued recovery in some patients in the relaxation group. Factors that seem to interfere with treatment responsiveness include the presence of comorbid anxiety disorder that probably was present before the depressive episode.

Family education and participation are necessary treatment components for children with depression, especially to promote more effective conflict resolution. Because the psychosocial function of depressed children can remain impaired for long periods, even after the depressive episode has remitted, long-term social support from families and (in some cases) social skills interventions are helpful. Modeling and role-playing techniques can be useful in fostering good problem-solving skills.

Pharmacotherapy

Pharmacologic agents from among the selective serotonin reuptake inhibitors (SSRIs) are widely accepted as first-line intervention for moderate to severe depressive disorders in children and adolescents. Acute randomized clinical trials have demonstrated the efficacy of fluoxetine, citalopram (Celexa), and sertraline (Zoloft) compared with placebo in the treatment of major depression in children and adolescents. In September 2004, the U.S. Food and Drug Administration (FDA) received information from their Psychopharmacologic Drug and Pediatric Advisory Committee indicating, based on their review of reported suicidal thoughts and behavior among depressed children and adolescents who participated in randomized clinical trials with nine different antidepressants, an increased risk of suicidality in those children on active antidepressant medications. Although no suicides were reported, the rates of suicidal thinking and behaviors were 2 percent for patients on placebo versus 4 percent among patients on antidepressant medications. The FDA, in accordance with the recommendation of their advisory committees, instituted a "black-box" warning for the health professional label of all antidepressant medications indicating the increased risk of suicidal thoughts and behaviors in children and adolescents being treated with antidepressant medications and the need for close monitoring for these symptoms.

Several reviews since then, however, have concluded that the data do not indicate a significant increase in the risk of suicide or serious suicide attempt after starting treatment with antidepressant drugs. Rather than a worsening effect, antidepressant use was associated with a protective effect against new-onset and ongoing suicidal ideation. One study showed that the rates of suicide attempts in patients treated with an antidepressant were one third of those observed for patients not treated with an antidepressant. A strongly worded editorial in the *Journal of the American Psychiatric Association* (July 2007) concluded, "It is much more likely that suicidal behavior leads to treatment than that treatment leads to suicidal behavior." There is pressure on the FDA to remove the black box warning, and if the evidence continues to mount, it is likely that this will happen. In the meantime, psychiatrists should not withhold antidepressant medication in suicidal children or adolescents. At the same time, they must remain vigilant and monitor their suicidal patients closely, regardless of the medication prescribed.

Fluoxetine is the only antidepressant that has FDA approval in the treatment of depression in children and adolescents. Common side effects observed with fluoxetine include headache, gastrointestinal symptoms, sedation, and insomnia.

Sertraline was shown to provide efficacy in two multicenter, double-blind, placebo-controlled trials of 376 children and adolescents who were treated with sertraline at doses that ranged from 50 to 200 mg per day or placebo. A response rate of greater than 40 percent decrease in depression rating scale scores was found in 69 percent of the patients treated with sertraline and 56 percent of the placebo group. Most common side effects are anorexia, vomiting, diarrhea, and agitation.

Citalopram was demonstrated in one RCT in the United States to be efficacious in 174 children and adolescents treated at doses of 20 to 40 mg per day or placebo for 8 weeks. Significantly more of the group on citalopram showed improvement compared with the placebo group on the depression rating scale (CDRS-R). A significantly increased response rate (response defined as less than 28 on CDRS-R) of 35 percent was found in the citalopram group, compared with 24 percent in the placebo group. Common side effects included headache, nausea, insomnia, rhinitis, abdominal pain, dizziness fatigue, and flu-like symptoms.

Similar to the literature for adult depression, as many negative as positive study findings have emerged in RCTs of the treatment of childhood and adolescent depression. RCTs that have not shown efficacy on primary outcome measures include those using paroxetine (Paxil), escitalopram (Lexapro), venlafaxine (Effexor), mirtazapine (Remeron), nefazodone (Serzone), and tricyclic antidepressants.

Bupropion (Wellbutrin) has demonstrated efficacy in adult depressed populations but has not been studied in a randomized, placebo-controlled trial of depression among children and adolescents. Starting doses of SSRIs for prepubertal children are lower than doses recommended for adults, and adolescents are generally treated at the same doses recommended for adults.

When first-line SSRI medications have not led to improvement, other antidepressant agents have been used clinically, although without proved efficacy. For example, bupropion has stimulant properties as well as antidepressant efficacy and has been used for youth with both ADHD and depression. It has few anticholinergic properties or other adverse effects such as sedation. Venlafaxine, which blocks both serotonin and norepinephrine uptake, has been used clinically in the treatment of depression in adolescents. Adverse effects are usually mild and include agitation, nervousness, and nausea. Mirtazapine is also a serotonin and norepinephrine uptake inhibitor with a relatively safe adverse-effect profile, but it has not been used as frequently because of its adverse effect of sedation.

Tricyclic antidepressants are not generally recommended for the treatment of depression in children and adolescents because of the lack of proved efficacy along with the potential risk of cardiac arrhythmia associated with their use.

One possible outcome of treating a depressed child or adolescent with an antidepressant agent is the emergence of behavioral activation or induction of hypomanic symptoms. In these cases, the medication should be discontinued to determine whether the activation resolves with discontinuation of the medication or evolves into a hypomanic or manic episode. Hypomanic symptom responses to antidepressants, however, do not necessarily predict that bipolar disorder has emerged.

Table 14.1–1 lists drugs used in the treatment of major depression in children and adolescents.

Duration of Treatment

Based on longitudinal data and the natural history of major depression in children and adolescents, recommendations include maintaining antidepressant treatment for 1 year in a depressed child who has achieved a good response and then discontinuing the medication at a time of relatively low stress for a medication-free period.

Pharmacologic Treatment Strategies for Resistant Depression

Based on the available data, pharmacologic recommendations, taking into account a consensus panel for the Texas Children's Medication Algorithm Project (TMAP), are to treat first with one of the SSRIs alone and, if no response occurs within a reasonable amount of time—perhaps, up to 3 months—change to another SSRI medication. If a child is not responsive to the second SSRI medication, then either a combination of antidepressants or augmentation strategies may be reasonable choices, as well as an antidepressant from another class of medications.

Electroconvulsive Therapy. Electroconvulsive therapy (ECT) has been used for a variety of psychiatric illnesses in adults—primarily severe depressive and manic mood disorders and catatonia. ECT rarely is used for adolescents, although published case reports indicate its efficacy in adolescents with depression and mania. Case reports suggest that ECT may be a relatively safe and useful treatment for adolescents who have persistent severe affective disorders, particularly with psychotic features, catatonic symptoms, or persistent suicidality.

SUICIDE

In the United States, suicide is the second-leading cause of death among adolescents, topped by accidental death and homicide. In all countries, suicide rarely occurs in children who have not reached puberty. In the last 15 years, the rates of both completed suicide and suicidal ideation have decreased among adolescents. This decrease appears to coincide with the increase in SSRI medications prescribed to adolescents with mood and behavioral disturbance. Suicidal ideation, gestures, and attempts are frequently, but not always, associated with depressive disorders. Reports indicate that as many as half of suicidal individuals express suicidal intentions to a friend or a relative within 24 hours before enacting suicidal behavior.

Suicidal ideation occurs in all age groups and with greatest frequency in children and adolescents with severe mood disorders. More than 12,000 children and adolescents are hospitalized in the United States each year because of suicidal threats or behavior, but completed suicide is rare in children younger than 12 years of age. A young child is hardly capable of designing and carrying out a realistic suicide plan. Cognitive immaturity seems to play a protective role in preventing even children who wish they were dead from committing suicide. Completed suicide occurs about five times more often in adolescent boys than in girls, although the rate of suicide attempts is at least three times higher among adolescent girls than among boys. Suicidal ideation is not a static phenomenon; it can wax and wane with time. The decision to engage in suicidal behavior may be made impulsively without much forethought, or the decision may be the culmination of prolonged rumination.

The method of the suicide attempt influences the morbidity and completion rates, independent of the severity of the intent to die at the time of the suicidal behavior. The most common method of completed suicide in children and adolescents is the use of firearms, which accounts for about two thirds of all suicides in boys and almost one half of suicides in girls. The second-most-common method of suicide in boys, occurring in about one fourth of all cases, is hanging; in girls, about one fourth commit suicide through ingestion of toxic substances. Carbon monoxide poisoning is the next-most-common method of suicide in boys, but it occurs in less than 10 percent; suicide by hanging and

Table 14.1–1
Pharmacotherapy for Children and Adolescents with Major Depression (MDD)

Generic Name	U.S. Trade Name	How Supplied (mg caps/tabs, intramuscular [IM] or liquid in mg/mL)	Half-Life (hrs)	Starting Dose (mg)	Target Dose (mg/day)	Side Effects	Precautions and Notes of Efficacy in Published Trials
Selective serotonin reuptake inhibitors (SSRIs)							
Fluoxetine	Prozac	10, 20, 40; 20 mg/5 mL	24–72 (acute); 96–144 (chronic)	10 (2.5–10 preadolescent)	20–60	Gastrointestinal symptoms, restlessness, diaphoresis, headaches, akathisia, decrease or increase in appetite, sleep changes (e.g., vivid dreams, nightmares, and impaired sleep), and decrease in libido **Serious (rare):** prolonged QT interval, hyponatremia, seizure, serotonin syndrome, increased suicidal ideation or behavior	Only FDA approved antidepressant to treat MDD in children younger than 7 years; three positive placebo-controlled clinical trials demonstrating efficacy; contraindicated with concomitant use of MAOIs or within 2 weeks of MAOI use (for all SSRIs)
Sertraline	Zoloft	25, 50, 100; 20 mg/mL	26	25 (12.5–25, preadolescent)	50–200	Same as fluoxetine	Ten percent separation between treatment and placebo groups; one of two trials positive for efficacy compared to placebo
Citalopram	Celexa	10, 20, 40; 10 mg/5 mL	35	10 (2.5–10 preadolescent)	20–40	Same as fluoxetine, flu-like, rhinitis, nausea, abdominal pain, fatigue, diarrhea, back pain	High drop-out rate when studied in inpatient with outpatient; one trial positive for efficacy compared to placebo
Escitalopram	Lexapro	5, 10, 20; 5 mg/5 mL	27–32	10	10–20	Same as fluoxetine	No published safety or efficacy data in more than 18 years
Paroxetine	Paxil	10, 20, 30, 40; 10 mg/5 mL	21–26	10 (2.5–10 preadolescent)	20–50	Same as fluoxetine, nausea, dizziness, dry mouth, somnolence	Negative outcome based on Hamilton Depression Rating Scale (HAM-D) scores but positive on secondary outcome measures (Clinical Global Impression-Improvement scale, CGI-1
Fluvoxamine	Luvox	25, 50, 100	15.6	25 (12.5–25 preadolescent)	50–300	Same as fluoxetine	No randomized, controlled trial on safety or efficacy in more than 18 years
Tricyclic antidepressants (TCAs)							
Amitriptyline	Elavil	10, 25, 50, 75, 100, 150; 10 mg/mL IM	15	25–50 (1–3 mg/kg/day divided three times daily [preadolescent])	100	Weight change, bloating, constipation, appetite loss, nausea, dry mouth, asthenia, dizziness, headache, somnolence, blurred vision, fatigue **Serious (rare):** cardiac dysrhythmia, myocardial infarction, sudden death, agranulocytosis, drug-induced eosinophilia, purpura, thrombocytopenia, decreased liver function, jaundice, stroke, worsening depression/suicidal ideation, seizure	Not significantly better than placebo; contraindicated with concomitant use of MAOIs or within 2 weeks of MAOI use (for all TCAs); ECG in patients with cardiac disease or hyperthyroidism
Nortriptyline	Pamelor	10, 25, 50, 75; 10 mg/5 mL	18	1–3 mg/kg/day divided in 3 or 4 doses	150	Same as amitriptyline	Not significantly better than placebo; same monitoring as amitriptyline

(*continued*)

Table 14.1–1 (Continued)

Generic Name	U.S. Trade Name	How Supplied (mg caps/tabs, intramuscular [IM] or liquid in mg/mL)	Half-Life (hrs)	Starting Dose (mg)	Target Dose (mg/day)	Side Effects	Precautions and Notes of Efficacy in Published Trials
Imipramine	Tofranil	10, 25, 50; 12.5 mg/mL IM	19	25–50 (1.5–5 mg/kg/day divided [preadolescent])	200	Same as amitriptyline	Not significantly better than placebo; ECG, monitor white blood cell count and differential cells in patients with fever, sore throat, signs of infection
Desipramine	Norpramin	10, 25, 50, 75, 100, 150	21–23	25–50 (1–3 mg/kg/day [preadolescent])	100–150	Same as amitriptyline	No randomized, controlled trial on safety or efficacy in more than 18 years; same monitoring as imipramine
Selective norepinephrine reuptake inhibitors (SNRI)							
Venlafaxine XR	Effexor XR	37.5, 75, 150	11	37.5	75 to 225	Tachycardia, hypertension, sweating, weight loss, loss of appetite, nausea, constipation, dizziness, headache, insomnia, somnolence, blurred vision, abnormal ejaculation **Serious (rare):** hyponatremia, hepatitis, neuroleptic malignant syndrome, seizure	Medication superior to placebo seen in adolescents but not in children
Other							
Trazodone	Desyrel	50, 100, 150, 300	3–6	25–50 (1.5–2 mg/kg/day divided [preadolescent])	100–150	Sedation, sweating, weight change, constipation, diarrhea, nausea, dizziness, headache, insomnia, lethargy, memory impairment, blurred vision **Serious (rare):** priapism in males, cardiac dysrhythmia, blood pressure change, hemolytic anemia, seizure	Not significantly better than placebo
Nefazodone	Serzone	50, 100, 150, 200, 250	2 to 4	100	600	Similar to trazodone; increased frequency of cough **Serious (rare):** orthostatic hypotension, fatal hepatic failure, seizure	Taken off the market because of one case of liver failure; not significantly better than placebo; contraindicated with MAOI therapy within 14 days
Mirtazapine	Remeron	7.5, 15, 30, 45	20–40 (greater in females than in males)	7.5–15	45	Sedation, increased appetite, weight gain, hypercholesterolemia, hypertriglyceridemia, constipation, increased liver function tests, dizziness **Serious (rare):** agranulocytosis, neurotropenia, seizure	Not significantly better than placebo; monitor CBC and lipid panel; contraindicated with MAOI therapy within 14 days
Bupropion SR	Wellbutrin SR	100, 150, 200	29	150	300	Hypertension, tachycardia, rash, urticaria, weight change, nausea, constipation, dry mouth, arthralgia/myalgia, headache, insomnia, dizziness, confusion, tremor, tinnitus **Serious (rare):** cardiac dysrhythmia, Stevens-Johnson syndrome, anaphylaxis, seizure	No published safety or efficacy data in more than 18 years; contraindicated with MAOI therapy within 14 days; contraindicated with presence of seizure disorder
Bupropion XL	Wellbutrin XL	150, 300	37	150	450	Same as bupropion SR	Same as Bupropion SR

CBC, complete blood count; ECG, electrocardiogram; FDA, U.S. Food and Drug Administration; MAOI, monoamine oxidase inhibitor.
Note: Children younger than 12 years may need lower doses than indicated.

carbon monoxide poisoning are equally frequent among girls and account for about 10 percent each. Additional risk factors in suicide include a family history of suicidal behavior, exposure to family violence, impulsivity, substance abuse, and availability of lethal methods.

Epidemiology

Suicide rates in the year 2000 among boys and girls 10 to 14 years of age were 2.3 and 0.6 per 100,000, whereas among late adolescent boys and girls the rates increased to 13.2 and 2.8 per 100,000. Large surveys indicate that, although up to 20 percent of high school students in the United States have experienced suicidal ideation and 10 percent have exhibited suicidal behaviors, only about 2 percent of adolescents who attempt suicide come to medical attention. In the last 15 years, the rates of both completed suicide and suicidal ideation have decreased.

The rate for suicide depends on age and increases significantly after puberty. Whereas less than 1 per 100,000 completed suicide occurs in persons younger than 14 years of age, about 10 per 100,000 completed suicides occur in adolescents between 15 and 19 years of age. In adolescents younger than 14 years of age, suicide attempts are at least 50 times more common than suicide completions. Between 15 and 19 years of age, however, the rate of suicide attempts is about 15 times greater than the rate of suicide completions. The number of adolescent suicides over the last several decades has tripled to quadrupled.

Etiology

Universal features in adolescents who resort to suicidal behaviors are the inability to synthesize viable solutions to ongoing problems and the lack of coping strategies to deal with immediate crises. Therefore, a narrow view of the options available to deal with recurrent family discord, rejection, or failure contributes to a decision to commit suicide.

Genetic Factors. Completed suicide and suicidal behavior are two to four times more likely to occur in individuals with a first-degree family member with similar behavior. Evidence of a genetic contribution to suicidal behavior is based on family suicide risk studies and the higher concordance for suicide among monozygotic twins than dizygotic twins.

Biological Factors. Recent studies have documented a reduction in the density of serotonin transporter receptors in the prefrontal cortex and serotonin receptors among individuals with suicidal behaviors. Neurochemical findings show some overlap between persons with aggressive, impulsive behaviors and those who complete suicide. Low levels of serotonin and its major metabolite, 5-hydroxyindoleacetic acid (5-HIAA), have been found postmortem in the brains of persons who completed suicide. Low levels of 5-HIAA have been found in the cerebrospinal fluid of depressed persons who attempted suicide by violent methods. Alcohol and other psychoactive substances may lower 5-HIAA levels, perhaps by increasing the vulnerability for suicidal behavior in an already predisposed person. Low serotonin may turn out to be a marker, rather than a cause, of aggression and suicidal propensity, influencing behavioral responses to stress.

Psychosocial Factors. Although major depressive illness is the most significant risk factor for suicide, increasing its risk by 20 percent, many severely depressed individuals are not suicidal. Various features, including a sense of hopelessness, impulsivity, recurrent substance use, and a history of aggressive behavior, have been associated with an increase risk of suicide. A wide range of psychopathologic symptoms can result from exposure to violent and abusive homes. Aggressive, self-destructive, and suicidal behaviors seem to occur with greatest frequency among youth who have endured chronically stressful family lives. Large community studies have provided data suggesting that sexual orientation is a risk factor, with increased rates of suicidal behavior of two to six times among youth who identify themselves as gay, lesbian, or bisexual. The mechanisms of this correlation are unknown; however, this population of adolescents has higher rates of depressive disorders, as well as of substance use disorders, which may contribute to this relationship.

Diagnosis and Clinical Features

The characteristics of adolescents who attempt suicide and those who complete suicides are similar, and as many as 40 percent of suicidal persons have made a previous attempt. Direct questioning of children and adolescents about suicidal thoughts is necessary because studies have consistently shown that parents are frequently unaware of such ideas in their children. Suicidal thoughts (i.e., children talking about wanting to harm themselves) and suicidal threats (e.g., children stating that they want to jump in front of a car) are more common than suicide completion.

Most suicidal youth meet diagnostic criteria for one or more psychiatric disorders, which often include major depressive disorder, manic episodes, and psychotic disorders. Those with mood disorders in combination with substance abuse and a history of aggressive behavior are particularly at high risk. Those without mood disorders who are violent, aggressive, and impulsive may be susceptible to suicide during family or peer conflicts. High levels of hopelessness, poor problem-solving skills, and a history of aggressive behavior are risk factors for suicide. Depression alone is a more serious risk factor for suicide in girls than in boys, but boys often have more severe psychopathology than girls who commit suicide. The profile of an adolescent who commits suicide is occasionally one of high achievement and perfectionistic character traits; such an adolescent may have been humiliated recently by a perceived failure, such as diminished academic performance.

In psychiatrically disturbed and vulnerable adolescents, suicide attempts typically are related to recent stressors. The precipitants of suicidal behavior include conflicts and arguments with family members and boyfriends or girlfriends. Alcohol and other substance use can further predispose an already vulnerable adolescent to suicidal behavior. In other cases, an adolescent attempts suicide in anticipation of punishment after being caught by the police or other authority figures for a forbidden behavior.

About 40 percent of youthful persons who complete suicide had previous psychiatric treatment, and about 40 percent had made a previous suicide attempt. A child who has lost a parent by any means before age 13 years is at high risk for mood disorders and suicide. The precipitating factors include loss of face with peers, a broken romance, school difficulties, unemployment, bereavement, separation, and rejection. Clusters of suicides among adolescents who know one another and go to the same school have been reported. Suicidal behavior can precipitate other such attempts within a peer group through identification—so-called copycat suicides. Some studies have found an increase in adolescent suicide after television programs in which the main theme was the suicide of a teenager. In general, however, many other factors are involved, including a necessary substrate of psychopathology.

One recent study investigated two clusters of teenage suicide in Texas. The researchers found that indirect exposure to suicide through the media was not significantly associated with suicide. Factors that were associated included previous suicidal threats or attempts, self-injury, exposure to someone who had died violently, recent romantic breakups, and a high frequency of moves and changes in schools attended and parental figures lived with.

The tendency of disturbed young persons to imitate highly publicized suicides has been called the *Werther syndrome*, after the protagonist in Johann Wolfgang von Goethe's novel, *The Sorrows of Young Werther*. The novel, in which the hero kills himself, was banned in some European countries after its publication more than 200 years ago because of a rash of suicides by young men who read it; some dressed like Werther before killing themselves or left the book open at the passage describing his death. In general, although imitation may play a role in the timing of suicide attempts by vulnerable adolescents, the overall suicide rate does not seem to increase when media exposure increases.

Treatment

The prognostic significance of suicidal behavior among adolescents ranges from relatively benign to heralding a grave risk of completed suicide. Adolescents who come to medical attention because of suicidal attempts must be evaluated before determining whether hospitalization is necessary. Those who fall into high-risk groups should be hospitalized until the acute suicidality is no longer present. Persons at high risk include those who have made previous suicide attempts; boys older than 12 years of age with histories of aggressive behavior or substance abuse; those who have made an attempt with a lethal method, such as a gun or a toxic ingested substance; those with major depressive disorder characterized by social withdrawal, hopelessness, and a lack of energy; girls who have run away from home, are pregnant, or have made an attempt with a method other than ingesting a toxic substance; and any person who exhibits persistent suicidal ideation. A child or an adolescent with suicidal ideation must be hospitalized if a clinician has any doubt about the family's ability to supervise the child or to cooperate with treatment in an outpatient setting. In such a situation, child protective services must be involved before the child can be discharged. When adolescents with suicidal ideation report that they are no longer suicidal, discharge can be considered only after a complete discharge plan is in place.

Relatively few adolescents evaluated for suicidal behavior in a hospital emergency room subsequently engage in ongoing psychiatric treatment. Factors that may increase the probability of psychiatric interventions include initiating psychoeducation for the family in the emergency room, diffusing acute family conflict, and setting up an outpatient follow-up during the emergency room visit. Frequent emergency room discharge plans include a written contract with the adolescent, outlining the adolescent's agreement not to engage in suicidal behavior and providing an alternative if suicidal ideation reoccurs, and a telephone hot-line number provided to the adolescent and the family in case suicidal ideation reappears.

Scant data exist to evaluate the efficacy of psychotherapy in reducing suicidal behavior among adolescents. Cognitive-behavioral therapy has been shown to be effective in the treatment of depression among adolescents; however, no evidence is available to assess its efficacy in preventing suicidal behavior per se. Dialectical behavior therapy (DBT), a long-term behavioral intervention that can be applied to individuals or groups of patients, has been shown to reduce suicidal behavior in adults but has yet to be investigated in adolescents. Components of DBT include mindfulness training to improve self-acceptance, assertiveness training, instruction on avoiding situations that may trigger self-destructive behavior, and increasing the ability to tolerate psychologic distress. This approach warrants investigation among adolescents.

Pharmacotherapy. Pharmacologic efficacy in the treatment of suicidal behavior has been shown in adults with depression and cluster B personality with SSRI antidepressants and in suicidal adults with bipolar disorder using lithium.

In children and adolescents with major depression, fluoxetine, citalopram, and sertraline have all been shown to have efficacy through randomized clinical trials; however, pharmacologic interventions targeting suicidal behavior have not been investigated in this population. Given the reduction in completed suicide among adolescents over the last decade during the same period in which SSRI antidepressant treatment in this population has markedly risen, it is possible that SSRI antidepressants have been instrumental in this effect. As mentioned earlier, close monitoring for suicidality is mandatory for any child or adolescent being treated with antidepressants.

▲ 14.2 Early-Onset Bipolar Disorders

Bipolar I disorder is being diagnosed with increasing frequency in prepubertal children, with the caveat that "classic" manic episodes are uncommon in this age group, even when depressive symptoms have already appeared. Because few prepubertal children with features of depression and mania or hypomania exhibit discrete mood "cycles," that these children satisfy diagnostic criteria for bipolar disorder remains controversial. These "atypical" manic episodes among prepubertal children are sometimes associated with family histories of classic bipolar I disorder. Features of the mood and behavior disturbances among prepubertal children who are currently diagnosed with bipolar disorder by some clinicians include extreme mood variability, intermittent aggressive behavior, high levels of distractibility, and poor attention span. This constellation of mood and behavior disturbance is often not clearly episodic but is fluctuating and appears to be less responsive to mood-stabilizing agents than classic episodes of depression or mania in older adolescents and adults. Children with atypical hypomanic episodes often have past histories of severe attention-deficit/hyperactivity disorder (ADHD), making the diagnosis of bipolar disorder even more complicated. In general, families with many relatives with ADHD do not have family histories with an increased rate of bipolar I disorder. Children with atypical bipolar disorder function poorly, often require hospitalization, exhibit symptoms of depression, and often have a history of ADHD. How many of these children will develop discrete mood cycling as they mature or whether their clinical pictures will remain consistent over time remains under investigation.

Among adults and older adolescents, a major depressive episode typically precedes a manic episode in the natural evolution of bipolar I disorder. A classic manic episode in an adolescent emerges as a distinct departure from a preexisting state often characterized by grandiose and paranoid delusions and hallucinatory phenomena. According to the text revision of the fourth edition of the *Diagnostic and Statistical Manual of Mental Disorders* (DSM-IV-TR), the diagnostic criteria for a manic episode are the same for children and adolescents as for adults. The diagnostic criteria for a manic episode include a distinct period of an abnormally elevated, expansive, or irritable mood that lasts at least 1 week or for any duration if hospitalization is necessary. In addition, during periods of mood disturbance, at least three of the following significant and persistent symptoms must be present: inflated self-esteem or grandiosity, decreased need for sleep, pressure to talk, flight of ideas or racing thoughts, distractibility, an increase in goal-directed activity, and excessive involvement in pleasurable activities that may result in painful consequences. The mood disturbance suffices to cause marked impairment, and it is not caused by the direct effect of a substance or a general medical condition. Thus, manic states precipitated by somatic medications (e.g., antidepressants) cannot be interpreted as indicating a diagnosis of bipolar I disorder.

When mania appears in an adolescent, there is a higher incidence of psychotic features than occurs in adults, and hospitalization is often necessary. Delusions and hallucinations of adolescents may involve grandiose notions about their power, worth, knowledge, family, or relationships. Persecutory delusions and flight of ideas are common. Overall, gross impairment of reality testing is common in adolescent manic episodes. In adolescents with major depressive disorder destined for bipolar I disorder, those at highest risk have family histories of bipolar I disorder and exhibit acute, severe depressive episodes with psychosis, hypersomnia, and psychomotor retardation.

EPIDEMIOLOGY

The prevalence of early-onset bipolar disorder is rare based on the diagnostic criteria in the DSM-IV-TR. Epidemiologic studies in older adolescents have reported lifetime prevalence of bipolar I and II disorders to be approximately 1 percent. A recent epidemiologic survey of current illness in children younger than 13 years of age found no cases of classic bipolar illness.

The most valid diagnosis for prepubertal children with mood lability, extreme irritability, or rapid mood cycling is controversial. Among adults with bipolar disorder, the 20 to 30 percent who exhibit "mixed mania" are most likely to have a chronic course, absence of discrete episodes, higher risk of suicidal behavior, onset of the disorder in childhood and adolescence, neuropsychologic features similar to those in children with ADHD, and show a poorer response to treatment. These phenomenologic features appear to be similar to the clinical presentation of the prepubertal children who are more frequently being described as having atypical bipolar disorders. Longitudinal studies are warranted to determine whether children with early-onset atypical bipolar disorders become adults with bipolar disorders with mixed mania.

ETIOLOGY

Genetic Factors

Family studies consistently demonstrate that offspring of a parent with bipolar I disorder have a 25 percent chance of having a mood disorder, and offspring of two parents with bipolar disorder have a 50 to 75 percent risk of developing a mood disorder. The high rates of comorbid ADHD among children with early-onset bipolar disorder has led to questions regarding the co-transmission of these disorders in family members. Offspring of parents with bipolar disorder have been found to have higher rates of ADHD than controls. In first-degree relatives of children with bipolar disorder, ADHD occurs with the same rate as in first-degree relatives of children with ADHD only. The combination of ADHD and bipolar disorder was not found as frequently in relatives of children with ADHD only, however, compared with first-degree relatives of children with the combination. These results suggest that childhood bipolar disorder may be distinguished as a subtype of bipolar disorder that emerges in children whose family histories are heavily loaded for bipolar disorder and psychiatric comorbidities, such as ADHD.

Neurobiologic Factors

The neurobiology of early-onset bipolar disorder is in its infancy, although an area of current investigation. Although brain volume reaches about 90 percent of its adult size by age 6 years, according to work done by J. N. Giedd, increasing white matter over the next 20 years has been shown using magnetic resonance imaging (MRI). The few studies with children with bipolar disorder suggest a dysfunction in neural circuitry in the amygdala, striatal, thalamic, and prefrontal structures of the brain.

Neuropsychologic Studies

A growing body of evidence suggests that children and adolescents with bipolar disorder make a greater number of emotion recognition errors than controls. Their overreporting of faces as "angry" occurred when they were presented with adult faces, whereas these errors did not occur when they were shown children's faces. Impaired perception of facial expression has also been reported in studies of adults with bipolar disorder. Preliminary data suggest that, on tasks of working memory, processing speed, and attention, children and adolescents with comorbid bipolar disorder and ADHD demonstrated more pronounced impairments than those without ADHD. Very preliminary findings suggest similarities between neuropsychologic profiles of child, adolescent, and adult bipolar disorder.

DIAGNOSIS AND CLINICAL FEATURES

Early-onset bipolar disorder is characterized by extreme irritability that is severe and persistent and may include aggressive outbursts and violent behavior. Between outbursts, children with this syndrome may continue to be angry or dysphoric. Occasionally, a child with early-onset bipolar disorder may exhibit grandiose thoughts or euphoric mood; for the most part, children with this disorder are predominantly intensely emotional with a fluctuating but overriding negative mood. Diagnostic criteria for bipolar disorders in children and adolescents in the DSM-IV-TR are the same as those used in adults. The clinical picture of early-onset bipolar disorder, however, is complicated by the prevalent comorbid psychiatric disorders.

Comorbidity with ADHD

One of the main sources of diagnostic confusion regarding children with early-onset bipolar disorder is the comorbid ADHD, which is present in 60 to 90 percent of cases. One of the reasons for the vast concurrence of these two disorders is that they share many diagnostic criteria, including distractibility, hyperactivity, and talkativeness. Even when the overlapping symptoms were removed from the diagnostic count, 89 percent of children with bipolar disorder continued to meet the full criteria for ADHD. This implies that both disorders with their own distinct features are present in many cases.

Comorbidity with Conduct Disorder

Rates of comorbid conduct disorder have been found to range from 48 to 69 percent among children and adolescents with bipolar disorder. Joseph Biederman found that the two manic symptoms more common in the comorbid group than in the bipolar-only group were *physical restlessness* and *poor judgment*.

Comorbidity with Anxiety Disorders

Children and adolescents with bipolar disorder have been reported to have higher-than-expected rates of panic and other anxiety disorders. Lifetime prevalence of panic disorder was found to be 21 percent among patients with bipolar disorder, compared with 0.8 percent in those without mood disorders. Patients with bipolar disorder with high levels of anxiety symptoms were reported to abuse alcohol and exhibit suicidal behavior.

PATHOLOGY AND LABORATORY EXAMINATION

No specific laboratory indices are helpful in making the diagnosis of bipolar disorders among children and adolescents.

DIFFERENTIAL DIAGNOSIS

A consensus of research studies in children diagnosed with early-onset bipolar disorder suggests that between 80 and 90 percent also meet diagnostic criteria for ADHD. Among youth with adolescent onset of mania, rates of ADHD have been found to be 60 percent, a rate that is markedly increased compared with controls. Although childhood ADHD tends to have its onset earlier than pediatric mania, evidence from family studies supports the presence of ADHD and bipolar disorders as highly comorbid in children, and the concurrence is not because of the overlapping symptoms that the two disorders share. In a recent study by S. Faraone and colleagues of more than 300 children and adolescents who attended a psychopharmacology clinic and received a diagnosis of ADHD, bipolar disorder was also evident in almost one third of those children with ADHD who had combined type and hyperactive types and occurred with much less frequency (i.e., in less than 10 percent) in children with ADHD, inattentive type.

COURSE AND PROGNOSIS

It is not known whether early-onset bipolar disorders have the same natural history over time as bipolar disorders with an onset during adolescence or early adulthood. Current investigations of

Table 14.2–1
Pharmacotherapy for Children and Adolescents with Bipolar Disorder (BPD)

Generic Name	U.S. Trade Name	How Supplied (mg)	Half-Life (hrs)	Pediatric Starting Dose (mg/kg)	Target Dose	Associated Side Effects	Precautions
Lithium	Lithobid	150, 300, 600	18	30 daily	Serum level of 0.8–1.2 mEq/L	Abnormal ECG, diarrhea, nausea/vomiting, muscle weakness, fine tremor, hyperreflexia, sedation, visual field scotoma, albuminuria, glycosuria, polyuria, hypothyroidism, acne **Serious (rare):** cardiac dysrhythmia, diabetes insipidus, tinnitus, blurred vision, ataxia, coma, pseudotumor cerebi, seizure, Ebstein's anomaly if fetal exposure in first trimester	Monitor complete blood count, creatinine, pregnancy status, thyroid function, blood urea nitrogen, urinalysis, and serum calcium biannually to quarterly; avoid in first trimester (Epstein anomaly); contraindicated if breastfeeding. **Signs of toxicity:** diarrhea, vomiting, tremor, mild ataxia, drowsiness, or muscular weakness and lack of coordination may be seen at concentrations <2 mEq/L
Valproate	Depakote	250, 500, liquid	8–16	20 daily	Serum level of 80–120 μg/mL	Alopecia, thrombocytopenia, liver toxicity, pancreatitis, polycystic ovary syndrome; seizures possible at higher doses	Monitor liver function test, complete blood counts, pregnancy status, and valproate levels; check baseline ECG and as doses increase
Clozapine	Clozaril	25, 100	12	25 twice daily	200–400	Weight gain/metabolic syndrome; agranulocytosis; cardiotoxicity	Monitor white blood cells weekly; avoid smoking (decreases levels); monitor metabolic parameters: fasting glucose, fasting lipid profile, body mass index, waist circumference, and blood pressure
Olanzapine	Zyprexa	2.5, 5, 7.5, 10, 15, 20 (Zydis 5)	30	2.5 twice daily	10–20	Weight gain/metabolic syndrome; hypotension with EtOH or benzodiazepines (IV)	Monitor weight, cholesterol; monitor metabolic parameters as in clozapine; assess for orthostatic hypotension; avoid IV use with benzodiazepines/EtOH; monitor for CYP 2D6 interactions
Quetiapine	Seroquel	25, 100, 200, 300	3	50 twice daily	400–600	Weight gain/metabolic syndrome; sedation; orthostatic hypotension	Monitor metabolic parameters as in clozapine
Risperidone	Risperdal Consta	0.25, 0.5, 1, 2, 3, 4	20	0.25 twice daily	1–2	Weight gain/metabolic syndrome; EPS at higher doses; gallactorrhea	Monitor for EPS and hyperprolactinemia; monitor metabolic parameters as in clozapine
Ziprasidone	Geodon	20, 40, 60, 80	7	20 twice daily	80–160	Weight gain/metabolic syndrome; activation at lower doses; QTc prolongation	Check baseline ECG and as dose increases; monitor metabolic parameters as in clozapine
Aripiprazole	Abilify	2.5, 5, 10, 15, 20, 30, liquid	75	2.5–5 at bedtime	10–30	Weight gain/metabolic syndrome	Monitor for PY450 interactions (CYP 3A4 and CYP 2D6); monitor metabolic parameters as in clozapine

ECG, electrocardiogram; EPS extrapyramidal symptoms, EtOH, ethanol; IV, intravenous; CYP, cytochrome P450.

the course of early-onset bipolar disorder have focused on rates of recovery, recurrence, changes in symptoms over time, and predictors of outcome. A recent longitudinal study of 263 child and adolescent inpatients and outpatients with bipolar disorders followed for an average of 2 years found that approximately 70 percent recovered from their index episode within that period. Half of these patients had at least one recurrence of a mood disorder during this time, more frequently a depressive episode than a mania. No differences were found in the rates of recovery for children and adolescents whose diagnosis was bipolar I disorder, bipolar II disorder, or bipolar disorder not otherwise specified; however, youth whose diagnosis was bipolar disorder not otherwise specified had a significant longer duration of illness before recovery, with less frequent recurrences once they recovered. About 19 percent of patients changed polarity once per year or less, 61 percent shifted 5 or more times per year, about half cycled more than 10 times per year, and about one third cycled more than 20 times per year. Predictors of more rapid cycling included lower socioeconomic status (SES), presence of lifetime psychosis, and diagnosis of bipolar disorder not otherwise specified. Over the follow-up period, about 20 percent of patients who were diagnosed with bipolar II disorder converted to bipolar I disorder, and 25 percent of the bipolar disorder not otherwise specified patients developed bipolar I disorder or bipolar II disorder during the follow-up period. Similar to the literature depicting the natural history of bipolar disorders in adults, the youth followed in this study had a wide range of symptom severity in manic and depressed episodes. The more frequent diagnostic conversion from bipolar II disorder to bipolar I disorder among the youth in this study and other investigations of bipolar disorders among children and adolescents than in the adult literature highlights the lack of stability of the bipolar II disorder diagnosis in youth. This is also the case in this study with respect to conversion from bipolar disorder not otherwise specified to other bipolar disorders.

All of the longitudinal literature on bipolar disorders in early childhood found that when the illness emerges in young children, recovery rates are lower. In addition, a greater likelihood is seen of mixed states and rapid cycling, as well as higher rates of polarity changes than in those who develop bipolar disorders in late adolescence or early adulthood. Further investigations are needed to understand the mechanisms by which low SES, psychosis, and less well-defined mood episodes predict more changes in polarity and a poorer prognosis.

TREATMENT

Few randomized, placebo-controlled treatment trials have been conducted with youth diagnosed with early-onset bipolar disorder. Therefore, clinical strategies for youth diagnosed with bipolar disorders continue to include downward extensions of the literature from older adolescent and adult treatment studies of bipolar disorders.

Pharmacotherapy

Mood-stabilizing agents, particularly lithium, has been demonstrated to be an effective treatment for adults with bipolar disorder for acute mania and bipolar depressive states and has been shown to have prophylactic properties in bipolar disorders. In childhood, controlled trials have provided evidence suggesting that lithium is efficacious in the management of aggression behavior disorders.

Open trials and retrospective chart reviews of children with early-onset bipolar disorder suggest that valproate (Depacon) is efficacious in the treatment of mania in childhood.

A recent randomized clinical trial comparing divalproex (Depakote) and quetiapine (Seroquel), an atypical antipsychotic, in the treatment of 50 adolescent patients with mania suggested that quetiapine is at least as effective as divalproex in the treatment of acute manic symptoms and may work more quickly. Placebo-controlled trials will be necessary to determine whether quetiapine is an effective monotherapy for child and adolescent mania.

An open-label trial of lamotrigine (Lamictal) in the treatment of bipolar depression among youth provides preliminary support for its use in children and adolescents. No significant weight changes, rash, or other adverse events were seen during the 8-week trial with 20 adolescents, whose mean final dose of lamotrigine was approximately 130 mg per day.

Open trials using atypical antipsychotics including risperidone (Risperdal) and others using risperidone in combination with either lithium or valproate suggest that these combinations may be efficacious in controlling symptoms of mania.

An open trial of olanzapine monotherapy in the treatment of childhood bipolar disorder found improvements in measures of both mania and depression after 8 weeks of treatment at doses ranging from 2.5 to 20 mg per day.

Psychosocial treatment intervention studies for bipolar disorder among youth include a pilot study by D. J. Miklowitz using an adjunctive family-focused psychoeducational treatment (FFT-A) modified for children and adolescents that had been shown to reduce relapse rate when used in adult bipolar patients. Results of this pilot investigation in children and adolescents treated with mood-stabilizing agents in addition to the psychosocial intervention included improvement in depressive symptoms, manic symptoms, and behavioral disturbance over 1 year.

In addition to managing manic and depressive symptoms in early-onset bipolar disorder, most children with bipolar disorder are likely to need treatment for comorbid ADHD. Chart reviews indicate that treatment of ADHD is significantly more successfully achieved after mood stabilization is accomplished.

More investigation is needed to determine the most efficacious treatments for early-onset bipolar disorder and its frequent comorbidities.

Table 14.2–1 lists medications used in children and adults with bipolar disorder.

15 Anxiety Disorders

▲ 15.1 Obsessive-Compulsive Disorder

Obsessive-compulsive disorder (OCD) is characterized by the presence of recurrent intrusive thoughts associated with anxiety or tension and/or repetitive purposeful mental or physical actions aimed at reducing fears and tensions caused by obsessions. It has become increasingly evident that the majority of cases of OCD begin in childhood or adolescence. The clinical presentation of OCD in childhood and adolescence is similar to that in adults, and the only alteration in diagnostic criteria in the text revision of the fourth edition of the *Diagnostic and Statistical Manual of Mental Disorders* (DSM-IV-TR) for children is that they do not necessarily demonstrate awareness that their thoughts or behaviors are unreasonable. Pediatric OCD has been investigated with respect to treatment with placebo-controlled trials of pharmacologic agents and cognitive-behavioral therapy (CBT), and it is the only childhood anxiety disorder with data showing optimal treatment to include a combination of serotoninergic agents and CBT treatment.

EPIDEMIOLOGY

Obsessive-compulsive disorder is common among children and adolescence, with a point prevalence of about 0.5 percent and a lifetime rate of 1 to 3 percent. The rate of OCD rises exponentially with increasing age among youth, with rates of 0.3 percent in children between the ages of 5 years and 7 years, rising to rates of 0.6 percent among teens. Rates of OCD among adolescents are greater than rates for disorders such as schizophrenia or bipolar disorder. Among young children with OCD there appears to be a slight male predominance, which diminishes with age.

ETIOLOGY

Genetic Factors

OCD is a heterogeneous disorder that has been recognized for decades to run in families. Family studies have documented an increased risk of at least fourfold in first-degree relatives of early-onset OCD. In addition, the presence of subclinical symptom constellations in family members appears to breed true. Molecular genetic studies have suggested linkage to regions of chromosomes 2 and 9 in certain pedigrees with multiple members exhibiting early-onset OCD. Candidate gene studies have been inconclusive. Family studies have pointed to a relationship between OCD and tic disorders such as Tourette's syndrome. OCD and tic disorders are believed to share susceptibility factors along with other conditions in a broader "obsessive-compulsive spectrum," including eating disorders and somatoform disorders, which may account for expression of repetitive and stereotyped symptoms.

Neuroimmunology

The association of emergence of OCD syndromes after a documented exposure to or infection with group A β-hemolytic *Streptococcus* in a subgroup of children and adolescents has led to the studies of immune responses in OCD. Cases of infection-triggered OCD have been termed pediatric autoimmune neuropsychiatric disorders associated with *Streptococcus* (PANDAS) and are believed to signify an autoimmune process such as that of Sydenham's chorea during rheumatic fever. It is hypothesized that exposure to streptococcal bacteria activates the immune system, leading to inflammation of the basal ganglia and resulting disruption of the cortical-striatal-thalamo-cortical function. Magnetic resonance imaging (MRI) has documented a proportional relationship between the size of the basal ganglia and the severity of OCD symptoms. The presentation of OCD in children and adolescence due to acute exposure to group A β-hemolytic *Streptococcus* represents a minority of OCD cases in this population.

Neurochemistry

Involvement of several neurotransmitter systems, including the serotonin system and the dopamine system, has been postulated to contribute to the emergence of OCD. The observation that selective serotonin reuptake inhibitors (SSRIs) diminish symptoms of OCD, along with the findings of altered sensitivity to the acute administration of 5-hydroxytryptamine (5-HT) agonists, supports the likelihood that the serotonin system plays a role in OCD. In addition, the dopamine system is believed to be influential in this disorder, especially in light of the frequent comorbidity of OCD with tic disorders in children. Clinical observations have indicated that obsessions and compulsions may be exacerbated during treatment of ADHD (another frequent comorbidity) with stimulant agents. Dopamine antagonists administered along with SSRIs may augment effectiveness of SSRIs in the treatment of OCD. It is most likely that multiple neurotransmitter systems play a role in OCD.

Neuroimaging

Both computed tomography (CT) and MRI of untreated children and adults with OCD have revealed smaller volumes of basal ganglia segments than in normal controls. In children, there is a suggestion that thalamic volume is increased. Adult studies have provided evidence of hypermetabolism of frontal cortical-striatal-thalamo-cortical networks in untreated individuals with OCD. Of interest, imaging studies before and after treatment have revealed that both medication and behavioral interventions lead to a reduction of orbit frontal and caudate metabolic rates in children and adults with OCD.

DIAGNOSIS AND CLINICAL FEATURES

Children and adolescents with obsessions or compulsions are often referred for treatment due to the excessive time that they devote to their intrusive thoughts and repetitive rituals. For some children their compulsive rituals are perceived as reasonable responses to their extreme fears and anxieties. Nevertheless, they are aware of their discomfort and inability to carry out usual daily activities in a timely manner due to the compulsions, such as getting ready to leave their homes to go to school each morning.

The most commonly reported obsessions in children and adolescents include extreme fears of contamination and exposure to dirt, germs, or disease, followed by worries related to harm befalling themselves or family members and fear of harming others due to losing control over aggressive impulses. Also commonly reported are obsessional need for symmetry or exactness, hoarding, and excessive religious or moral concerns. Typical compulsive rituals among children and adolescents involve cleaning, checking, counting, repeating behaviors, and arranging items. Associated features in children and adolescents with OCD include avoidance, indecision, doubt, and a slowness to complete tasks. In most cases of OCD among youth, obsessions and compulsions are present. According to the DSM-IV-TR, diagnosis of OCD is identical to that of adults, with the modification that children are not required, as are adults, to recognize that their obsessions or compulsions are excessive or irrational. Table 15.1–1 gives the DSM-IV-TR diagnostic criteria for OCD.

The majority of children who develop OCD have an insidious presentation and may hide their symptoms when possible, whereas a minority of children, particularly boys with early onset, may have a rapid unfolding of multiple symptoms within a few months. OCD is commonly comorbid with other psychiatric disorders, especially other anxiety disorders. There are also higher-than-expected rates of attention-deficit/hyperactivity disorder (ADHD) and tic disorders, including Tourette's syndrome, among children and adolescents with OCD. Children with comorbid OCD and tic disorders are more likely to exhibit counting, arranging, and ordering compulsions and less likely to manifest excessive washing and cleaning compulsions. The high comorbidity of OCD, Tourette's syndrome, and ADHD has led investigators to postulate a common genetic vulnerability to all three of these disorders. It is important to search for comorbidity in children and adolescents with OCD so that optimal treatments can be administered.

John, a 9-year-old boy in the third grade, was brought for evaluation by his parents, who expressed concerns over his repeated questioning and anxious and sad moods. The parents described John as a previously happy and well-adjusted boy who abruptly developed unusual behaviors approximately 2 to 3 months before the evaluation. These behaviors included John's concern about contracting illness, washing rituals, uncertainty over his own behavior, needing reassurance, repeating rituals, and avoidance.

Specifically, John had begun to express the worry that he may have been exposed to human immunodeficiency virus (HIV) whenever he would observe another person in public who he believed may be suffering with acquired immune deficiency syndrome (AIDS). For example, while riding in the car, if John saw someone who appeared to him to be poor or ill-kempt, he would begin asking his parents if they thought it possible that he may have been exposed to germs even from quite a distance. Although his parents' reassurances had some effect, John usually insisted on vigorously washing himself once home. John also had begun to express doubts over his control of his own behavior. He would often ask his parents, "Did I use the s___ word? Did I use the f___ word?" Reassurance was only temporarily calming. Of much concern to John was his new-found difficulty with schoolwork. Reading passages from assigned materials, John would frequently get to the end of a sentence, only to question whether he might have missed a word or content of the sentence and need to reread the material. Completing a page could take up to 15 to 30 minutes. Over several weeks, he was less and less capable of completing assignments, and as a result he was very distressed over his dropping grades.

Examination of the family history suggested that John's older sister may have had similar traits but with less interference in functioning, and she had never received any treatment for those behaviors.

At the intake interview, John appeared as a quiet and sad boy who was cooperative with questioning. He did not volunteer as much information as his parents regarding the nature and extent of his symptoms but did not deny what his parents reported. He acknowledged that he felt his mind was "tricking" him and that it led to his need to ask for reassurance from his parents. John met full criteria for OCD.

Table 15.1–1
DSM-IV-TR Diagnostic Criteria for Obsessive-Compulsive Disorder

A. Either obsessions or compulsions:
Obsessions as defined by (1), (2), (3), and (4):
(1) Recurrent and persistent thoughts, impulses, or images that are experienced, at some time during the disturbance, as intrusive and inappropriate and that cause marked anxiety or distress
(2) The thoughts, impulses, or images are not simply excessive worries about real-life problems
(3) The person attempts to ignore or suppress such thoughts, impulses, or images, or to neutralize them with some other thought or action
(4) The person recognizes that the obsessional thoughts, impulses, or images are a product of his or her own mind (not imposed from without as in thought insertion)
Compulsions as defined by (1) and (2):
(1) Repetitive behaviors (e.g., hand washing, ordering, checking) or mental acts (e.g., praying, counting, repeating words silently) that the person feels driven to perform in response to an obsession, or according to rules that must be applied rigidly
(2) The behaviors or mental acts are aimed at preventing or reducing distress or preventing some dreaded event or situation; however, these behaviors or mental acts either are not connected in a realistic way with what they are designed to neutralize or prevent or are clearly excessive

B. At some point during the course of the disorder, the person has recognized that the obsessions or compulsions are excessive or unreasonable. **Note:** This does not apply to children.

C. The obsessions or compulsions cause marked distress, are time consuming (take more than 1 hour a day), or significantly interfere with the person's normal routine, occupational (or academic) functioning, or usual social activities or relationships.

D. If another Axis I disorder is present, the content of the obsessions or compulsions is not restricted to it (e.g., preoccupation with food in the presence of an eating disorder; hair pulling in the presence of trichotillomania; concern with appearance in the presence of body dysmorphic disorder; preoccupation with drugs in the presence of a substance use disorder; preoccupation with having a serious illness in the presence of hypochondriasis; preoccupation with sexual urges or fantasies in the presence of a paraphilia; or guilty ruminations in the presence of major depressive disorder).

E. The disturbance is not due to the direct physiologic effects of a substance (e.g., a drug of abuse, a medication) or a general medical condition.

Specify if:
With poor insight: if, for most of the time during the current episode, the person does not recognize that the obsessions and compulsions are excessive or unreasonable

From American Psychiatric Association. *Diagnostic and Statistical Manual of Mental Disorders.* 4th ed. Text rev. Washington, DC: American Psychiatric Association; copyright 2000, with permission.

Some symptoms of depression were present but not sufficient for major depressive disorder.

An initial attempt at cognitive-behavioral therapy (CBT) was attempted, but John continued to feel overwhelmed and discouraged by these behaviors. He began to try to refuse school, apparently due to his increasing distress associated with reading. Given limited progress during the first 2 months of cognitive-behavioral therapy, fluoxetine (Prozac) was added and increased up to 40 mg per day, with good improvement. After three more months of CBT and SSRI treatment, John was able to stop cognitive-behavioral therapy and maintain substantial improvement. Follow-up over the next year showed John to be able to retain all of his gains from initial treatment and to show minimal interference from occasional OCD symptoms. (Courtesy of James T. McCracken, M.D.)

Pathology and Laboratory Examination

No specific laboratory measures are useful in the diagnosis of obsessive-compulsive disorder.

When the onset of obsessions or compulsions is believed to be associated with an exposure to or recent infection with group A β-hemolytic *Streptococcus*, antigens and antibodies to the bacteria can be obtained, although a diagnosis of OCD cannot be confirmed on the basis of positive results.

DIFFERENTIAL DIAGNOSIS

Developmentally appropriate rituals in the play and behavior of young children must be differentiated from obsessive-compulsive disorder in this age group. Preschoolers often engage in ritualistic play and request a predictable routine such as bathing, reading stories, or selecting the same stuffed animal at bedtime to promote a sense of security and comfort. These routines allay developmentally normal fears and lead to reasonable completion of daily activities, contrary to obsessions or compulsions, which are driven by extreme fears and interfere with normative daily function due to the excessive time that they consume and the extreme distress when not fully completed. The rituals of preschoolers generally become less rigid by the time they enter grade school, and school-aged children usually do not have a surge of anxiety when they encounter small changes in their routine.

Children and adolescents with anxiety disorders such as generalized anxiety disorder, separation anxiety disorder, and social phobia experience more intense worries than children without any anxiety disorders and may express their concerns repeatedly, but these are differentiated from typical obsessions by their more mundane content, whereas obsessions are so excessive that they approach seeming bizarre. A child with generalized anxiety disorder might worry repeatedly about performance on academic examinations, whereas a child with OCD is likely to have intrusive concerns about losing control and harming a loved one. The compulsions of OCD are not exhibited in other anxiety disorders, but children and adolescents with pervasive developmental disorders often display repetitive behaviors that resemble those of OCD. In contrast with the rituals of OCD, however, children with pervasive developmental disorder are not responding to anxiety but are more often manifesting stereotyped behaviors that are self-stimulating or self-comforting.

Children and adolescents with tic disorders such as Tourette's syndrome may exhibit complex repetitive compulsive behaviors that are similar to the compulsions seen in OCD. In fact, children and adolescents with tic disorders are at higher risk for the development of concurrent OCD.

In severe cases of OCD, it may be difficult to establish whether psychosis is present, given the extreme and bizarre nature that obsessions and compulsions can have. In adults and often in children and adolescents with OCD, despite the inability to control the obsessions or the irresistible drive to complete the compulsions, insight about their lack of reasonableness is preserved. When insight is present and underlying anxiety can be described, even in the face of significant dysfunction due to bizarre obsessions and compulsion, the diagnosis of OCD is suspect.

COURSE AND PROGNOSIS

OCD with an onset in childhood and adolescence is characterized as a chronic, albeit waxing and waning disorder with a great variation in severity and outcome. Follow-up studies suggest that up to 50 percent of affected children and adolescents experience recovery from OCD with minimal remaining symptoms. In a recent study of childhood OCD, treatment with sertraline resulted in close to 50 percent of patients experiencing complete remission and another 25 percent with partial remission with a follow-up time of 1 year. Predictors of the best outcome were in children and adolescents without comorbid disorders including tic disorders and ADHD. Overall, the prognosis is hopeful for most children and adolescents with mild to moderate OCD. In a minority of cases, however, the OCD diagnosis may be considered a prodrome of a psychotic disorder, which has been found to emerge in up to 10 percent in some samples of children and adolescents with OCD. In children with subthreshold symptoms of OCD, there is a high risk of the development of the full OCD disorder within 2 years. In the majority of studies of childhood OCD, treatments result in improvement if not complete remission in the majority of cases.

TREATMENT

Results from multiple randomized, placebo-controlled trials of both medication and cognitive-behavioral interventions in children and adolescents with OCD show the most evidence for successful treatment of this disorder than of any of the other anxiety disorders of childhood. A recent multisite National Institute of Health–funded investigation of sertraline and cognitive-behavioral therapy each alone and in combination for the treatment of childhood onset OCD—the Pediatric OCD Treatment Study (POTS)—revealed that the combination was superior to either treatment alone. Each treatment alone also provided encouraging levels of response. Mean daily dose of sertraline was 133 mg in the group administered the combination treatment and 170 mg for the sertraline-alone group.

A meta-analysis of 13 studies of SSRIs, including sertraline, fluvoxamine, fluoxetine, and paroxetine, provided evidence of efficacy of SSRI medications with a moderate effect size. There have been no apparent differences in the rate of response for the individual SSRIs.

Three SSRIs—sertraline (children at least 6 years of age), fluoxetine (at least 7 years), and fluvoxamine (at least 8 years)—have received U.S. Federal Drug Administration (FDA) approval for the treatment of OCD. The black box warning for antidepressants used in children for any disorder, including OCD, is applicable, so that close monitoring for suicidal ideation or behavior is mandated when these agents are used in the treatment of childhood OCD.

Typical side effects that emerge with the use of SSRI agents include insomnia, nausea, agitation, tremor, and fatigue. Dose ranges for the various SSRIs found to have efficacy in randomized clinical trials are fluoxetine, 20 to 60 mg; sertraline, 50 to 200 mg; fluvoxamine, up to 200 mg; and paroxetine, up to 50 mg.

Clomipramine was the first SSRI studied in the treatment of OCD in childhood and the only tricyclic antidepressant that has FDA approval for the treatment of anxiety disorders in childhood. Clomipramine was found to be efficacious in doses up to 200 mg, or 3 mg per kg, whichever is less, and may be chosen for children or adolescents who cannot tolerate other SSRIs due to insomnia, significant appetite suppression, or activation. Nevertheless, clomipramine is not recommended as a first-line treatment due to its greater potential risks than other SSRI agents, including cardiovascular risk of hypotension and arrhythmia and seizure risk.

Cognitive-behavioral therapy (CBT) geared toward children of varying ages is based on the principle of developmentally appropriate exposure to the feared stimuli coupled with response prevention, leading to diminishing anxiety over time experienced on exposure to feared situations. CBT manuals have been developed to ensure that developmentally appropriate interventions are made and that comprehensive education is provided to the child and parents.

Most treatment guidelines for children and adolescents with mild to moderate OCD recommend a trial of CBT prior to initiating medication, although there is evidence from one large investigation (POTS) that optimal treatment includes the combination of SSRI medication and CBT. In terms of pharmacologic interventions, remission of childhood OCD has been shown to occur within 8 to 12 weeks of acute treatment. The vast majority of children and adolescents who experienced a remission with acute treatment using SSRIs were still responsive over a period of 1 year. Given the lack of data on discontinuation, recommendations for maintaining medication include stabilization, education about relapse risk, and tapering medication during the summer to minimize academic compromise in case of relapse. For children and adolescents with more severe or multiple episodes of significant exacerbation of symptoms, treatment for a longer period of time—more than 1 year—is recommended.

Augmentation strategies enhancing serotonergic effects, such as use of atypical antipsychotics like risperidone, have demonstrated increased response when partial response has been achieved with SSRI agents.

Overall, efficacy of treatment for children and adolescents with OCD is high with appropriate choices of SSRI agents and CBT therapy.

Pharmacotherapy

Pharmacotherapy is not indicated in this disorder unless there is a comorbid condition (i.e., anxiety or depression) that is a contributing factor to the disorder or results from it.

▲ 15.2 Posttraumatic Stress Disorder

Posttraumatic stress disorder (PTSD) is characterized by a set of symptoms such as reexperiencing symptoms, distressing recollections, persistent avoidance, and hyperarousal in response to exposure to one or more traumatic events. PTSD is the only disorder described in the text revision of the fourth edition of the *Diagnostic and Statistical Manual of Mental Disorders* (DSM-IV-TR) in which the etiologic factors—exposure to an extreme traumatic stressor either directly or as a witness—is the first diagnostic criterion. Many children and adolescents are exposed to traumatic events, such as direct experience with physical or sexual abuse, domestic violence, motor vehicle accidents, severe medical illnesses, and natural or human-created disasters, that lead to full-blown PTSD in some cases and at least some PTSD symptoms in many others. Although the presence of posttraumatic stress symptoms has been described among adults for more than a century, it was first officially recognized as a psychiatric disorder in 1980 with the publication of the third edition of the DSM (DSM-III). Recognition of its frequent emergence in children and adolescence has broadened over the last decade. PTSD occurs frequently in children and adolescents, with up to 6 percent of youth meeting criteria for this diagnosis at some point. Developmental factors strongly influence the manifestation of symptoms, many of which reflect internal states that are identified mainly through verbal articulation by the patient. In children and adolescents, reexperiencing of a traumatic event is often observed through play, recurrent nightmares without recall of the traumatic events, and behaviors that reenact the traumatic situation, along with agitation, fear, or disorganization.

EPIDEMIOLOGY

Epidemiologic studies have reported lifetime prevalence rates of PTSD ranging from 1.3 to 8 percent in adults in the United States. A recent epidemiologic survey of preschoolers aged 4 to 5 years found a rate of 1.3 percent of PTSD, whereas among children 2 to 3 years of age, the full criteria for PTSD were not met. Epidemiologic studies of children from 9 to 17 years of age have found 3-month prevalence rates of PTSD ranging from 0.5 to 4 percent. Among trauma-exposed samples of persons not referred for treatment, a wide range, 25 to 90 percent, were reported to exhibit the full diagnosis of PTSD. Children exposed chronically to trauma, such as child abuse or other traumas resulting in the dissolution of the family or ongoing exposure to broader disruption of entire communities, such as in war, have the greatest risk for the development of PTSD. In addition to the staggering rate of the full-blown disorder of PTSD among youth, several studies indicate that most children exposed to severe or chronic trauma develop PTSD symptoms sufficiently severe to disrupt functioning, even in the absence of the full diagnosis.

ETIOLOGY

Biological Factors

Some children exposed to significant traumatic events do not develop PTSD, and investigations have documented that risk factors in children for developing PTSD include preexisting anxiety disorders, which suggests that a genetic predisposition for anxiety disorders, as well as a family history with increased risk of depressive disorders, may predispose a trauma-exposed child to develop PTSD. Children with PTSD have been found to exhibit increased excretion of adrenergic and dopaminergic metabolites, smaller intracranial volume and corpus callosum, memory deficits, and lower intelligence quotients (IQs) than age-matched controls. Adults with PTSD have been found to have overactive amygdale regions of the brain and decreased hippocampal volume.

Long-Term Impact of Childhood Trauma. Studies of adult patients who experienced childhood trauma found that there were long-lasting physiologic effects resulting from those experiences. Compared with a no-trauma group, the childhood-trauma group had greater eye-blink response and greater skin conductance (i.e., startle) response. They also had a higher risk for mood and anxiety disorders, even after 20 years.

Psychologic Factors

Although the exposure to trauma is the initial etiologic factor in the development of PTSD, the enduring symptoms typical of PTSD, such as avoidance of the place where the trauma occurred, can be conceptualized, in part, as the result of both classic and operant conditioning. An extreme physiologic response that accompanies fear of a given traumatic event, such as in an adolescent who was terrorized by an attack by a group of students near school who then develops an extreme negative physiologic reaction each time he or she is near the school, is an example of classic conditioning, in that a neutral cue (the school) has become paired with an intensely fearful past event. Operant conditioning occurs when a child learns to avoid traumatic reminders to prevent distressing feelings from arising. For example, if a child was in a motor vehicle accident, the child may then refuse to ride in cars altogether to prevent negative physiologic reactions and fear from occurring.

Another conceptualization in developing and maintaining symptoms of PTSD is through the mechanism of modeling, which is a form of learning. For example, when parents and children are exposed to traumatic events, such as natural disasters, children may emulate parental responses, such as avoidance, withdrawal, or extreme expressions of fear, and "learn" to respond to their own memories of the traumatic event in the same manner.

Social Factors

Family support and reactions to traumatic events in children may play a significant role in the development of PTSD, in that adverse parental emotional reactions to a child's abuse may increase that child's risk of developing PTSD. Lack of parental support and psychopathology among parents—especially maternal depression—have been identified as risk factors in the development of PTSD after a child has been exposed to a traumatic event.

DIAGNOSIS AND CLINICAL FEATURES

For PTSD to ensue, exposure to a traumatic event consisting of either a direct personal experience or witnessing of an event involving the threat of death, serious injury, or serious harm must occur. The most common traumatic exposures for children and adolescents include physical or sexual abuse; domestic, school, or community violence; being kidnapped; terrorist attacks; motor vehicle or household accidents; and disasters, such as floods, hurricanes, tornadoes, fires, explosions, and airline crashes. The child's response must involve intense fear, terror, helplessness, horror, or disorganized or agitated behavior.

Symptoms of PTSD include *reexperiencing* the traumatic event in at least one of the following ways. Children may have intrusive thoughts that they perceive as recurrently coming into their head, memories, images, or body sensations that remind them of the event. In very young children, it is common to observe play that includes elements of the traumatic event or behaviors, such as sexual behaviors, that are not developmentally expected. Children may experience periods during which they either act or feel that the event is taking place presently, which is a dissociative event usually described by adults as "flashbacks."

Another critical symptom characteristic of PTSD is *avoidance and numbing*. Children with PTSD exhibit avoidance, either by making active physical efforts to avoid the places that would present traumatic reminders to them of the event or being unable to recall important aspects of the traumatic event. The inability to remember parts of a traumatic event is termed *psychological amnesia*. After a traumatic event, children may experience a sense of detachment from their usual play activities ("psychological numbing") or a diminished capacity to feel emotions, whereas older adolescents may express a fear of dying young (sense of foreshortened future).

Other typical responses to traumatic events include symptoms of hyperarousal that were not present before the traumatic exposure, such as difficulty falling asleep or staying asleep; hypervigilance regarding safety and increased checking that doors are locked; and exaggerated startle reaction. In some children, hyperarousal can present as a generalized inability to relax, with increased irritability, outbursts, and impaired ability to concentrate.

To meet the diagnostic criteria for PTSD according to the DSM-IV-TR, the symptoms must be present for at least 1 month and cause distress and impairment in important functional areas of life. When all of the diagnostic symptoms of PTSD are met but resolve within 3 months, acute PTSD is diagnosed. When the full syndrome of PTSD persists beyond 3 months, it is designated as chronic PTSD. In some cases, the PTSD symptoms increase over time, and it is not until more than 6 months have elapsed after the exposure to the trauma that the whole syndrome emerges; in that case, the diagnosis is PTSD, delayed onset. DSM-IV-TR criteria are described in Table 15.2–1.

It is not uncommon for children and adolescents with PTSD to experience feelings of guilt, especially if they survived the trauma and others in the situation did not. They may blame themselves for the demise of the others and may go on to develop a comorbid depressive episode. Childhood PTSD is also associated with increased rates of other anxiety disorders in addition to depressive episodes, substance use disorders, and attentional difficulties.

Pathology and Laboratory Examination

Although reports indicate some alterations in both neurophysiologic and neuroimaging studies of children and adolescents with PTSD, no laboratory test can help in making this diagnosis.

Differential Diagnosis

A number of overlapping symptoms are seen in childhood presentations of anxiety disorders, such as obsessive-compulsive

Table 15.2–1
DSM-IV-TR Diagnostic Criteria for Posttraumatic Stress Disorder

A. The person has been exposed to a traumatic event in which both of the following were present:
   (1) the person experienced, witnessed, or was confronted with an event or events that involved actual or threatened death or serious injury, or a threat to the physical integrity of self or others
   (2) the person's response involved intense fear, helplessness, or horror. **Note**: In children, this may be expressed instead by disorganized or agitated behavior.

B. The traumatic event is persistently reexperienced in one (or more) of the following ways:
   (1) recurrent and intrusive distressing recollections of the event, including images, thoughts, or perceptions. **Note**: In young children, repetitive play may occur in which themes or aspects of the trauma are expressed.
   (2) recurrent distressing dreams of the event. **Note**: In children, there may be frightening dreams without recognizable content.
   (3) acting or feeling as if the traumatic event were recurring (includes a sense of reliving the experience, illusions, hallucinations, and dissociative flashback episodes, including those that occur on awakening or when intoxicated). **Note**: In young children, trauma-specific reenactment may occur.
   (4) intense psychologic distress at exposure to internal or external cues that symbolize or resemble an aspect of the traumatic event
   (5) physiologic reactivity on exposure to internal or external cues that symbolize or resemble an aspect of the traumatic event

C. Persistent avoidance of stimuli associated with the trauma and numbing of general responsiveness (not present before the trauma), as indicated by three (or more) of the following:
   (1) efforts to avoid thoughts, feelings, or conversations associated with the trauma
   (2) efforts to avoid activities, places, or people that arouse recollections of the trauma
   (3) inability to recall an important aspect of the trauma
   (4) markedly diminished interest or participation in significant activities
   (5) feeling of detachment or estrangement from others
   (6) restricted range of affect (e.g., unable to have loving feelings)
   (7) sense of a foreshortened future (e.g., does not expect to have a career, marriage, children, or a normal life span)

D. Persistent symptoms of increased arousal (not present before the trauma), as indicated by two (or more) of the following:
   (1) difficulty falling or staying asleep
   (2) irritability or outbursts of anger
   (3) difficulty concentrating
   (4) hypervigilance
   (5) exaggerated startle response

E. Duration of the disturbance (symptoms in Criteria B, C, and D) is more than 1 month.

F. The disturbance causes clinically significant distress or impairment in social, occupational, or other important areas of functioning.

Specify if:
Acute: if duration of symptoms is less than 3 months
Chronic: if duration of symptoms is 3 months or more

Specify if:
With delayed onset: if onset of symptoms is at least 6 months after the stressor

From American Psychiatric Association. *Diagnostic and Statistical Manual of Mental Disorders*. 4th ed. Text rev. Washington, DC: American Psychiatric Association; copyright 2000, with permission.

disorder (OCD) and social phobia, in which recurrent intrusive thoughts and avoidance occur in social phobia of situations in which the given child may experience anxiety. Children with depressive disorders often exhibit withdrawal and a sense of isolation from peers, as well as guilt about life events over which they realistically have no control. Irritability, poor concentration, sleep disturbance, and decreased interest in usual activities can also be observed in both PTSD and major depressive disorder.

Children who have lost a loved one in a traumatic event may go on to experience both PTSD and a major depressive disorder when bereavement persists beyond its expected course. Children with PTSD may also be confused with children who have disruptive behavior disorders, because they often show poor concentration, inattention, and irritability. It is critical to elicit a history of traumatic exposure and evaluate the chronology of the trauma and the onset of the symptoms to make an accurate diagnosis of PTSD.

Course and Prognosis

Many studies have documented the presence of both partial PTSD syndromes and the full syndrome in children who have been exposed to traumatic events. A wide range of outcomes exists, depending on the severity and intensity of the trauma and the preexisting emotional and psychiatric state of the child. For many children and adolescents with milder forms of PTSD, symptoms may persist for 1 to 2 years, after which they diminish. In more severe circumstances, however, PTSD syndromes persist for many years or decades in children and adolescents, with spontaneous remission in only a portion of them.

The prognosis of untreated PTSD has become an issue of growing concern for researchers and clinicians, who have documented a variety of serious comorbidities and psychobiologic abnormalities associated with PTSD. In one study, children and adolescents with severe PTSD were at risk for decreased intracranial volume, diminished corpus callosum area, and lower

IQs than with children without PTSD. Children and adolescents with histories of physical and sexual abuse exhibit higher rates of depression and suicidality, and subsequently so do their offspring. This highlights the importance of early recognition and treatment of PTSD among youth that may significantly improve their long-term outcome.

TREATMENT

Trauma-Focused Cognitive-Behavior Therapy

Several randomized clinical trials have provided evidence for the efficacy of trauma-focused cognitive-behavior therapy (CBT) in the treatment of PTSD in children and adolescents. This treatment is generally administered over 10 to 16 treatment sessions and includes a number of components. The first component of trauma-focused CBT is *psychoeducation* regarding the nature of typical emotional and physiologic reactions to traumatic events and PTSD. Next is *stress inoculation*, in which children are guided to use muscle relaxation, focused breathing, affective modulation, thought stopping, and cognitive coping techniques to diminish feelings of helplessness and distress. *Gradual exposure* may then be introduced as a technique for a child to recall, first in small segments and then in increasing amounts, the details of the traumatic exposure and describe the thoughts, feelings, and physical sensations experienced during the trauma, as well as in the retelling of the event. *Cognitive processing* is the next step in identifying those associated thoughts, feelings, and ideas that may be inaccurate and serve to cause additional impairment to the victim, so that reframing of the thoughts and feelings can help them alleviate the sense of being incapacitated by them. At this time, during the cognitive processing, a *parental treatment component* is added that provides parent management strategies for the parent to use to enhance the child's ability to communicate proactively and elicit support from the parents. This set of therapeutic strategies is considered by experts to be the first line of treatment of PTSD symptoms. They can be adapted for use in group settings in school, with entire families who have been traumatized, and in groups of adolescents.

A variant of trauma-focused CBT for PTSD is called *eye movement desensitization and reprocessing* (EMDR), in which exposure and cognitive reprocessing interventions are paired with directed eye movements. This technique is not as well accepted as the more extensive trauma-focused CBT.

Crisis Intervention/Psychologic Debriefing

Crisis intervention/psychologic debriefing typically consists of several sessions immediately after an exposure to a traumatic event in which a traumatized child or adolescent is encouraged to describe the traumatic event in the context of a supportive environment. Psychoeducation is provided, as may guidance about the management of initial emotional reactions. Anecdotal reports suggest that this intervention may be helpful, but no controlled studies have provided evidence that it leads to a more positive outcome.

Psychopharmacologic Treatment

Serotonin reuptake inhibitors (SSRIs) are frequently used in children with PTSD in the absence of evidence demonstrating efficacy. Citalopram (Celexa) from 20 to 40 mg has been reported to be helpful in the management of PTSD in children and adolescents according to the results of an open trial over an 8-week period. Most of the SSRI efficacy data have been obtained through open trials with adults that suggested that they are beneficial.

In adults, clonidine (Catapres) and propranolol (Inderal) have been used to treat symptoms of PTSD, especially nightmares and exaggerated startle response, with a suggestion of improvement. One report of propranolol treatment in 11 pediatric patients with PTSD based on sexual or physical abuse, with a mean age of 8.5 years, who exhibited agitation and hyperarousal indicated some decrease in symptoms in 8 of the children. Another open study of transdermal clonidine treatment of preschoolers with PTSD suggested that clonidine may be efficacious in this population in decreasing activation and hyperarousal. An additional open trial of oral clonidine with doses of 0.05 to 0.1 mg twice daily similarly suggested that this medication may provide some relief for the symptoms of hyperarousal, impulsivity, and agitation in young children with PTSD.

One open study used imipramine (Tofranil) in the treatment of acute stress disorder symptoms in 25 children with burns and suggested that this medication provided benefit for sleep. A case report indicated that guanfacine (Tenex) successfully treated PTSD nightmares in a child.

No randomized, placebo-controlled trials of medication for youth in the treatment of PTSD are being conducted; in general, extrapolation from adult studies points to the likelihood that SSRI medications may provide relief for some symptoms of PTSD among youth.

Pharmacotherapy. Pharmacotherapy is not indicated in this disorder unless there is a comorbid condition (i.e., anxiety or depression) that is a contributing factor to the disorder or results from it.

▲ 15.3 Separation Anxiety Disorder, Generalized Anxiety Disorder, and Social Phobia

Anxiety disorders are among the most common disorders in youth, affecting more than 10 percent of children and adolescents at some point in their development. Separation anxiety is a universal human developmental phenomenon emerging in infants less than 1 year of age and marking a child's awareness of a separation from his or her mother or primary caregiver. Normative separation anxiety peaks between 9 and 18 months and diminishes by about 2.5 years of age, enabling young children to develop a sense of comfort away from their parents in preschool. Separation anxiety, or stranger anxiety as it has been termed, most likely evolved as a human response that has survival value. The expression of transient separation anxiety is also normal in young children entering school for the first time. Approximately 15 percent of young children display intense and persistent fear, shyness, and social withdrawal when faced with unfamiliar settings and people. Young children with this pattern of behavioral inhibition are at higher risk for the development of separation anxiety disorder, generalized anxiety disorder, and social phobia. Behaviorally inhibited children, as a group, exhibit characteristic physiologic traits, including higher-than-average resting heart rates, higher morning cortisol levels than average, and low heart rate variability. Separation anxiety disorder is diagnosed when developmentally inappropriate and excessive anxiety emerges related to separation from the major attachment figure. According to the text revision of the fourth edition of the *Diagnostic and Statistical Manual of Mental Disorders* (DSM-IV-TR), separation anxiety disorder requires the presence of at least three symptoms related to excessive worry about separation from the major attachment figures. The worries may take the form of refusal to go to school, fears and distress on separation, repeated complaints of such physical symptoms as headaches and stomachaches when separation is anticipated, and nightmares related to separation issues.

Separation anxiety disorder and *selective mutism* are the two anxiety disorders found in the child and adolescent section of the DSM-IV-TR, although childhood onset of all of the anxiety disorders is frequent. Children who exhibit recurrent excessive worries pertaining to their performance in school and social settings and experience at least one physiologic symptom, such as restlessness, poor concentration, or irritability related to their fears, may be diagnosed with generalized anxiety disorder. Children with generalized anxiety disorder tend to feel fearful in multiple settings and expect more negative outcomes when faced with academic or social challenges than do peers. Children who experience recurrent extreme anxiety and avoid social situations in which they fear scrutiny or humiliation may meet the DSM-IV-TR diagnostic criteria for *social phobia*, a disorder that also occurs in adolescents and adults. Children with social phobia experience distress and discomfort in the presence of peers as well as adults. Separation anxiety disorder, generalized anxiety, and social phobia in children are often considered together in a differential diagnosis and in developing treatment strategies because they are highly comorbid and have overlapping symptoms. A child with separation anxiety disorder, generalized anxiety disorder, or social phobia has a 60 percent chance of also having at least one of the other two disorders. Of children with one of the aforementioned anxiety disorders, 30 percent have all three of them. Children and adolescents may also have other anxiety disorders described among the adult disorders of DSM-IV-TR, including specific phobia, panic disorder, obsessive-compulsive disorder (OCD), and posttraumatic stress disorder (PTSD).

EPIDEMIOLOGY

The prevalence of anxiety disorders has varied with the age group of the children surveyed and the diagnostic instruments used. Lifetime prevalence of any anxiety disorder in children and adolescents ranges from 8.3 to 27 percent. A recent epidemiologic survey using the *Preschool* Age Psychiatric Assessment (PAPA) found that 9.5 percent of preschoolers met DSM-IV-TR criteria for any anxiety disorder, with 6.5 percent exhibiting generalized anxiety disorder, 2.4 percent meeting criteria for separation anxiety disorder, and 2.2 percent meeting criteria for social phobia. Separation anxiety disorder is estimated to be about 4 percent in children and young adolescents. Separation anxiety disorder is more common in young children than in adolescents and has been reported to occur equally in boys and girls. The onset may occur during preschool years but is most common in children 7 to 8 years of age. The rate of generalized anxiety disorder in school-age children is estimated to be approximately 3 percent, the rate of social phobia is 1 percent, and the rate of simple phobias is 2.4 percent. In adolescents, lifetime prevalence for panic disorder was found to be 0.6 percent; the prevalence for generalized anxiety disorder was 3.7 percent.

ETIOLOGY

Biopsychosocial Factors

In very young children, psychosocial factors in conjunction with temperament may influence the degree of separation anxiety that emerges in situations of brief separation and exposure to unfamiliar environments. The relation between temperamental traits and the predisposition to develop anxiety symptoms has been investigated. The temperamental tendency to be unusually shy or to withdraw in unfamiliar situations seems to be an enduring response pattern, and young children with this propensity are at higher risk of developing separation anxiety disorder, generalized anxiety disorder, social anxiety disorders, or all three during their next few years of life.

Neurophysiologic correlation is found with behavioral inhibition (extreme shyness); children with this constellation are shown to have a higher resting heart rate and an acceleration of heart rate with tasks requiring cognitive concentration. Additional physiologic correlates of behavioral inhibition include elevated salivary cortisol levels, elevated urinary catecholamine levels, and greater papillary dilation during cognitive tasks. The quality of maternal attachment also appears to play a role in the development of anxiety disorder in children. Mothers with anxiety disorders who are observed to show insecure attachment to their children tend to have children with higher rates of anxiety disorders. It is difficult to separate the contribution of the relationship between mother and child from the mother's potential genetic contribution to anxiety. Families in which a child manifests separation anxiety disorder may be close-knit and caring, and the children often seem to be the objects of parental overconcern. External life stresses often coincide with development of the disorder. The death of a relative, a child's illness, a change in a child's environment, or a move to a new neighborhood or school is frequently noted in the histories of children with separation anxiety disorder. In a vulnerable child, these changes probably intensify anxiety.

Social Learning Factors

Fear in response to a variety of unfamiliar or unexpected situations may be unwittingly communicated from parents to children by direct modeling. If a parent is fearful, the child will probably have a phobic adaptation to new situations, especially to a school environment. Some parents appear to teach their children to be anxious by overprotecting them from expected dangers or by exaggerating the dangers. For example, a parent who cringes in a room during a lightning storm teaches a child to do the same. A parent who is afraid of mice or insects conveys the affect of fright to a child. Conversely, a parent who becomes angry with a child when the child expresses fear of a given situation, for example, when exposed to animals, may promote a phobic concern in the child by exposing the child to the intensity of the anger expressed by the parent. Social learning factors in the development of anxiety reactions are magnified when parents have anxiety disorders. These factors may be pertinent in the development of separation anxiety disorder, as well as in that of generalized anxiety disorder and social phobia. In a recent study of adverse psychosocial events, such as ongoing family conflict, no association was found between psychosocial hardships and behavioral inhibition among young children. It appears that temperamental predisposition to anxiety disorders emerges as a highly heritable constellation of traits and is not created by psychosocial stressor.

Genetic Factors

Genetic studies of families suggest that genes account for at least one third of the variance in the development of anxiety disorders in children. Thus, temperamental constellation of behavioral inhibition, excessive shyness, the tendency to withdraw from unfamiliar situations, and the eventual emergence of anxiety disorders has a genetic contribution; however, approximately two thirds of young children with behavioral inhibition do not appear to go on to develop anxiety disorders. Family studies have shown that the biological offspring of adults with anxiety disorders are susceptible to parents with panic disorder with agoraphobia, who appear to have an increased risk of having a child with separation anxiety disorder. Separation anxiety disorder and depression in children overlap, and the presence of an anxiety disorder increases the risk of a future episode of a depressive disorder. Consensus on the genetics of anxiety disorders suggests that what is inherited is a general predisposition toward anxiety, with resulting heightened levels of arousability, emotional reactivity, and increased negative affect, all of which increase the risk for the development of separation anxiety disorder, generalized anxiety disorder, and social phobia.

DIAGNOSIS AND CLINICAL FEATURES

Separation anxiety disorder, generalized anxiety disorder, and social phobia are highly related in children and adolescence because, in most children, if one occurs, another is present as well. Generalized anxiety disorder is the most common anxiety disorder in childhood, but in 30 percent of cases, a child with generalized anxiety disorder also exhibits the other two disorders. Separation anxiety disorder and selective mutism are the two anxiety disorders in the childhood section of the DSM-IV-TR; however, most anxiety disorders originate in childhood or adolescence. Diagnostic criteria for separation anxiety disorder according to DSM-IV-TR include three of the following symptoms for at least 4 weeks: persistent and excessive worry about losing, or possible harm befalling, major attachment figures; persistent and excessive worry that an untoward event can lead to separation from a major attachment figure; persistent reluctance or refusal to go to school or elsewhere because of fear of separation; persistent and excessive fear or reluctance to be alone or without major attachment figures at home or without significant adults in other settings; persistent reluctance or refusal to go to sleep without being near a major attachment figure or to sleep away from home; repeated nightmares involving the theme of separation; repeated complaints of physical symptoms, including headaches and stomachaches, when separation from major attachment figures is anticipated; and recurrent excessive distress when separation from home or major attachment figures is anticipated or involved (Tables 15.3–1 through 15.3–3).

Alan W was an 8-year-old boy referred for outpatient evaluation by his family physician. He was having trouble sleeping in his room alone at night and was refusing to go to school. Alan expressed recurrent fears that something bad would happen to his mother. He worried that she would get into a car accident or that there would be a fire at home and his mother would be killed. Developmental history showed Alan was anxious and irritable as an infant and toddler. He had trouble adjusting to babysitters in the preschool years. There was a history of panic disorder, with agoraphobia in the mother and major depression in the father.

Nighttime was a particularly difficult time at home. While Mrs. W would read to her son and talk with him before bedtime, Alan would often whine and cry, asking to have mother lie in bed with him until he fell asleep. He also expected his mother to be in the master bedroom across the hall from his room throughout the evening. Mrs. W reported that some evenings her son would get up and peek through the crack in the master bedroom door, as frequently as every 10 minutes, to be certain that she was still there. Alan reported

Table 15.3–1
DSM-IV-TR Diagnostic Criteria for Separation Anxiety Disorder

A. Developmentally inappropriate and excessive anxiety concerning separation from home or from those to whom the individual is attached, as evidenced by three (or more) of the following:
   (1) recurrent excessive distress when separation from home or major attachment figures occurs or is anticipated
   (2) persistent and excessive worry about losing, or about possible harm befalling, major attachment figures
   (3) persistent and excessive worry that an untoward event will lead to separation from a major attachment figure (e.g., getting lost or being kidnapped)
   (4) persistent reluctance or refusal to go to school or elsewhere because of fear of separation
   (5) persistently and excessively fearful or reluctant to be alone or without major attachment figures at home or without significant adults in other settings
   (6) persistent reluctance or refusal to go to sleep without being near a major attachment figure or to sleep away from home
   (7) repeated nightmares involving the theme of separation
   (8) repeated complaints of physical symptoms (such as headaches, stomachaches, nausea, or vomiting) when separation from major attachment figures occurs or is anticipated

B. The duration of the disturbance is at least 4 weeks.

C. The onset is before age 18 years.

D. The disturbance causes clinically significant distress or impairment in social, academic (occupational), or other important areas of functioning.

E. The disturbance does not occur exclusively during the course of a pervasive developmental disorder, schizophrenia, or other psychotic disorder and, in adolescents and adults, is not better accounted for by panic disorder with agoraphobia.

Specify if:
Early onset: if onset occurs before age 6 years

From American Psychiatric Association. *Diagnostic and Statistical Manual of Mental Disorders.* 4th ed. Text rev. Washington, DC: American Psychiatric Association; copyright 2000, with permission.

frequent bad dreams that his parents were killed or that monsters caught him and took him away from his family forever.

During the daytime, he would shadow his mother around the house. Alan would agree to play a game with his sister in the lower level of the house only if his mother was close by. When Mrs. W went upstairs, he would interrupt the game and follow her upstairs. He was reluctant to sleep at a friend's house; a couple of times he attempted to do this. However, as the evening progressed, he described a queasy sensation in his stomach, a feeling of sadness, and missing his mother. Subsequently Alan would call home and his parents would pick him up.

Table 15.3–2
DSM-IV-TR Diagnostic Criteria for Generalized Anxiety Disorder

A. Excessive anxiety and worry (apprehensive expectation), occurring more days than not for at least 6 months, about a number of events or activities (such as work or school performance).

B. The person finds it difficult to control the worry.

C. The anxiety and worry are associated with three (or more) of the following six symptoms (with at least some symptoms present for more days than not for the past 6 months). **Note:** Only one item is required in children.
   (1) Restlessness or feeling keyed up or on edge
   (2) Being easily fatigued
   (3) Difficulty concentrating or mind going blank
   (4) Irritability
   (5) Muscle tension
   (6) Sleep disturbance (difficulty falling or staying asleep, or restless unsatisfying sleep)

D. The focus of the anxiety and worry is not confined to features of an Axis I disorder, e.g., the anxiety or worry is not about having a panic attack (as in panic disorder), being embarrassed in public (as in social phobia), being contaminated (as in obsessive-compulsive disorder), being away from home or close relatives (as in separation anxiety disorder), gaining weight (as in anorexia nervosa), having multiple physical complaints (as in somatization disorder), or having a serious illness (as in hypochondriasis), and the anxiety and worry do not occur exclusively during posttraumatic stress disorder.

E. The anxiety, worry, or physical symptoms cause clinically significant distress or impairment in social, occupational, or other important areas of functioning.

F. The disturbance is not due to the direct physiologic effects of a substance (e.g., a drug of abuse, a medication) or a general medical condition (e.g., hyperthyroidism) and does not occur exclusively during a mood disorder, psychotic disorder, or a pervasive developmental disorder.

From American Psychiatric Association. *Diagnostic and Statistical Manual of Mental Disorders.* 4th ed. Text rev. Washington, DC: American Psychiatric Association; 2000, with permission.

Table 15.3–3
DSM-IV-TR Diagnostic Criteria for Social Phobia

A. A marked and persistent fear of one or more social or performance situations in which the person is exposed to unfamiliar people or to possible scrutiny by others. The individual fears that he or she will act in a way (or show anxiety symptoms) that will be humiliating or embarrassing. **Note:** In children, there must be evidence of capacity for age-appropriate social relationships with familiar people and the anxiety must occur in peer settings, not just in interactions with adults.
B. Exposure to the feared social situation almost invariably provokes anxiety, which may take the form of a situationally bound or situationally predisposed panic attack. **Note:** In children, the anxiety may be expressed by crying, tantrums, freezing, or shrinking from social situations with unfamiliar people.
C. The person recognizes that the fear is excessive or unreasonable. **Note:** In children, this feature may be absent.
D. The feared social or performance situations are avoided, or else endured with intense anxiety or distress.
E. The avoidance, anxious anticipation, or distress in the feared social or performance situation(s) interferes significantly with the person's normal routine, occupational (academic) functioning, or social activities or relationships with others, or there is marked distress about having the phobia.
F. In individuals under age 18 years, the duration is at least 6 months.
G. The fear or avoidance is not due to the direct physiologic effects of a substance (e.g., a drug of abuse, a medication) or a general medical condition, and is not better accounted for by another mental disorder (e.g., panic disorder with or without agoraphobia, separation anxiety disorder, body dysmorphic disorder, a pervasive developmental disorder, or schizoid personality disorder).
H. If a general medical condition or other mental disorder is present, the fear in Criterion A is unrelated to it, (e.g., the fear is not of stuttering, trembling in Parkinson's disease, or exhibiting abnormal eating behavior in anorexia nervosa or bulimia nervosa).

Specify if:
Generalized: If the fears include most social situations (also consider the additional diagnosis of avoidant personality disorder).

From American Psychiatric Association. *Diagnostic and Statistical Manual of Mental Disorders.* 4th ed. Text rev. Washington, DC: American Psychiatric Association; 2000, with permission.

On school days, Alan had stomachaches and tried to stay home. He appeared quite distressed and panicky when it was time to separate from his mother. Once at school, he seemed calmer and less anxious, but occasionally was seen in the nurse's office, complaining of nausea and seeking to be sent home. (Courtesy of Gail A. Bernstein, M.D., and Anne E. Layne, Ph.D.)

The essential feature of separation anxiety disorder is extreme anxiety precipitated by separation from parents, home, or other familiar surroundings, whereas in generalized anxiety disorder, fears are extended to negative outcomes for all kinds of events, including academic, peer relationship, and family activities. In generalized anxiety disorder, a child or adolescent experiences at least one recurrent physiologic symptom, such as restlessness, poor concentration, irritability, or muscle tension. In social phobia, the child's fears peak during performance situations involving exposure to unfamiliar people or situations. Children and adolescents with social phobia have extreme concerns about being embarrassed, humiliated, or negatively judged. In each of the aforementioned anxiety disorders, the child's experience can approach terror or panic. The distress is greater than that normally expected for the child's developmental level and cannot be explained by any other disorder. Morbid fears, preoccupations, and ruminations characterize separation anxiety disorder. Children with anxiety disorders overestimate the probability of danger and the likelihood of negative outcome. Children with separation anxiety disorder and generalized anxiety disorder become overly fearful that someone close to them will be hurt or that something terrible will happen to them or their families, especially when they are away from important caring figures. Many children with anxiety disorders are preoccupied with health, and worry that their families or friends will become ill. Fears of getting lost, being kidnapped, and losing the ability to be in contact with their families are predominant among children with separation anxiety disorder.

Adolescents with anxiety disorders may not directly express their worries, however; their behavior patterns often reflect either separation anxiety or other anxiety if they exhibit discomfort about leaving home, engage in solitary activities because of fears about how they will perform in front of peers, or have distress when away from their families. Separation anxiety disorder in children is often manifested at the thought of travel or in the course of travel away from home. Children may refuse to go to camp, a new school, or even a friend's house. Frequently, a continuum exists between mild anticipatory anxiety before separation from an important figure and pervasive anxiety after the separation has occurred. Premonitory signs include irritability, difficulty eating, whining, staying in a room alone, clinging to parents, and following a parent everywhere. Often, when a family moves, a child displays separation anxiety by intense clinging to the mother figure. Sometimes, geographic relocation anxiety is expressed in feelings of acute homesickness or psychophysiologic symptoms that break out when the child is away from home or is going to a new country. The child yearns to return home and becomes preoccupied with fantasies of how much better the old home was. Integration into the new life situation may become extremely difficult. Children with anxiety disorders may retreat from social or group activities and express feelings of loneliness because of their self-imposed isolation.

Sleep difficulties are frequent in children and adolescents with any anxiety disorder or in severe separation anxiety; a child or adolescent may require having someone remain with him or her until he or she falls asleep. An anxious child may awaken and go to a parent's bed or even sleep at the parents' door in an effort to diminish anxiety. Nightmares and morbid fears may be expressions of anxiety.

Associated features of anxiety disorders include fear of the dark and imaginary, bizarre worries. Children may have the feeling that eyes are staring at them and monsters are reaching out for them in their bedrooms. Children with anxiety disorders often complain of somatic symptoms and are very sensitive to changes in their bodies. They are often more sensitive than peers and more easily brought to tears. Frequent somatic complaints include gastrointestinal symptoms, nausea, vomiting, and stomachaches; unexplained pain in various parts of the body; sore throats; and flu-like symptoms. Older children typically complain of somatic experiences classically reported by adults with anxiety, such as cardiovascular and respiratory symptoms—palpitations, dizziness, faintness, and feelings of strangulation. Physiologic signs of anxiety are a part of the diagnostic criteria for generalized anxiety disorder, but they are more often also experienced by children with separation anxiety and social phobia than the general population. The most common anxiety disorder that coexists with separation anxiety disorder is specific phobia, which occurs in about one third of referred cases of separation anxiety disorder.

Julie T was an 11-year-old girl referred for an evaluation by her pediatrician based on concern that the source of her chronic gastrointestinal complaints was anxiety. On interview, Julie was meek but responsive to questions. She endorsed a number of worries that included concerns about her health, her parents' safety, her school performance, and her peer relationships. Julie's greatest worries were related to threats to her health and safety. Julie's mother, Mrs. T, reported that Julie had recently been very reluctant to play outside, because she feared she would contract Lyme disease from a tick bite or West Nile virus from a mosquito bite. Mrs. T reported that Julie was also very distressed by news reports about negative events locally and around the world (e.g., kidnapping, crime, terrorism) and that they no longer have the news on when Julie is home. Mrs. T described her as overly conscientious about her schoolwork and as often being concerned about adult matters (e.g., finances, parents' job security). Symptoms that accompanied Julie's worries primarily involved stomach pain and problems falling asleep. Julie's mother stated that, when worrying about something, Julie tended to be quite perseverative, worrying even after reassurance was given. Julie said that she worried often and could not "turn off" her worried thoughts.

Julie was the product of a normal pregnancy and delivery. Her medical history was unremarkable, with the exception of frequent gastrointestinal pain since kindergarten. Julie was described as irritable and difficult to soothe as an infant. Developmental milestones were met within normal limits. She was described as very obedient and had no history of externalizing behavior problems. She was very concerned about her academic performance from an early age and earned A's with an occasional B. Julie was somewhat shy in social situations but well liked by her peers. Family history included depression in her maternal grandmother and a maternal history of separation anxiety disorder as a child. Julie had two younger siblings who were high functioning and without notable problems. (Courtesy of Gail A. Bernstein, M.D., and Ann E. Layne, Ph.D.)

Tina is an 11-year-old 6th grader who lives with her biological parents and two sisters, age 9 and 14 years. Tina is a very articulate girl who has always been a good student, although she never volunteers answers in school unless she is called on by her teacher. She gets along well with her sisters when at home, but since she entered middle school this school year, she has declined invitations to go to friend's homes, has turned down opportunities to go to parties, and has even stopped going on outings with her sisters to the neighborhood mall and the movies. Tina reports that she gets too nervous, and blushes when she is with friends outside of the classroom at school because she can't think of anything to say to them. She reports that she is embarrassed to go shopping or to the movies with her sisters because they often run into neighborhood peers along the way, stop to chat, and this makes her feel "stupid" because she does not say anything, and believes that her sisters' friends will laugh at her shyness. Recently, one of her best friends from the 5th grade confronted her about why she had stopped "hanging out" with her and their other friends. Tina stopped eating lunch with her friends in school because she felt humiliated when they would talk about their weekend plans and even when they invited her to join, she would just look the other way and ignore the conversation. Tina was becoming more isolated, even in school, and admitted to her sister that she was lonely. Tina was brought for an evaluation after her older sister told her mother that Tina was spending all of her time alone whenever her sisters saw their friends, and that she looked sad and stressed out whenever she was around peers. Tina was in good spirits and had fun whenever her sisters stayed home and played with her, but this was becoming rarer because both of her sisters liked being with their own friends. On various occasions Tina's older sister had offered to accompany Tina to parties or to friend's homes, but Tina had declined and burst into tears.

Tina was evaluated by a child psychiatrist who made the diagnosis of social phobia and described a range of treatment options, including cognitive-behavioral therapy (CBT) and a trial of a serotonin reuptake inhibitor agent such as fluvoxamine (Luvox). Tina and her family discussed the options and decided to try the medication. Tina was started on 50 mg of fluvoxamine and over the next month was titrated to a dose of 200 mg. By the third week of the medication trial,

Tina was noticeably less resistant to going out with her sisters to places where they were likely to encounter peers. Her sisters noticed that she did not seem as stressed, and started to eat lunch with her friends in the school cafeteria. She stated that she did not feel as self-conscious as she used to in class and was willing to go to a friend's house. She still declined to go to a birthday party of a classmate that she didn't know very well. Tina continued on this dose of medication and within 2 months, she was significantly less anxious in social situations. She complained occasionally of a stomachache, but overall tolerated the medication well. Her family was impressed when she requested they plan a large birthday party for her 12th birthday and decided to invite 25 peers.

Pathology and Laboratory Examination

No specific laboratory measures help in the diagnosis of separation anxiety disorder.

DIFFERENTIAL DIAGNOSIS

Because some degree of separation anxiety is a normal phenomenon in a very young child, clinical judgment must be used in distinguishing normal anxiety from separation anxiety disorder in this age group. In older school-age children, it is apparent when a child is experiencing more than normal distress when school is refused on a regular basis. For children who resist school, it is important to distinguish whether fear of separation, general worry about performance, or more specific fears of humiliation in front of peers or the teacher are driving the resistance. In many cases in which anxiety is the primary obstacle, all three of the aforementioned feared scenarios come into play. In generalized anxiety disorder, anxiety is not focused on separation. In pervasive developmental disorders and schizophrenia, anxiety about separation may occur but is viewed as caused by these conditions rather than being a separate disorder. When depressive disorders occur in children, the comorbid diagnosis of separation anxiety disorder should also be made when the criteria for both disorders are met; the two diagnoses often coexist. Panic disorder with agoraphobia is uncommon before 18 years of age; the fear is of being incapacitated by a panic attack rather than of separation from parental figures. In some adult cases, however, many symptoms of separation anxiety disorder may be present. In conduct disorder, truancy is common, but children stay away from home and do not have anxiety about separation. School refusal is a frequent symptom in separation anxiety disorder, but is not pathognomonic of it. Children with other diagnoses, such as simple phobias, social phobias, or fear of failure in school because of learning disorder, also evidence school refusal. When school refusal occurs in an adolescent, the severity of the dysfunction is generally greater than when separation anxiety emerges in a young child. Similar and distinguishing characteristics of childhood separation anxiety disorder, generalized anxiety disorder, and social phobia are presented in Table 15.3–4.

COURSE AND PROGNOSIS

The course and the prognosis of separation anxiety disorder, generalized anxiety, and social phobia are varied and are related to the age of onset, the duration of the symptoms, and the development of comorbid anxiety and depressive disorders. Young children who can maintain attendance in school, after-school activities, and peer relationships generally have a better prognosis than children or adolescents who refuse to attend school or drop out of social activities. A follow-up study of children and adolescents with anxiety disorders over a 3-year period reported that up to 82 percent no longer met criteria for the anxiety disorder at follow-up. Of the group followed, 96 percent of those with separation anxiety disorder had a remission at follow-up. Most children who recovered did so within the first year. Early age of onset and later age at diagnosis were factors that predicted slower recovery. Close to one third of the group studied, however, had developed another psychiatric disorder within the follow-up period, and 50 percent of these children developed another anxiety disorder. Reports have indicated a significant overlap of separation anxiety disorder and depressive disorders. In these complicated cases, the prognosis is guarded. Most follow-up studies have methodologic problems and are limited to hospitalized, school-phobic children, not children with separation anxiety disorder per se. Little is reported about the outcome of mild cases whether children are seen in outpatient treatment or receive no treatment. Notwithstanding the limitations of the studies, reports indicate that some children with severe school phobia continue to resist attending school for many years.

During the 1970s, it was reported that many adult women with agoraphobia had suffered from separation anxiety disorder in childhood. Research indicates that children with anxiety disorders are at increased risk for adult anxiety disorders, although the specific link between separation anxiety disorder in childhood and agoraphobia in adulthood has not been established clearly. Studies do indicate that anxious parents are at increased risk of having children with anxiety disorders. In recent years, some cases of children with both panic disorder and separation anxiety disorder have been reported.

TREATMENT

The treatments of separation anxiety disorder, generalized anxiety disorder, and social phobia are often considered together, given the frequent comorbidity and overlapping symptomatology of these disorders. A multimodal comprehensive treatment approach may include CBT, family education, family psychosocial intervention, and pharmacologic interventions. A trial of CBT may be applied first, if available, when a child is able to function sufficiently well to engage in daily activities while obtaining this treatment. Evidence from a recent large multisite National Institute of Mental Health investigation (Research Units in Pediatric Psychopharmacology [RUPP]) confirms the safety and efficacy of fluvoxamine (Luvox) in the treatment of

Table 15.3–4
Common Characteristics of Selected Anxiety Disorders That Occur in Children

Criteria	Separation Anxiety Disorder	Social Phobia	Generalized Anxiety Disorder
Minimal duration to establish diagnosis	At least 4 weeks	No minimum	At least 6 months
Age of onset	Preschool to 18 years	Not specified	Not specified
Precipitating stresses	Separation from significant parental figures, other losses, travel	Pressure for social participation with peers	Unusual pressure for performance, damage to self-esteem, feelings of lack of competence
Peer relationships	Good when no separation is involved	Tentative, overly inhibited	Overly eager to please, peers sought out and dependent relationships established
Sleep	Reluctance or refusal to go to sleep, fear of dark, nightmares	Difficulty in falling asleep at times	Difficulty in falling asleep
Psychophysiologic symptoms	Complaints of stomachaches, nausea, vomiting, flu-like symptoms, headaches, palpitations, dizziness, faintness	Blushing, body tension	Stomachaches, nausea, vomiting, lump in the throat, shortness of breath, dizziness, palpitations
Differential diagnosis	Generalized anxiety disorder, schizophrenia, depressive disorders, conduct disorder, pervasive developmental disorders, major depressive disorder, panic disorder with agoraphobia	Adjustment disorder with depressed mood, generalized anxiety disorder, separation anxiety disorder, major depressive disorder, dysthymic disorder, avoidant personality disorder, borderline personality disorder	Separation anxiety disorder, attention-deficit/hyperactivity disorder, social phobia, adjustment disorder with anxiety, obsessive-compulsive disorder, psychotic disorders, mood disorders

Adapted from Sidney Werkman, M.D.

childhood separation anxiety disorder, generalized anxiety disorder, and social phobia. This double-blind, placebo-controlled study of 128 children and adolescents revealed 76 percent of children in the group treated with fluvoxamine showed significant improvement, compared with 29 percent of those in the placebo group. Response to medication was noticeable after as little as 2 weeks of treatment. Fluvoxamine doses ranged from 50 to 250 mg per day in children and up to 300 mg per day in adolescents. Children and adolescents with less-comorbid depressive symptoms had the best response. Children and adolescents who responded to this medication were continued on fluvoxamine for a period of 6 months, and almost all of them continued to be responders at the 6-month mark. Several other randomized clinical trials have also supported the efficacy of selective serotonin reuptake inhibitor (SSRI) medications in the treatment of child and adolescent anxiety disorders. A recent trial showed fluoxetine at a dose of 20 mg per day to be safe and effective for children with these disorders, with minor side effects, including gastrointestinal distress, headache, and drowsiness. In addition, a randomized clinical trial for the treatment of generalized anxiety disorder in children lent support for the efficacy of sertraline (Zoloft). Finally, a large industry randomized clinical trial of paroxetine (Paxil) in the treatment of children with social phobia found that paroxetine was associated with response in 78 percent of children treated. Paroxetine was used at doses of 10 to 50 mg per day. The U.S. Food and Drug Administration (FDA) has placed a black box warning on antidepressants, including all of the SSRI agents, used in the treatment of any childhood disorder because of concerns about increased suicidality; however, no individual childhood anxiety study has found a statistically significant increase in suicidal thoughts or behaviors. Clearly, SSRI medications have been shown to be both safe and efficacious in the treatment of childhood anxiety disorders, yet the evidence is not yet in on whether the optimal treatment approach is to administer CBT first, medication first, or both simultaneously. The ongoing National Institute of Mental Health (NIMH)–funded Child/Adolescent Anxiety Multimodal Treatment Study (CAMS) is investigating these questions. This double-blind, placebo-controlled study includes more than 300 children and adolescents with separation anxiety disorder, generalized anxiety disorder, or social phobia who are being treated with either sertraline alone, CBT alone, both CBT and medication, or placebo. This is the first large-scale study to investigate the combination of therapeutic interventions compared with each condition alone in the treatment of child and adolescent anxiety disorders. The data from this study will be available within the next few years so that optimal treatment strategies can be designed for anxiety disorders in childhood. Without evidence to support clinical decisions, pharmacologic interventions have historically been recommended as second-line treatments when psychosocial strategies have not been effective. Cognitive-behavioral therapy is widely accepted as a first-line treatment for a variety of anxiety disorders for children, including separation anxiety disorder, social phobia, and selective mutism. Specific cognitive strategies and relaxation exercises may also be added components of treatment for some children as self-contained strategies to control their anxiety. Family interventions are also frequently critical in the management of separation anxiety disorder, especially in children who refuse to attend school, so that firm encouragement of school attendance is maintained while appropriate support is also provided.

Pharmacologic management of childhood anxiety disorders in clinical practice often includes the use of agents even when no evidence base exists for such management. Widely recommended SSRIs include fluoxetine, fluvoxamine, sertraline, paroxetine, and citalopram (Celexa). Tricyclic drugs are not recommended due to their potentially serious cardiac adverse effects. β-Adrenergic receptor antagonists, such as propranolol (Inderal) and buspirone (BuSpar), have been used clinically in children with anxiety disorders, but no data support their efficacy. Diphenhydramine (Benadryl) may be used in the short term to control sleep disturbances in children with anxiety disorders. Open trials and one double-blind, placebo-controlled study suggested that alprazolam (Xanax), a benzodiazepine, may help to control anxiety symptoms in separation anxiety disorder. Clonazepam (Klonopin) has been studied in open trials and may be useful in controlling symptoms of panic and other anxiety symptoms.

School refusal associated with separation anxiety disorder can be viewed as a psychiatric emergency. A comprehensive treatment plan involves the child, the parents, and the child's peers and school. The child should be encouraged to attend school, but when a return to a full school day is overwhelming, a program should be arranged so the child can progressively increase the time spent at school. Graded contact with an object of anxiety is a form of behavior modification that can be applied to any type of separation anxiety. Some severe cases of school refusal require hospitalization. Cognitive-behavioral modalities include exposure to feared separations and cognitive strategies, such as coping self-statements aimed at increasing a sense of autonomy and mastery.

Pharmacotherapy

Pharmacotherapy is not indicated in this disorder unless there is a comorbid condition (i.e., anxiety or depression) that is a contributing factor to the disorder or results from it.

▲ 15.4 Selective Mutism

Selective mutism is characterized in a child by persistent failure to speak in one or more specific social situations, most typically including the school setting. A child with selective mutism may remain completely silent or near silent, in some cases whispering instead of speaking out loud. The most recent conceptualization of selective mutism highlights the relationship between underlying social anxiety and the resulting failure to speak. Most children with the disorder are completely silent during the stressful situations, whereas some may almost inaudibly verbalize single-syllable words. Children with selective mutism are fully capable of speaking competently when not in a socially anxiety-producing situation. Some children with the disorder communicate with eye contact or nonverbal gestures. These children speak fluently in other situations, such as at home and in certain familiar settings. Selective mutism is believed to be an expression of social phobia because of its expression in selective social situations.

EPIDEMIOLOGY

The prevalence of selective mutism varies with age, with younger children at increased risk for the disorder. One epidemiologic study using criteria from the text revision of the fourth edition of the *Diagnostic and Statistical Manual of Mental Disorders* (DSM-IV-TR) reported the rate of selective mutism in preschoolers to be 0.6 percent. Another large epidemiologic survey in the United Kingdom reported a prevalence rate of selective mutism to be 0.69 percent in children 4 to 5 years of age, which dropped to 0.8 percent near the end of the same academic year. Another survey in the United Kingdom identified 0.06 percent of 7-year-olds as having selective mutism. Selective mutism has been estimated to range between 3 and 8 per 10,000 children. Some surveys indicate that it may occur in up to 0.5 percent of school children in the community. Young children are more vulnerable to the disorder than older ones. Selective mutism appears to be more common in girls than in boys.

ETIOLOGY

Genetic Contribution

Over the last two decades, the conceptualization of selective mutism has evolved from one that focused on oppositionality or childhood trauma as possible contributing factors to the current consensus that it has the same etiologic factors, including genetic factors, that lead to the emergence of social phobia and other comorbid anxiety disorders. Such children have histories of delayed onset of speech or speech abnormalities that may be contributory. In a recent survey, 90 percent of children with selective mutism met diagnostic criteria for social phobia. These children showed high levels of social anxiety without notable psychopathology in other areas, according to parent and teacher ratings. Thus, selective mutism may not represent a distinct disorder but may be better conceptualized as a subtype of social phobia. Similar to families with children who exhibit other anxiety disorders, maternal anxiety, depression, and heightened dependence needs are often noted in families of children with selective mutism.

Parental Interactions

Given the likely higher levels of anxiety disorders in parents of children with selective mutism, anxiety-tinged interpersonal interactions between parents and child may unwittingly serve to promote social anxiety in children with selective mutism.

Maternal overprotection and an overly close but ambivalent relationship between parents and a selectively mute child may promote symptoms. Children with selective mutism usually speak freely at home and only exhibit symptoms when under social pressure either in school or other social situations. Some children seem predisposed to selective mutism after early emotional or physical trauma; thus, some clinicians refer to the phenomenon as *traumatic mutism* rather than selective mutism.

Speech and Language Factors

Selective mutism is a psychologically determined inhibition or refusal to speak, yet a higher-than-expected proportion of children with the disorder have a history of speech delay. An interesting finding suggests that children with selective mutism are at higher risk for a disturbance in auditory processing, which may interfere with efficient processing of incoming sounds. For the most part, however, speech and language problems in children with selective mutism are subtle and are exclusionary criteria for the diagnosis of selective mutism.

DIAGNOSIS AND CLINICAL FEATURES

Table 15.4–1 gives the DSM-IV-TR diagnostic criteria. The diagnosis of selective mutism is not difficult to make after it is clear that a child has adequate language skills in some environments but not in others. The mutism may have developed gradually or suddenly after a disturbing experience. The age of onset can range from 4 to 8 years. Mute periods are most commonly manifested in school or outside the home; in rare cases, a child is mute at home but not in school. Children who exhibit selective mutism may also have symptoms of separation anxiety disorder, school refusal, and delayed language acquisition. Because social anxiety is almost always present in children with selective mutism, behavioral disturbances, such as temper tantrums and oppositional behaviors, may also occur in the home.

Table 15.4–1
DSM-IV-TR Diagnostic Criteria for Selective Mutism

A. Consistent failure to speak in specific social situations (in which there is an expectation for speaking, e.g., at school) despite speaking in other situations.
B. The disturbance interferes with educational or occupational achievement or with social communication.
C. The duration of the disturbance is at least 1 month (not limited to the first month of school).
D. The failure to speak is not due to a lack of knowledge of, or comfort with, the spoken language required in the social situation.
E. The disturbance is not better accounted for by a communication disorder (e.g., stuttering) and does not occur exclusively during the course of a pervasive developmental disorder, schizophrenia, or other psychotic disorder.

From American Psychiatric Association. *Diagnostic and Statistical Manual of Mental Disorders.* 4th ed. Text rev. Washington, DC: American Psychiatric Association; copyright 2000, with permission.

Beth is a 5-year-old Vietnamese-American girl who lives with her biological mother, father, and siblings. Beth's parents reported a 2-year history of not speaking at school (preschool) or to any children or adults outside of her family, despite speaking normally at home. At home, she reportedly is animated and quite talkative with her immediate family and a few young cousins as well. Although she speaks to adult relatives outside of her immediate family, her communication is often limited to one-word responses to their questions. By her parents' report, Beth also exhibits extreme social anxiety, to the point of "freezing" in certain situations when attention is focused on her. At the time of her evaluation, Beth had not received prior treatment for selective mutism or any other emotional or behavioral disorders. Beth speaks fluent English, as well as Vietnamese, and, according to her parents, met all developmental milestones on time and appears to have above-average intelligence. They also reported that Beth enjoys dancing, singing, and imaginative play with her sisters.

During initial evaluation, Beth failed to make eye contact or respond in any way to the intake clinician. Beth's parents reported that this behavior is typical of her when in a new situation with new people but that she communicates nonverbally and makes eye contact with most people once she "gets to know them." On request, Beth's parents provided a videotaped recording of Beth playing at home with her sisters. In this video, Beth appeared animated and was speaking spontaneously and fluently without obvious impairment. Beth received diagnoses of selective mutism (severe) and social phobia (moderately severe). Behavioral treatment was recommended at this time.

Behavioral treatment was initiated after the intake evaluation. Initially, the therapist instructed Beth and her mother to come up with lists of easy, medium, and hard speaking situations and lists of small, medium, and large rewards. These lists then became the basis for assignments (and reinforcement) for speaking tasks that gradually increased in difficulty. In general, sessions included time with Beth and her mother together to review past and future assignments and time with Beth and the therapist alone.

When treatment began, Beth did not communicate at all verbally or nonverbally with the therapist. The therapist gradually increased rapport (via unstructured play) while having Beth try increasingly difficult tasks, such as first whispering to her mother with the therapist in the corner, then nodding yes or no, pointing, whispering to a stuffed animal, whispering to her mother while facing the therapist, and then subsequently responding to the therapist directly. A successful technique in working with Beth was the use of pretend play; the therapist often used several puppets as additional "participants" in the treatment. Talking to, for, or about these animals in the context of pretend play provided Beth with a good "warm-up" period and facilitated talking. After three sessions, Beth consistently and spontaneously talked to the therapist. Beth received stickers for completing each speaking assignment, and, after filling up sticker charts, she received rewards (small toy or treat from reward list).

Beth was also given assignments that involved her teacher and classmates. These were implemented in gradual fashion and included waving to the teacher, playing an audiotape of her saying "hello" to the teacher, whispering "hello" to the teacher, speaking "hello" to the teacher in a regular voice, and so on. After approximately 14 sessions, Beth spoke a complete sentence in front of the class when called on and spoke to her teacher in front of several other students.

During the last few sessions, which were tapered over several weeks, Beth's mother took an increasingly primary role in assigning and following up on speaking assignments. Beth entered kindergarten and, after only a few days, began regularly speaking to her teacher (both privately and in front of peers) and to most peers in class. After completion of therapy, the mother continued to monitor Beth's speaking behaviors and to promote speaking in new situations by encouraging (and rewarding) Beth's gradual successes with novel people and situations. (Courtesy of R. Lindsey Bergman, Ph.D., and John Piacentini, Ph.D.)

Pathology and Laboratory Examination

No specific laboratory measures are useful in the diagnosis or treatment of selective mutism.

DIFFERENTIAL DIAGNOSIS

Differential diagnosis of children who are silent in social situations emphasizes ruling out pervasive developmental disorders, such as autism. Once it is confirmed that the child is fully capable of speaking in certain situations that are comfortable but not in school and other social situations, the possibility of an anxiety-related disorder is raised. Shy children may exhibit a transient muteness in new, anxiety-provoking situations. These children often have histories of not speaking in the presence of strangers and of clinging to their mothers. Most children who are mute on entering school improve spontaneously and may be described as having transient adaptational shyness. Selective mutism must also be distinguished from mental retardation, pervasive developmental disorders, and expressive language disorder. In these disorders, the symptoms are widespread, and no one situation exists in which the child communicates normally; the child may have an inability, rather than a refusal, to speak. In mutism secondary to conversion disorder, the mutism is pervasive. Children introduced into an environment in which a different language is spoken may be reticent to begin using the new language. Selective mutism should be diagnosed only when children also refuse to converse in their native language and when they have gained communicative competence in the new language but refuse to speak it.

COURSE AND PROGNOSIS

Many very young children with early symptoms of selective mutism in the transitional period when entering preschool may have a spontaneous improvement over a number of months and never fulfill criteria for the full disorder. Children with selective mutism are often abnormally shy during preschool years, but the onset of the full disorder is usually not until age 5 or 6 years. The most common pattern is that children speak almost exclusively at home with the nuclear family but not elsewhere, especially not at school. Consequently, they may have academic difficulties and even failure. Children with selective mutism are generally shy, anxious, and vulnerable to the development of depression. Most children with mild forms of anxiety disorder, including selective mutism, remit with or without treatment. With recent data suggesting that fluoxetine (Prozac) may influence the course of selective mutism, recovery may be enhanced. Children in whom the disorder persists often have difficulty in forming social relationships. Teasing and scapegoating by peers may cause them to refuse to go to school. Some children with this severe social phobia are characterized by rigidity, compulsive traits, negativism, temper tantrums, and oppositional and aggressive behavior at home. Other children with the disorder tolerate the feared situation better by communicating with gestures, such as nodding, shaking the head, and saying "Uh-huh" or "No." Most cases last for only a few weeks or months, but some cases persist for years. In one follow-up study, about one half of the children improved within 5 to 10 years. Children who do not improve by age 10 years appear to have a long-term course and a worse prognosis than those who do improve by age 10 years. As many as one third of children with selective mutism, with or without treatment, may develop other psychiatric disorders, particularly other anxiety disorders and depression.

TREATMENT

Published data on the successful treatment of children with selective mutism are very scant, yet solid evidence indicates that children with social phobia respond to various selective serotonin reuptake inhibitor agents (SSRIs), and cognitive-behavioral treatments are under investigation in a multisite, randomized, placebo-controlled trial of children with anxiety disorders.

In the absence of data to support an approach using therapy or medication alone or in combination, a multimodal approach using psychoeducation for the family, cognitive-behavioral therapy, and SSRI medication as needed is recommended. Preschool children may also benefit from a therapeutic nursery. For school-age children, individual cognitive-behavioral therapy is recommended as a first-line treatment. Family education and cooperation are beneficial. SSRI medication is an accepted component of treatment when psychosocial interventions do not suffice to manage symptoms.

A recent report of 21 children with selective mutism treated in an open trial with fluoxetine suggested that this medication may be effective for childhood selective mutism. Reports have confirmed the efficacy of fluoxetine in the treatment of adult social phobia and in at least one double-blind, placebo-controlled study using fluoxetine with children with mutism. A large National Institute of Mental Health–funded study of anxiety disorders in children and adolescents, including social phobia—Research Units in Pediatric Psychopharmacology (RUPP)—showed distinct superiority of fluvoxamine over placebo in the treatment of childhood anxiety. Children with selective mutism may benefit similarly to those with social phobia, given the current belief that it is a subgroup of social phobia. SSRI medications that have been shown in randomized, placebo-controlled trials to have benefit in the treatment of children with social phobia include fluoxetine (20 to 60 mg per day), fluvoxamine (Luvox) (50 to 300 mg per day), sertraline (Zoloft) (25 to 200 mg per day), and paroxetine (Paxil) (10 to 50 mg per day).

Other medications, such as phenelzine (Nardil), reportedly improve symptoms of social phobia in adults but are rarely recommended for mutism in school-age children, given the choice of multiple SSRI agents with significantly safer side-effect profiles.

Pharmacotherapy

Pharmacotherapy is not indicated in this disorder unless there is a comorbid condition (i.e., anxiety or depression) that is a contributing factor to the disorder or results from it.

16

Early-Onset Schizophrenia

Childhood-onset schizophrenia (COS) is a rare and severe form of schizophrenia characterized by an onset of psychotic symptoms by age 12 years and is believed to represent a subgroup of affected individuals with an increased heritable etiology. Children diagnosed with COS have high rates of premorbid developmental abnormalities that appear to be nonspecific markers of severe early impaired neurodevelopment. Recent imaging studies provided data suggesting that children with COS have decreased anterior cingulated gyrus (ACG) volumes with age, unlike controls, and an absence of the normal decreased left- to right-ACG volume asymmetry. These structural differences are hypothesized to be related to abnormal neurodevelopment influencing attention and emotion regulation, which are characteristic of some cognitive impairments in psychosis. The frequency of COS is reported to be less than 1 case in 10,000 children, whereas among adolescents between the ages of 13 and 18 years, the frequency of schizophrenia is markedly increased. Schizophrenia with childhood onset has the same core phenomenologic features as schizophrenia in adolescence and adulthood; however, extremely high rates are seen of comorbid psychiatric disorders, including attention-deficit/hyperactivity disorder (ADHD), depressive disorders, and separation anxiety disorder in children and adolescents with COS.

Psychosocial stressors are known to influence the course of schizophrenia, and the same stressors may possibly interact with biological risk factors in the emergence of the disorder, given that children who are diagnosed with COS have marked neuropsychologic deficits in a wide range of brain functions, including attention, working memory, and executive functions. Similar defects have been demonstrated in adolescents and adults with schizophrenia; however, children with schizophrenia have been shown to have more significant deficits in measures of intelligence quotient (IQ) and memory and tests of perceptuomotor skills than individuals with adolescent-onset or adult-onset schizophrenia. Differences in these cognitive measures in persons with schizophrenia of different ages of onset suggest that these deficits may not be sequelae of the disorder but are markers of brain dysfunction even before the onset of the illness. Furthermore, the brain dysfunction in schizophrenia occurs on a continuum with COS, reflecting the most severe neuropsychologic deficits. In addition, a study comparing the severity of cognitive deficits between adolescents and adults early in the course of schizophrenia concluded that, although greater cognitive deficits are seen in earlier-onset schizophrenia, a waning may occur of the development of certain cognitive domains influencing working memory and attention after the onset of schizophrenia in adolescent patients. The clinical presentation of schizophrenia, however, taking into consideration the developmental level of the child, remains remarkably similar across ages. Schizophrenia in prepubertal children includes the presence of at least two of the following: hallucinations, delusions, grossly disorganized speech or behavior, and severe withdrawal for at least 1 month. Social or academic dysfunction must be present, and continuous signs of the disturbance must persist for at least 6 months. The diagnostic criteria for schizophrenia in children are identical to the criteria for the adult form, except that instead of showing deteriorating functioning, children may fail to achieve their expected levels of social and academic functioning.

Before the 1960s, the term *childhood psychosis* was applied to a heterogeneous group of pervasive developmental disorders without hallucinations and delusions. In the 1960s and 1970s, children with evidence of a profound psychotic disturbance early in life often were observed to have mental retardation, be socially dysfunctional with severe communication and language impairments, and not have a family history of schizophrenia. In children with psychoses that emerged after the age of 5 years, however, auditory hallucinations, delusions, inappropriate affects, thought disorder, and normal intelligence were manifest, and these children often had a family history of schizophrenia; they were viewed as exhibiting schizophrenia, whereas the younger children were identified as having an entirely different disorder—either autistic disorder or a pervasive developmental disorder.

In the 1980s, schizophrenia with childhood onset was formally separated from autistic disorder. This change reflected evidence accrued during the 1960s and 1970s that the clinical picture, family history, age of onset, and course of the two disorders differed. After the separation of the disorders, two controversies ensued. First, a few researchers remained of the opinion that a subgroup of autistic children will eventually have schizophrenia, as evidence shows for a small group. The diagnosis of schizophrenia is specifically differentiated from autistic disorder. Many children with early onset schizophrenia have neurodevelopmental abnormalities, some of which are also evident in children with autistic disorder. Children with autistic disorder are impaired in multiple areas of adaptive functioning from early life onward. The onset is almost always before 3 years of age, whereas the onset of childhood schizophrenia occurs before early adolescence but often is not apparent in children until after the age of 3 years. COS is more rare than onset in adolescence or young adulthood, and practically no reports are found of an onset of schizophrenia before 5 years of age. According to the text revision of the fourth edition of the *Diagnostic and Statistical Manual of Mental Disorders* (DSM-IV-TR), schizophrenia can be diagnosed in the presence of autistic disorder.

One of the challenges in applying adult diagnostic criteria to COS is that some very young children who report hallucinations and apparent thought disorders in conjunction with developmental immaturities in language and in differentiating reality from fantasy may be manifesting phenomena that are better accounted for by immaturity than psychosis.

EPIDEMIOLOGY

Schizophrenia in prepubertal children is exceedingly rare; it is estimated to occur in less than 1 of 10,000 children. In adolescents, the prevalence of schizophrenia is estimated to be 50 times that in younger children, with probable rates of 1 to 2 per 1,000. Boys seem to have a slight preponderance among children diagnosed with schizophrenia, with an estimated ratio of about 1.67 boys to 1 girl. Boys often become identified at a younger age than girls. It has been estimated that 0.1 to 1 percent present before age 10 years, with 4 percent presenting before 15 years of age. The rate of onset increases sharply during adolescence. Schizophrenia rarely is diagnosed in children younger than 5 years of age. Psychotic symptoms usually emerge insidiously, and the diagnostic criteria are met gradually over time. Occasionally, the onset of schizophrenia is sudden and occurs in a previously well-functioning child. Schizophrenia also may be diagnosed in a child who has had chronic difficulties and then experiences a significant exacerbation. The prevalence of schizophrenia among the parents of children with schizophrenia is about 8 percent, which is close to twice the prevalence in the parents of patients with adult-onset schizophrenia.

Schizotypal personality disorder is similar to schizophrenia in its inappropriate affects, excessive magical thinking, odd beliefs, social isolation, ideas of reference, and unusual perceptual experiences, such as illusions. Schizotypal personality disorder, however, does not have psychotic features; still, the disorder seems to aggregate in families with adult-onset schizophrenia. The relation between the two disorders is unclear.

ETIOLOGY

The etiology of COS has multiple contributing factors, and estimates of its heritability are as high as 80 percent. COS is a severe form of schizophrenia, which may increase its likelihood of heritability to among the highest of estimates. Genetic studies provide substantial evidence for a significant genetic basis in the development of schizophrenia. The precise mechanisms of transmission of schizophrenia are not well understood. Schizophrenia is known to be up to eight times more prevalent among first-degree relatives of those with schizophrenia than in the general population. Adoption studies of patients with adult-onset schizophrenia have shown that schizophrenia occurs in the biological relatives, not the adoptive relatives. Additional genetic evidence is supported by higher concordance rates for schizophrenia in monozygotic twins than in dizygotic twins. Higher rates of schizophrenia have been established among relatives of those with COS than in the relatives of those with adult-onset schizophrenia. A recent case report identified a rare genetic occurrence in which an offspring received two chromosome homologues from the same parent (uniparental isodisomy) of chromosome 5, already implicated in several linkage studies to be associated with schizophrenia in a child with COS.

No reliable method can identify persons at the highest risk for schizophrenia in a given family. Neurodevelopmental abnormalities and higher-than-expected rates of neurologic soft signs and impairments in sustaining attention and in strategies for information processing appear among children at high risk. Increased rates of disturbed communication styles are found in families with a member with schizophrenia. Recent reports have documented marked neuropsychologic deficits in attention, working memory, and premorbid IQ among children who develop schizophrenia and its spectrum disorders. High expressed emotion, characterized by overly critical responses in families, has been shown to be correlated with increased relapse rates among patients with schizophrenia.

Recent studies have documented gray matter loss in the brains of children with COS that started in the parietal region and proceeded frontally to dorsolateral prefrontal and temporal cortices, including superior temporal gyri. Magnetic resonance imaging (MRI) studies of 12 children with COS at baseline and at follow-up 5 years later were compared with normal controls. Children with COS showed severe bilateral frontal gray matter loss over the 5-year period that occurred in a dorsal-to-ventral pattern across the medial hemispheres. Frontal regions were most affected, whereas cingulated-limbic regions were less vulnerable, which correlates with the brain areas responsible for the cognitive and metabolic dysfunction typically observed in schizophrenia. Children and adolescents with schizophrenia are more likely to have a premorbid history of social rejection, poor peer relationships, clingy withdrawn behavior, and academic trouble than those with adult-onset schizophrenia. Some children with schizophrenia first seen in middle childhood have early histories of motor milestones and delayed language acquisition that are similar to some symptoms of autistic disorder. The mechanisms of biological vulnerability and environmental influences producing manifestations of schizophrenia are under investigation.

DIAGNOSIS AND CLINICAL FEATURES

All of the symptoms included in adult-onset schizophrenia may be manifest in children with the disorder. The onset is frequently insidious; after first exhibiting inappropriate affects of unusual behavior, a child may take months or years to meet all of the diagnostic criteria for schizophrenia. Children who eventually meet the criteria often are socially rejected and clingy and have limited social skills. They may have histories of delayed motor and verbal milestones and do poorly in school, despite normal intelligence. Although children with schizophrenia and autistic disorder may be similar in their early histories, children with schizophrenia have normal intelligence and do not meet the criteria for a pervasive developmental disorder.

According to the DSM-IV-TR, a child with schizophrenia may experience deterioration of function along with the emergence of psychotic symptoms, or the child may never achieve the expected level of functioning. Auditory hallucinations commonly occur in children with schizophrenia. They may hear several voices making an ongoing critical commentary, or command hallucinations may tell children to kill themselves or others. The voices may be bizarre, identified as "a computer in my head," Martians, or the voice of someone familiar, such as a relative. Visual hallucinations are experienced by a significant number of children with schizophrenia and often are frightening; the children may see the devil, skeletons, scary faces, or space creatures. Transient phobic visual hallucinations also occur in traumatized children who do not eventually have a major psychotic disorder.

Delusions are present in more than one half of children with schizophrenia; the delusions take various forms, including persecutory, grandiose, and religious. Delusions increase in frequency with increased age. Blunted or inappropriate affects appear almost universally in children with schizophrenia. Children with schizophrenia may giggle inappropriately or cry without being able to explain why. Formal thought disorders, including loosening of associations and thought blocking, are common features among children with schizophrenia. Illogical thinking and poverty of thought are also often present. Unlike adults with schizophrenia, children with schizophrenia do not have poverty of speech content, but they speak less than other children of the same intelligence and are ambiguous in the way they refer to persons, objects, and events. The communication deficits observable in children with schizophrenia include unpredictably changing the topic of conversation without introducing the new topic to the listener (loose associations). Children with schizophrenia also exhibit illogical thinking and speaking and tend to underuse self-initiated repair strategies to aid in their communication. When an utterance is unclear or vague, normal children attempt to clarify their communication with repetitions, revision, and more detail. Children with schizophrenia, on the other hand, fail to aid communication with revision, fillers, or starting over. These deficits may be conceptualized as negative symptoms in childhood schizophrenia.

The core phenomena for schizophrenia seem to be the same among various age groups, but a child's developmental level influences the presentation of the symptoms. Delusions of young children are less complex than those of older children. Age-appropriate content, such as animal imagery and monsters, is likely to be a source of delusional fear in children. Other features that seem to occur frequently in children with schizophrenia are poor motor functioning, visuospatial impairments, and attention deficits.

The DSM-IV-TR delineates five types of schizophrenia: paranoid, disorganized, catatonic, undifferentiated, and residual.

A 12-year-old boy developed concerns that his parents might be poisoning his food. Over the next year, his symptoms progressed with increased fearfulness, preoccupation with food, and beliefs that Satan and voices from the radio and television were sending him bad thoughts. During this time, his parents also observed bizarre behaviors, including talking and yelling to himself, perseverating about devils and demons, assaulting family members because he thought they were evil, and attempting to hurt himself because he believed it would please God. No predominant mood symptoms or any history of substance abuse were found.

Developmentally, he was the product of a full-term pregnancy complicated by a difficult labor and forceps delivery. His early motor and speech milestones were normal. As a younger child, he tended to be quiet and socially awkward. His intelligence was felt to be in the normal range, but academic testing was consistently below grade level.

He has had no significant medical problems. An organic work-up included normal serum chemistries, thyroid functions, toxicology screen, ceruloplasmin, and brain MRI. His family psychiatric history was significant for depression in a maternal aunt and a completed suicide in a maternal great-grandparent. His symptoms have not significantly improved in the 5 years subsequent to the onset of his illness. He has been hospitalized nine times, including placement in a long-term residential program. He has been on numerous antipsychotic medications, both traditional neuroleptics and atypical agents, and numerous other agents, including selective serotonin reuptake inhibitors (SSRIs) and mood stabilizers. His mental status examination continued to display tangential and disorganized thinking, paranoid delusions, loose associations, perseverative speech patterns, and a flat, at times inappropriate, affect. His time has generally been spent pacing and muttering to himself, with no social interaction with others unless initiated by adults. Some improvement was finally noted with clozapine (Clozaril) therapy, although he remained symptomatic. (Courtesy of Jon M. McClellan, M.D.)

PATHOLOGY AND LABORATORY EXAMINATIONS

No specific laboratory tests are diagnostically specific for COS. Although neuroimaging studies are converging to suggest that children with COS have decreased ACG volumes with age and an absence of the normal decreased left- to right-ACG volume asymmetry, this research cannot be used as an index for diagnosis. High incidences of pregnancy and birth complications have been reported in the histories of children with schizophrenia, but no specificity has been found in these risks for childhood schizophrenia. Electroencephalogram (EEG) studies have not been helpful in distinguishing children with schizophrenia from other children. Although data exist to suggest that hypoprolinemia is associated with the risk of schizoaffective disorder because of an alteration on chromosome 22q11, no association has been found of hyperprolinemia with COS.

DIFFERENTIAL DIAGNOSIS

The differential diagnosis of COS includes autistic disorder, bipolar disorders, depressive psychotic disorders, multicomplex developmental syndromes, Asperger's syndrome, drug-induced psychosis, and psychotic states caused by organic disorders. Children with COS have been shown to have multiple frequently occurring concurrent disorders, including ADHD, oppositional defiant disorder, and depression. Children with schizotypal personality disorder have some traits in common with children who meet diagnostic criteria for schizophrenia. Blunted affect, social isolation, eccentric thoughts, ideas of reference, and bizarre behavior can be seen in both disorders; however, in schizophrenia, overt psychotic symptoms, such as hallucinations, delusions, and incoherence, must be present at some point. When they are present, they exclude a diagnosis of schizotypal personality disorder. Hallucinations alone, however, are not evidence of schizophrenia; patients must show either a deterioration of function or an inability to meet an expected developmental level to warrant the diagnosis of schizophrenia. Auditory and visual hallucinations can appear as self-limited events in nonpsychotic young children who are faced with extreme psychosocial stressors, such as the breakup of their parents, and in children experiencing a major loss or significant change in lifestyle.

Psychotic phenomena are common among children with major depressive disorder, in which both hallucinations and, less commonly, delusions may occur. The congruence of mood with psychotic features is most pronounced in depressed children, although children with schizophrenia may also seem sad. The hallucinations and delusions of schizophrenia are more likely to have a bizarre quality than those of children with depressive disorders. In children and adolescents with bipolar I disorder, it often is difficult to distinguish a first episode of mania with psychotic features from schizophrenia if the child has no history of previous depressions. Grandiose delusions and hallucinations are typical of manic episodes, but clinicians often must follow the natural history of the disorder to confirm the presence of a mood disorder. Pervasive developmental disorders, including autistic disorder with normal intelligence, often share some features with schizophrenia. Most notably, difficulty with social relationships, an early history of delayed language acquisition, and ongoing communication deviance occur in both disorders; however, hallucinations, delusions, and formal thought disorder are core features of schizophrenia and are not expected features of pervasive developmental disorders. Pervasive developmental disorders usually are diagnosed by 3 years of age, but schizophrenia with childhood onset can rarely be diagnosed before 5 years of age.

Alcohol and other substance abuse sometimes can result in a deterioration of function, psychotic symptoms, and paranoid delusions. Amphetamines, lysergic acid diethylamide (LSD), and phencyclidine (PCP) may lead to a psychotic state. A sudden, flagrant onset of paranoid psychosis is more suggestive of substance-induced psychotic disorder than an insidious onset. Medical conditions that can induce psychotic features include thyroid disease, systemic lupus erythematosus, and temporal lobe disease.

COURSE AND PROGNOSIS

Important predictors of the course and outcome of early-onset schizophrenia include the child's level of functioning before the onset of schizophrenia, the age of onset, IQ, response to pharmacologic interventions, how much functioning the child regained after the first episode, and the amount of support available from the family. Children with developmental delays, learning disorders, lower IQ, and premorbid behavioral disorders such as ADHD and conduct disorder seem to respond less well to medication treatment of schizophrenia and are likely to have the most guarded prognoses. In a long-term outcome study of patients with schizophrenia with onset before 14 years of age, the worst prognoses occurred in children with schizophrenia that was diagnosed before they were 10 years of age and who had preexisting personality disorders.

An additional issue in outcome studies is the stability of the diagnosis of schizophrenia. In one study, one third of children who received a diagnosis of schizophrenia were diagnosed with bipolar disorder in adolescence. Children and adolescents with bipolar I disorder may have a better long-term prognosis than children and adolescents with schizophrenia. In adult-onset schizophrenia, family interactions, such as high expressed emotion, may be associated with increased relapse rates. No clear-cut data are available regarding childhood schizophrenia, but the degree of supportiveness, as opposed to critical and overinvolved family responses, probably influences the prognosis.

Childhood-onset schizophrenia appears to be a more malignant type of schizophrenia, which presents a greater challenge to treatment with pharmacology and psychosocial interventions. It seems to respond less to medication than schizophrenia with adult onset or adolescent onset, and the prognosis may be poorer. Positive symptoms—that is, hallucinations and delusions—are likely to be more responsive to medication than negative symptoms such as withdrawal. In a recent report of 38 children with schizophrenia who had been hospitalized, two-thirds required placement in residential facilities, and only one third improved sufficiently to return home.

TREATMENT

The treatment of COS requires a multimodal approach, including pharmacologic interventions, family education, social skills interventions, and appropriate educational placement. Research suggests that in adolescents and young adults early interventions during the prodrome of schizophrenia with atypical antipsychotics and psychosocial support may improve symptoms and delay or prevent progression to full-blown schizophrenia. Investigation is needed on the recognition of prodromal states of COS to assess the benefits of very early interventions. Treatments for COS are based on very limited data. Antipsychotic medications are indicated, given the degree of impairment in both social relationships and academic function exhibited by children with schizophrenia. Children with COS may have less robust responses to antipsychotic medications than adolescents and adults with the same disorder. Family education and ongoing family interventions are critical to maximize the level of support that the family can give to the patient. The proper educational setting for the child is also important because social skills deficits, attention deficits, and academic difficulties often accompany childhood schizophrenia.

Pharmacotherapy

Atypical antipsychotics—serotonin-dopamine antagonists—are current first-line treatment for children and adolescents with schizophrenia, having replaced the dopamine receptor antagonists because of their more favorable side effect profiles. The serotonin-dopamine agonists, including risperidone (Risperdal), olanzapine (Zyprexa), and clozapine (Clozaril), differ from the conventional antipsychotics in that they act as serotonin-receptor antagonists with some dopamine (D2) activity but without a predominance of D2-receptor antagonism. They are hypothesized to be more effective in reducing positive and negative symptoms of schizophrenia and incur less risk of causing extrapyramidal adverse effects. Additional atypical antipsychotics, such as quetiapine (Seroquel), ziprasidone (Geodon), and aripiprazole (Abilify), are also serotonin-dopamine antagonists that are used in clinical practice for children and adolescents with psychotic disorders who do not respond to other atypical antipsychotics. A limited evidence base exists to inform the treatment of COS with the atypical antipsychotics, and there a need for randomized clinical trials in this patient population.

A recent double-blind, randomized, 8-week controlled trial compared the efficacy and safety of olanzapine to clozapine in COS. Children with COS who were resistant to at least two previous treatments with antipsychotics were randomized to treatment for 8 weeks with either olanzapine or clozapine followed by a 2-year open-label follow-up. Based on the use of the Clinical Global Impression of Severity of Symptoms Scale and Schedule for the Assessment of Negative/Positive Symptoms, clozapine was found to be associated with a significant reduction in all outcome measures, whereas olanzapine showed improvement on some measures but not on all. The only statistically significant measure in which clozapine was superior to olanzapine was in alleviating negative symptoms compared with baseline. Clozapine was associated with more adverse events, such as lipid abnormalities and a seizure in one patient.

Several recent studies have provided evidence that risperidone, a benzisoxazole derivative, is as effective as the older high-potency conventional antipsychotics, such as haloperidol (Haldol), and causes less frequent severe side effects in the treatment of schizophrenia in older adolescents and adults. Published case reports and limited larger controlled studies have supported the efficacy of risperidone in the treatment of psychosis in children and adolescents. Risperidone has been reported to cause weight gain and dystonic reactions and other extrapyramidal adverse effects in children and adolescents. Olanzapine is generally well tolerated with respect to extrapyramidal adverse effects compared with conventional antipsychotics and risperidone but is associated with moderate sedation and significant weight gain.

High-potency conventional antipsychotics, such as haloperidol and trifluoperazine (Stelazine), are available as second-line treatments; however, lower-potency antipsychotics, such as chlorpromazine (Thorazine), may be preferable for young children because of their decreased risk of dystonic reaction. Acute dystonic reactions do occur in children, and 1 to 2 mg per day of benztropine (Cogentin) usually is sufficient to treat the extrapyramidal adverse effects.

Children and adolescents who are treated with antipsychotic medications are at risk for withdrawal dyskinesia. The long-term adverse effects, including tardive dyskinesia, are perpetual risks for any patients treated with an antipsychotic medication.

Psychotherapy

Psychosocial interventions aimed at family education and patient and family support are recognized as critical component of the treatment plan for COS. Psychotherapists who work with children with schizophrenia must take into account a child's developmental level. They must continually support the child's good reality testing and be sensitive to the child's sense of self. Long-term intensive and supportive psychotherapy combined with pharmacotherapy is the most effective approach to this disorder.

17 Adolescent Substance Abuse

Adolescent substance use and abuse includes a wide range of substances, such as alcohol, marijuana, nicotine, cocaine, heroin, inhalants, phencyclidine (PCP), lysergic acid diethylamide (LSD), dextromorphan, anabolic steroids, and various "club" drugs, including 3,4-methylenedioxymethamphetamine (MDMA or Ecstasy), flunitrazepam (Rohypnol), γ-hydroxybutyrate (GHB), and ketamine (Ketalar). It is estimated that approximately 20 percent of 8th-graders in the United States have tried illicit drugs and that about 30 percent of 10th- through 12th-graders have used an illicit substance. Alcohol is the most common substance used and abused by adolescents. Binge drinking occurs in about 6 percent of adolescents, and teens with alcohol use disorders are at greater risk of problems with other substances as well.

Many risk and protective factors influence the age of onset and severity of substance use among adolescents. Psychosocial risk factors mediating the development of substance use disorders include parent modeling of substance use, family conflict, lack of parental supervision, peer relationships, and individual stressful life events. Protective factors that mitigate substance use among adolescents include variables such as a stable family life, strong parent–child bond, consistent parental supervision investment in academic achievement, and a peer group that models prosocial family and school behaviors. Interventions that diminish risk factors are likely to mitigate substance use.

Approximately 1 of 5 adolescents has used marijuana or hashish. Approximately one third of adolescents have used cigarettes by age 17 years. Studies of alcohol use among adolescents in the United States have shown that by 13 years of age, one third of boys and almost one fourth of girls have tried alcohol. By 18 years of age, 92 percent of boys and 73 percent of girls reported trying alcohol and 4 percent reported using alcohol daily. Of high school seniors, 41 percent reported using marijuana; 2 percent reported using the drug daily. Emergency room visits for heroin use among those 18 to 25 years of age increased more than 50 percent from 1997 to 2000.

Drinking among adolescents follows adult demographic drinking patterns: The highest proportion of alcohol use occurs among adolescents in the Northeast; whites are more likely to drink than are other groups; among whites, Roman Catholics are the least likely nondrinkers. The four most common causes of death in persons between the ages of 10 and 24 years are motor vehicle accidents (37 percent), homicide (14 percent), suicide (12 percent), and other injuries or accidents (12 percent). Of adolescents treated in pediatric trauma centers, more than one third are treated for alcohol or drug use.

Studies considering alcohol and illicit drug use by adolescents as psychiatric disorders have demonstrated a greater prevalence of substance use, particularly alcoholism, among biological children of alcoholics than among adopted youngsters. This finding is supported by family studies of genetic contributions, by adoption studies, and by observing children of substance users reared outside of the biological home.

Numerous risk factors influence the emergence of adolescent substance abuse. These include parental belief in the harmlessness of substances, lack of anger control in families of substance abusers, lack of closeness and involvement of parents with children's activities, maternal passivity, academic difficulties, comorbid psychiatric disorders such as conduct disorder and depression, parental and peer substance use, impulsivity, and early onset of cigarette smoking. The greater the number of risk factors, the more likely it is that an adolescent will be a substance user.

EPIDEMIOLOGY

Alcohol

A recent survey showed that drinking was a significant problem for 10 to 20 percent of adolescents. In the age range of 13 to 17 years in the United States there are 3 million problem drinkers and 300,000 adolescents with alcohol dependence. The gap between male and female alcohol consumers is narrowing. Drinking was reported by 70 percent of 8th-grade students: 54 percent reported drinking within the prior year, 27 percent reported having gotten drunk at least once, and 13 percent reported binge drinking in the 2 weeks before the survey. By the 12th grade, 88 percent of high school students reported drinking, and 77 percent drank within the prior year; 5 percent of 8th-grade students, 1.3 percent of 10th-grade students, and 3.6 percent of 12th-grade students reported daily alcohol use.

Marijuana

Marijuana is the most widely used illicit drug among high school students. It has been termed a "gateway drug" because the strongest predictor of future cocaine use is frequent marijuana use during adolescence. Of 8th-grade, 10th-grade, and 12th-grade students, 10, 23, and 36 percent, respectively, reported using marijuana, a slight decrease from the year preceding the survey. Of 8th-grade, 10th-grade, and 12th-grade students, 0.2, 0.8, and 2 percent, respectively, reported daily marijuana use. Prevalence rates for marijuana are highest among male and female Native Americans; these rates are nearly as high in male and female whites and male Mexican-Americans. The lowest annual rates are reported by female Latin Americans, female African-Americans, and male and female Asian-Americans. Among juvenile arrests for illicit drug use in 2000, marijuana was the most commonly used drug by both boys (55 percent) and girls (60 percent).

Cocaine

The annual cocaine use reported by high school seniors decreased more than 30 percent between 1990 and 2000. About 0.5 percent of 8th-grade students, 1 percent of 10th-grade students, and 2 percent of 12th-grade students are estimated to have used cocaine. The prevalence rate for crack cocaine use, however, is increasing and is most common among those between the ages of 18 and 25 years.

Crystal Methamphetamine

Crystal methamphetamine, or "ice," was at a relative low level of use in adolescence about one decade ago, at 0.5 percent, and has steadily increased to a recent rate of 1.5 percent among 12th graders.

Lysergic Acid Diethylamide

Lysergic acid diethylamide has reportedly been used by 2.7 percent of 8th-grade students, 5.6 percent of 10th-grade students, and 8.8 percent of 12th-grade students. Of 12th-grade students, 0.1 percent report daily use. The current LSD rates are lower than rates of LSD use during the last two decades.

3,4-Methylenedioxymethamphetamine

The popularity of MDMA has increased over the last decade, and current rates of use in the United States are about 5 percent for 10th graders and 8 percent of 12th graders, despite the fact that the perceived harmfulness of this drug has increased over the last decade to almost 50 percent among 12th graders. Accidental adolescent deaths have been associated with the use of MDMA.

γ-Hydroxybutyrate

γ-Hydroxybutyrate, a club drug, has been found in surveys to have a annual prevalence rate of 1.1 percent for 8th graders, 1.0 percent rate for 10th graders, and 1.6 percent for 12th graders.

Ketamine (Ketalar)

Ketamine, another club drug, recently was found to have an annual prevalence rate of 1.3 percent for 8th graders, 2.1 percent for 10th graders, and 2.5 percent for 12th graders.

Flunitrazepam (Rohypnol)

Flunitrazepam (Rohypnol), a third club drug, has been found to have an annual prevalence rate of about 1 percent for all high school grades combined.

Anabolic Steroids

Despite reported knowledge of the risks of anabolic steroids among high school students, surveys over the last 5 years have found rates of anabolic steroid use to be 1.6 percent among 8th graders and 2.1 percent among 10th graders. Up to 45 percent of 10th and 12th graders reported knowledge of the risks of anabolic steroids; however, over the last decade it appears that high school seniors reported less disapproval of their use.

Inhalants

The use of inhalants in the form of glue, aerosols, and gasoline is relatively more common among younger than older adolescents. Among 8th-grade, 10th-grade, and 12th-grade students, 17.6, 15.7, and 17.6 percent, respectively, reported using inhalants; 0.2 percent of 8th-grade students, 0.1 percent of 10th-grade students, and 0.2 percent of 12th-grade students reported daily use of inhalants.

Multiple Substance Use

Among adolescents enrolled in substance abuse treatment programs, 96 percent are polydrug users; 97 percent of adolescents who abuse drugs also use alcohol.

ETIOLOGY

Genetic Factors

The concordance for alcoholism is reportedly higher among monozygotic than dizygotic twins. Considerably fewer studies have been conducted on families of drug abusers. One twin study of drug users showed that the drug abuse concordance for male monozygotic twins was twice that for dizygotic twins. Studies of children of alcoholics reared away from their biological homes have shown that these children have about a 25 percent chance of becoming alcoholics.

Psychosocial Factors

A recent study concluded that children in families with the lowest measures of parental supervision and monitoring initiated alcohol, tobacco, and other drug use earlier than children from families with more supervision. The risk was greatest for children younger 11 years of age. With more rigorous parental monitoring, young adolescents might be delayed in, or prevented from, initiating drug and alcohol use. Furthermore, increased supervision during middle childhood years may diminish drug and alcohol sampling and ultimately diminish the risk of using marijuana, cocaine, or inhalants in the future.

Comorbidity

Rates of alcohol and drug use are reportedly higher in relatives of children with depression and bipolar disorders. On the other hand, mood disorders are common among those with alcoholism. Evidence indicates a strong link among early antisocial behavior, conduct disorder, and substance abuse. Substance abuse can be viewed as one form of behavioral deviance that, unsurprisingly, is associated with other forms of social and behavioral deviance. Early intervention with children who show early signs of social deviance and antisocial behavior may conceivably impede the processes that contribute to later substance abuse.

Comorbidity, the occurrence of more than one substance use disorder or the combination of a substance use disorder and another psychiatric disorder, is common. It is important to know about all comorbid disorders, which may show differential responses to treatment. Surveys of adolescents with alcoholism show rates of 50 percent or higher for additional psychiatric disorders, especially mood disorders. A recent survey of adolescents who used alcohol found that more than 80 percent met criteria for another disorder. The disorders most frequently present were depressive disorders, disruptive behavior disorders, and drug use disorders. These rates of comorbidity are even higher than those for adults. The diagnosis of alcohol abuse or dependence was likely to follow, rather than precede, other disorders; that a large proportion of adolescents with alcoholism have a previous childhood disorder may have both etiologic and treatment implications. In this survey, the onset of alcohol disorders did not systematically precede drug abuse or dependence. In 50 percent of cases, alcohol use followed drug use. Alcohol use may be a gateway to drug use, but is not in most cases. The presence of other psychiatric disorders was associated with an earlier onset of alcohol disorder, but it did not seem to indicate a more protracted course of alcoholism.

DIAGNOSIS AND CLINICAL FEATURES

According to the text revision of the fourth edition of the *Diagnostic and Statistical Manual of Mental Disorders* (DSM-IV-TR), substance-related disorders include substance dependence, substance abuse, substance intoxication, substance withdrawal, and various substance-induced disorders (e.g., alcohol-induced anxiety disorder). Substance dependence refers to a cluster of cognitive, behavioral, and physiologic symptoms indicating that a person continues the use of a substance, despite significant substance-related problems. A pattern of repeated self-administration can result in tolerance, withdrawal, and compulsive drug-taking behavior. Dependence can be applied to every substance, with the exception of caffeine. It requires the presence of at least three symptoms of the maladaptive pattern, which can occur at any time during the same 12-month period. Symptoms of dependence can include tolerance, withdrawal, heavier use of the substance than was intended, an unsuccessful desire to cut down or control use, and reduction of social or occupational activities because of substance use. In addition, the user knows that the substance causes significant impairment but does not give it up. Physiologic dependence (evidence of tolerance or withdrawal) may or may not be present.

Substance abuse refers to a maladaptive pattern of substance use leading to clinically significant impairment or distress, manifested by one or more of the following symptoms within a 12-month period: recurrent substance use in situations that cause physical danger to the user, recurrent substance use in the face of obvious impairment in school or work situations, recurrent substance use despite resulting legal problems, or recurrent substance use despite social or interpersonal problems. To meet the criteria for substance abuse, the symptoms must never have met the criteria for substance dependence for this class of substance.

Substance intoxication refers to the development of a reversible, substance-specific syndrome caused by use of a substance. Clinically significant maladaptive behavioral or psychologic changes must be present.

Substance withdrawal refers to a substance-specific syndrome caused by the cessation of, or reduction in, prolonged substance use. The substance-specific syndrome causes clinically significant distress or impairs social or occupational functioning.

The diagnosis of alcohol or drug use in adolescents is made through careful interview, observations, laboratory findings, and history provided by reliable sources. Many nonspecific signs may point to alcohol or drug use, and clinicians must be careful to corroborate hunches before jumping to conclusions. Substance use can be viewed on a continuum with experimentation (the mildest use), regular use without obvious impairment, abuse, and, finally, dependence. Changes in academic performance, nonspecific physical ailments, changes in relationships with family members, changes in peer group, unexplained phone calls, or changes in personal hygiene may indicate substance use in an adolescent. Many of these indicators, however, also can be consistent with the onset of depression, adjustment to school, or the prodrome of a psychotic illness. It is important, therefore, to keep the channels of communication with an adolescent open when substance use is suspected.

Nicotine

Nicotine is one of the most addictive substances known, involving cholinergic receptors and enhancing acetylcholine, serotonin, and β-endorphin release. Young teens who smoke cigarettes are also exposed to other drugs more frequently than are nonsmoking peers.

Alcohol

Alcohol use in adolescents rarely results in the sequelae observed in adults with chronic abuse of alcohol, such as withdrawal seizures, Korsakoff's syndrome, Wernicke's aphasia, or cirrhosis of the liver. R. DeBellis, however, reported that adolescent exposure to alcohol may result in diminished hippocampal brain volume. Because the hippocampus is involved with attention, it is conceivable that adolescent alcohol use could result in compromised cognitive function, especially with respect to attention.

Marijuana

The short-term effects of the active ingredient in marijuana, tetrahydrocannabinol (THC), include impairment in memory and learning, distorted perception, diminished problem-solving ability, loss of coordination, increased heart rate, anxiety, and panic attacks. Abrupt cessation of heavy marijuana use by adolescents has been reported to result in a withdrawal syndrome characterized by insomnia, irritability, restlessness, drug craving, depressed mood, and nervousness followed by anxiety, tremors, nausea, muscle twitches, increased sweating, myalgia, and general malaise. Typically, the withdrawal syndrome begins 24 hours after the last use, peaks at 2 to 4 days, and diminishes after 2 weeks.

Cocaine

Cocaine can be sniffed or snorted, injected, or smoked. *Crack* is the term given to cocaine after it has been changed to a free base for smoking. Cocaine's effects include constriction of peripheral blood vessels, dilated pupils, hyperthermia, increased heart rate, and hypertension. High doses or prolonged use of cocaine can induce paranoid thinking. The immediate risk of death can occur secondary to cardiac arrest or from seizures followed by respiratory arrest. In contrast to stimulants used to treat attention-deficit/hyperactivity disorder (ADHD), such as methylphenidate, cocaine quickly crosses the blood–brain barrier and moves off the dopamine transporter within 20 minutes, unlike methylphenidate, which remains bound to dopamine for long periods of time.

Heroin

Heroin, a derivative of morphine, is produced from a poppy plant. Heroin usually appears as a white or brown powder that can be snorted, but more commonly it is used intravenously. Withdrawal symptoms include restlessness, muscle and bone pain, insomnia, diarrhea and vomiting, cold flashes with goose bumps, and kicking movements. Withdrawal occurs within a few hours after use, and symptoms peak between 48 and 72 hours later and remit within about 1 week.

Club Drugs

Adolescents who frequent nightclubs, "raves," bars, or music clubs also frequently use MDMA, GHB, Rohypnol, and ketamine. GHB, Rohypnol (a benzodiazepine) and ketamine (an anesthetic) are primarily depressants and can be added to drinks without detection because they are often colorless, tasteless, and odorless. The Drug-Induced Rape Prevention and Punishment Act of 1996 was passed after these were found to be associated with date rape. MDMA is a derivative of methamphetamine, a synthetic with both stimulant and hallucinogenic properties. MDMA can inhibit serotonin and dopamine reuptake. MDMA can result in dry mouth, increased heart rate, fatigue, muscle spasm, and hyperthermia.

Lysergic Acid Diethylamide

Lysergic acid diethylamide is odorless, colorless, and has a slightly bitter taste. Higher doses of LSD can produce visual hallucinations and delusions and, in some cases, panic. The sensations experienced after ingestion of LSD usually diminishes after 12 hours. Flashbacks can occur up to 1 year after use. LSD can produce tolerance; that is, after multiple uses, more is needed to provide the same degree of intoxication.

Substance use is related to a variety of high-risk behaviors, including early sexual experimentation, risky driving, destruction of property, stealing, occasionally, preoccupation with cults or Satanism. Although none of these behaviors necessarily predicts substance use, at the extreme, these behaviors reflect alienation from the mainstream of developmentally expected social behavior. Adolescents with inadequate social skills may use a substance as a modality to join a peer group. In some cases, adolescents begin their substance use at home with their parents, who also use substances to enhance their social interactions. Although there is no evidence on what determines a typical adolescent user of alcohol or drugs, many substance users seem to have underlying social skills deficits, academic difficulties, and less-than-optimal peer relationships.

TREATMENT

Treatment of substance use disorders in adolescents is designed directly to prevent the substance use behaviors, provide education for the patient and family, and address cognitive, emotional, and psychiatric factors that influence the substance use; treatment occurs in a variety of settings, such as a residential milieu or group and individual psychosocial sessions.

The Child and Adolescent Levels of Care Utilization System (CALOCUS) is a validated instrument for guiding clinicians in the treatment of adolescent substance use. It designates six symptom-appropriate levels of care:

Level 0: Basic services (prevention)
Level 1: Recovery maintenance (relapse prevention)
Level 2: Outpatient (once-per-week visits)
Level 3: Intensive outpatient (two or more visits per week)
Level 4: Intensive integrated services (day treatment, partial hospitalization, wraparound services)
Level 5: Nonsecure, 24-hour medically monitored service (group home, residential treatment facility)
Level 6: Secure 24-hour medical management (inpatient psychiatric or highly programmed residential facility)

Treatment settings that serve adolescents with alcohol or drug use disorders include inpatient units, residential treatment facilities, halfway houses, group homes, partial hospital programs, and outpatient settings. Basic components of adolescent alcohol or drug use treatment include individual psychotherapy, drug-specific counseling, self-help groups (Alcoholics Anonymous [AA], Narcotics Anonymous [NA], Alateen, Al-Anon), substance abuse education and relapse prevention programs, and random urine drug testing. Family therapy and psychopharmacologic intervention may be added.

Before deciding on the most appropriate treatment setting for a particular adolescent, a screening process must take place in which structured and unstructured interviews help to determine the types of substances being used and their quantities and frequencies. Determining coexisting psychiatric disorders is also critical. Rating scales are typically used to document pretreatment and posttreatment severity of abuse. The Teen Addiction Severity Index (T-ASI), the Adolescent Drug and Alcohol Diagnostic Assessment (ADAD), and the Adolescent Problem Severity Index (APSI) are severity-oriented rating scales. The T-ASI is broken down into dimensions that include family functioning, school or employment status, psychiatric status, peer social relationships, and legal status.

After most of the information about substance use and the patient's overall psychiatric status has been obtained, a treatment strategy must be chosen and an appropriate setting must be determined. Two very different approaches to the treatment of substance abuse are embodied in the Minnesota model and the multidisciplinary professional model. The Minnesota model is based on the premise of AA; it is an intensive 12-step program with a counselor who functions as the primary therapist. The program uses self-help participation and group processes. Inherent in this treatment strategy is the need for adolescents to admit that substance use is problematic and that help is necessary. Furthermore, they must be willing to work toward altering their lifestyle to eradicate substance use. The multidisciplinary professional model consists of a team of mental health professionals that usually is led by a physician. Following a case-management model, each member of the team has specific areas of treatment for which he or she is responsible. Interventions may include cognitive-behavioral therapy, family therapy, and pharmacologic intervention. This approach usually is suited for adolescents with comorbid psychiatric diagnoses.

Cognitive-behavioral approaches to psychotherapy for adolescents with substance use generally require that adolescents be motivated to participate in treatment and refrain from further substance use. The therapy focuses on relapse prevention and maintaining abstinence.

Psychopharmacologic interventions for adolescent alcohol and drug users are still in their early stages. The presence of mood disorders clearly indicates the need for antidepressants, and, generally, the selective serotonin reuptake inhibitors are the first line of treatment. Some pharmacologic interventions are aimed at aiding the abstinence process. For example, disulfiram (Antabuse) is used in alcoholism to cause an aversive reaction if alcohol is ingested. In certain instances, administration of a medication is used to block the reinforcing effect of the illicit drug, for instance, giving naltrexone (ReVia) for opioid or alcohol abuse. Some medications mitigate the craving or withdrawal symptoms for a drug that is no longer being used. Clonidine (Catapres) has been used transiently during heroin withdrawal. Occasionally, an intervention is made to substitute the illicit drug with another drug that is more amenable to the treatment situation—for example, using methadone instead of heroin. Adolescents are required to have two documented attempts at detoxification and consent from an adult before they can enter such a treatment program.

Fred, a 16-year-old male, was admitted to substance abuse treatment for the second time, following a relapse and threats of suicide. He was initially admitted to an inpatient program following a serious suicide attempt. He reported a long history of disruptive behavior and academic failure since childhood. He was increasingly truant and difficult for his family to control. During his first treatment episode, he reported an onset of substance use at age 11 years, rapid progression in substance involvement since age 13 years, then current use of marijuana on a daily basis, drinking alcohol up to several times a week, frequent trips on LSD, and experimentation with a variety of substances. Fred attended group sessions focusing on his initial denial of a substance use problem and then learned the process of recovery while attending other groups and AA and NA meetings. Family group sessions showed him and his parents the need for better communication and more adaptive interactions. Fred gradually responded to the structure of the treatment program, although he had frequent problems with anger control when confronted by peers or staff or when frustrated. Depressive symptoms failed to remit following 2 weeks of abstinence, and Fred was given fluoxetine (Prozac). He showed rapid improvement in mood and treatment compliance. On discharge, he was attending NA meetings and out-patient therapy. Family conflict soon recurred, however, and Fred became noncompliant with outpatient treatment, medication, and meetings. He resumed old relationships with deviant peers and relapsed into daily marijuana use and occasional alcohol use. (Courtesy of Oscar G. Bukstein, M.D.)

Efficacious treatments for cigarette smoking cessation include nicotine-containing gum, patches, or nasal spray or inhaler. Bupropion (Zyban) aids in diminishing cravings for nicotine and is beneficial in the treatment of smoking cessation.

Because comorbidity influences treatment outcome, it is important to pay attention to other disorders, such as mood disorders, anxiety disorders, conduct disorder, or ADHD, during the treatment of substance use disorders.

18

Additional Conditions That May Be a Focus of Clinical Attention

BORDERLINE INTELLECTUAL FUNCTIONING

Intellectual functioning of a child or adolescent is influenced by multiple factors, including birth history of full-term gestation, neonatal head circumference, learning, nutritional status, and brain development after birth. Brain parameters, parental head circumference, and prenatal nutrition are most highly correlated with the head circumference of the newborn. In a sample of Chilean school-age children, those born with small head circumference of at least two standard deviations below the mean (microcephalic) were most likely to present with lower overall brain volume, compromised intellectual and scholastic functions, and poor nutrition. Although intellectual quotients (IQs) are generally believed to be stable over time, in some cases, a single measurement of intellectual functioning does not accurately predict intellectual function in all areas over the long term. For example, a follow-up study conducted to investigate the stability of IQ measurement in a group of dyslexic adolescents and young adults who were tested at age 12 years and retested after a mean interval of 6.5 years found the following differences over time. Compared with first IQ tests, for the teens and young adults, the retests showed a significant relative decrease in verbal IQ (VIQ), which was interpreted as either poor reliability of the test or a loss of ability based on diminished experience with reading and writing compared with same-age peers over time. Performance IQ (PIQ), however, was found to be significantly increased, leading to the hypothesis that a compensatory process had been naturally developed by these children with dyslexia, such as a more visual or creative way to process information, leading to greater success on performance test items. The conclusion was that a single IQ test in childhood may not be a fully accurate predictor of later abilities and that potential interventions to help children with disabilities such as dyslexia keep up academically with peers may have implications for final IQ and intellectual functioning.

Borderline intellectual functioning, according to the text revision of the fourth edition of the *Diagnostic and Statistical Manual of Mental Disorders* (DSM-IV-TR), is a category that can be used when the focus of clinical attention is on a child's or adolescent's IQ in the 71 to 84 range. The intellectual functioning of children plays a major role in their adjustment to school, social relationships, and family function. Children who cannot quite understand class work and may also be slow in understanding rules of games and the "social" rules of their peer group are often bitterly rejected. Some children with borderline intellectual functioning can mingle socially better than they can keep up academically in class. In these cases, the strengths of these children may be peer relationships, especially if they excel at sports, but eventually their academic struggles will take a toll on self-esteem if they are not appropriately remediated.

Impaired adaptive functioning is diagnosed when difficulties in academic, social, or vocational areas pertaining to borderline intellectual functioning become the focus of clinical attention.

Clinicians must assess a patient's intellectual level and current and past levels of adaptive functioning to diagnose borderline intellectual functioning. In patients with major mental disorders whose current level of adaptive functioning has deteriorated, the diagnosis of borderline intellectual functioning may not be clearly evident. In such situations, clinicians must evaluate the patient's history to determine whether the level of adaptive functioning was compromised even before the onset of the mental disorder.

Only about 6 to 7 percent of the population has a borderline IQ as determined by the Stanford-Binet test or the Wechsler scales. The premise behind the inclusion of borderline intellectual functioning in the DSM-IV-TR is that persons may experience difficulties in their adaptive capacities as a result of their intellectual deficits and thus may require attention. In the absence of specific intrapsychic conflicts, developmental traumas, biochemical abnormalities, and other factors linked to any other mental disorder, such persons may experience severe emotional distress. Frustration and embarrassment over their difficulties may shape their life choices and lead to circumstances warranting psychiatric intervention.

Etiology

Genetic factors are increasingly found to play a role in intellectual deficits. Environmental deprivation and infectious and toxic exposures can also contribute to cognitive impairment. Twin and adoption studies support the hypothesis that many genes contribute to the development of a particular IQ. Specific infectious processes (e.g., congenital rubella), prenatal exposures (e.g., fetal alcohol syndrome), and specific chromosomal abnormalities (e.g., fragile X syndrome) result in mental retardation.

Diagnosis

The DSM-IV-TR contains the following statement about borderline intellectual functioning:

> This category can be used when the focus of clinical attention is associated with borderline intellectual functioning, that is, an IQ in the 71 to 84 range. Differential diagnosis between Borderline Intellectual Functioning and Mental Retardation (an IQ of 70 or below) is especially difficult when the coexistence of certain mental disorders (e.g., Schizophrenia) is involved. Coding note: This is categorized on a V Code.

A 13-year-old boy was referred to a partial hospital program because of anger outbursts, temper tantrums, and moodiness in the home. He was in a regular classroom setting, and his grades were marginal. He appeared passive, but, when given adult attention and guidance in school and at home, his overall demeanor and performance brightened. In addition to the psychiatric assessment, evaluation included a pediatric medical examination, blood tests, and urine screening for illicit drugs. School psychologic testing was reviewed. Results were generally unremarkable.

There were no medical problems. However, verbal IQ was 75, performance IQ was 80, and adaptive skills proficiency was several years below that expected for his age. A primary diagnosis of borderline intellectual functioning was made. Treatment included heavy emphasis on special help with resource room and accommodations in school, psychoeducation for the family, and brief individual, group, and behavior modification for the patient. Mood and behavior at home significantly improved, self-esteem was enhanced, and school performance—academically and socially—strengthened. (Courtesy of Frank John Ninivaggi, M.D.)

Treatment

The goals of treatment are to maximize educational and vocational placements so that individuals can develop the most optimal practical adaptive skills, social skills, and self-esteem. The goal is to improve the match between the person's capabilities and lifestyle. After the underlying problem becomes known to the therapist, psychiatric treatment can be useful. Many persons with borderline intellectual functioning can function at a superior level in some areas while being markedly deficient in others. By directing such persons to appropriate areas of endeavor, by pointing out socially acceptable behavior, and by teaching them living skills, the therapist can help improve to their self-esteem.

ACADEMIC PROBLEM

Academic difficulties in children and adolescents can accompany a wide range of psychosocial conditions related to family life, the environment, mood and behavioral problems, and connection with certain peer groups. In the absence of a specific learning disorder or a direct result of a psychiatric disorder, academic function is related to scholastic strengths, motivation, ability to apply oneself to the work, and stressful life events. A recent investigation of the effects of students' perception of support from parents, teachers, and peers showed a correlation with adolescent academic achievement. That is, adolescents' perception of support from their teachers and parents was directly related to their academic achievement; whereas perceived peer support was indirectly related to actual academic achievement, it contributed to an adolescent's overall perception of support, which was correlated to achievement.

Behavioral choices and life events can also exacerbate academic problems in the absence of learning disorder and can interfere with lessening academic failures. For example, once a student perceives that he or she is falling behind academically, a greater temptation is to replace academic pursuits with other activities, such as drug use. A recent study assessed the level of, and deterioration in, academic achievement in relation to initiation of marijuana use among young teens. In a sample of rural teens, 36 percent of boys and 23 percent of girls initiated use of marijuana by the end of the 9th grade, and deteriorating academic performance was a significant predictor of initiating marijuana use. The hypothesis remaining to be tested is whether timely intervention to improve academic standing would lower the risk of beginning drug use.

The DSM-IV-TR refers to an academic problem as a problem that is not caused by a mental disorder or, if caused by a mental disorder, is sufficiently severe to warrant clinical attention. This diagnostic category is used when a child or adolescent is having significant academic difficulties that are not deemed to be caused by a specific learning disorder or communication disorder or directly related to a psychiatric disorder. Nevertheless, intervention is necessary because the child's achievement in school is significantly impaired. A child or adolescent of normal intelligence who is free of a learning disorder or a communication disorder but is failing in school or doing poorly falls into this category.

Etiology

Many psychologic factors contribute to a child's confidence, competence, and academic success. In the absence of a specific learning disorder to account for the academic difficulty or primary psychiatric disorder responsible for the academic compromise, subclinical states of anxiety or depression and peer and family stressors such as divorce, marital discord, abuse, or mental illness in a family member may interrupt academic production. Children who are troubled by social isolation, identity issues, preoccupation with sexuality, or extreme shyness may withdraw from full participation in academic activities. Academic problems may be the result of a confluence of multiple contributing factors and may occur in adolescents who were previously high academic achievers. School is the main social and educational venue for children and adolescents. Success and acceptance in the school setting depend on children's physical, cognitive, social, and emotional adjustment. Children's general coping mechanisms in many developmental tasks usually are reflected in their academic and social success in school. Boys and girls must cope with the process of separation from parents, adjustment to new environments, adaptation to social contacts, competition, assertion, intimacy, and exposure to unfamiliar attitudes. A corresponding relation often exists between school performance and how well these tasks are mastered.

Anxiety can play a major role in interfering with children's academic performances. Anxiety can hamper their abilities to perform well on tests, speak in public, and ask questions when they do not understand something. Some children are so concerned about the way others view them that they cannot attend to their academic tasks. For some children, conflicts about success and fears of the consequences imagined to accompany the attainment of success can hamper academic success. Sigmund Freud described persons with such conflicts as "those wrecked by success." For example, an adolescent girl may be unable to succeed in school because she fears social rejection or the loss of femininity or both, and she may perceive success as being involved with aggression and competition with boys.

Depressed children also may withdraw from academic pursuits; they require specific interventions to improve their academic performances and to treat their depression. Children who do not have major depressive disorder but are consumed by family problems, such as financial troubles, marital discord in their parents, and mental illness in family members, may be distracted and unable to attend to academic tasks. Children who receive mixed messages from their parents about accepting criticism and redirection from their teachers can become confused and unable to perform well in school. The loss of the parents as the primary and predominant teachers in a child's life can result in identity conflicts for some children. Some students lack a stable sense of self and cannot identify goals for themselves, a situation that leads to a sense of boredom or futility.

Cultural and economic background can play a role in how well accepted a child feels in school and can affect the child's academic achievement. Familial socioeconomic level, parental education, race, religion, and family functioning can influence a child's sense of fitting in and can affect preparation to meet school demands.

Schools, teachers, and clinicians can share insights about how to foster productive and cooperative environments for all students in a classroom. Teachers' expectations about their students' performance influence these performances. Teachers serve as agents whose varying expectations can shape the differential development of students' skills and abilities. Such conditioning early in school, especially when negative, can disturb academic performance. A teacher's affective response to a child, therefore, can prompt the appearance of an academic problem. Most important is a teacher's humane approach to students at all levels of education, including medical school.

Diagnosis

The DSM-IV-TR contains the following statement about academic problem:

> This category can be used when the focus of clinical attention is an academic problem that is not due to a mental disorder or, if due to a mental disorder, is sufficiently severe to warrant independent clinical attention. An example is a pattern of failing grades or of significant underachievement in a person with adequate intellectual capacity in the absence of a learning or a communication disorder or any other mental disorder that would account for the problem.

A 15-year-old boy was admitted to an intensive outpatient program for evaluation of insidiously declining grades at school, isolative behavior, and anhedonia occurring for the first time over the course of the last semester at high school. The patient had no previous psychiatric history and was in good health. School reports showed his full-scale IQ to be 100 and revealed no previous behavior or academic problems. Interviews with family and patient revealed that the boy had an intact family with no apparent or unusual conflicts noted and that his mother found evidence of drug paraphernalia—cigarette papers, small pipe, matches, and a suspicious-looking dried substance in his bedroom. When confronted, the patient revealed a 6-month use of marijuana. A primary diagnosis of cannabis abuse, in addition to academic problem, was made. Referral to a therapeutic drug and alcohol program was immediately implemented. (Courtesy of Frank John Ninivaggi, M.D.)

Treatment

The initial step in determining a useful intervention for an academic problem is a comprehensive diagnostic evaluation. Identifying and addressing family-, school-, and peer-related stressors are critical. Substance use disorders must be carefully ruled out, as well as concurrent psychiatric disorders that may require treatment before improvement in academic function. An individualized educational plan evaluation and meeting may be requested in writing to the school so that specific educational testing can be integrated into the assessment of the overall academic problem and educational accommodations can be considered.

Psychosocial intervention may be applied successfully for scholastic difficulties related to poor motivation, poor self-concept, and underachievement. Early efforts to relieve the problem are critical: Sustained problems in learning and school performance frequently are compounded and precipitate severe difficulties. Feelings of anger, frustration, shame, loss of self-respect, and helplessness—emotions that most often accompany school failures—damage self-esteem emotionally and cognitively, disabling future performance and clouding expectations for success. Generally, children with academic problems require either school-based intervention or individual attention.

Tutoring is an effective technique for dealing with academic problems and should be considered in most cases. Tutoring has proved of value in preparing for objective multiple-choice examinations, such as the Scholastic Aptitude Test (SAT) and Medical College Aptitude Test (MCAT). Taking such examinations repetitively and using relaxation skills are two behavioral techniques of great value in diminishing anxiety.

CHILDHOOD OR ADOLESCENT ANTISOCIAL BEHAVIOR

Antisocial behaviors are the most common reasons for a child or adolescent to be referred for a psychiatric evaluation. Antisocial behaviors, however, are so varied in severity and frequency and occur in children and adolescents of such a wide range of ages and developmental levels that it would be difficult to identify a single etiology. Prospective studies of youth at risk for antisocial behavior have shown that meaningful subtypes exist of antisocial behavior. One way to classify these behaviors is by separating them into authority-defying behaviors and overt and covert antisocial acts. Less serious antisocial behaviors in childhood tend to be characterized as defiance, or defying authority figures. Covert antisocial behaviors, such as stealing, typically occur in later childhood, whereas the most severe overt antisocial acts, such as violent behaviors, do not usually emerge until adolescence. Youth with the poorest prognoses tend to exhibit overt antisocial acts at younger ages and display a pattern of overt, covert, and authority-defying behaviors over time.

Some of the most striking displays of antisocial behavior among youth in recent times have been the shootings of students and staff at Columbine High School in Colorado and at Santana High School in California. The relationship of antisocial behavior to psychopathology is complex, in that a given act of violence is not always equitably directly related to a specific psychiatric disorder. Data on the etiology of antisocial behavior fit best into a cumulative risk factor model in which the likelihood of antisocial acts increases as the risks accumulate.

This complex mechanism seems to perpetuate itself in the following way. A vulnerable child interacts with his or her immediate family, environment, and peer group to develop a pattern of impulsivity, aggression, and a disregard for the feelings and rights of others. When children with these negative behavioral patterns and cognitions then develop a second tier of negative interactions through rejection by peers, teachers, and parents, and especially when additional adverse life events or losses occur, even more negative behaviors ensue. A recent investigation by the U.S. Secret Service and the Department of Education found that youth who perpetrate attacks in schools were often shunned by peer groups, coped poorly with personal losses, and experienced academic and other failures. An additional typical factor in the profile is the regular access in their home environments to weapons. So, although no clear profile can predict who specifically may turn out to be a violent threat to a school, the data found that youth who have committed violent acts in schools were generally characterized as socially isolated, exhibited signs and symptoms of social and emotional stress, and had access to weapons, mainly guns.

According to the DSM-IV-TR, child or adolescent antisocial behavior refers to behavior that is not caused by a mental disorder and includes isolated antisocial acts, not a pattern of behavior. This category covers many acts by children and adolescents that violate the rights of others, such as overt acts of aggression and violence and covert acts of lying, stealing, truancy, and running away from home. Certain antisocial acts, such as fire setting, possession of a weapon, or a severe act of aggression toward another child, require intervention for even a single occurrence. Sometimes, children without a pattern of recurrent aggression or antisocial behavior become involved in occasional less severe behaviors that nevertheless require some intervention. The DSM-IV-TR definition of conduct disorder requires a repetitive pattern of at least three antisocial behaviors for at least 6 months, but childhood or adolescent antisocial behavior may consist of isolated events that do not constitute a mental disorder but do become the focus of clinical attention. The emergence of occasional antisocial symptoms is common among children who have a variety of mental disorders, including psychotic disorders, depressive disorders, impulse control disorders, disruptive behavior, and attention-deficit disorders, such as attention-deficit/hyperactivity disorder (ADHD) and oppositional defiant disorder.

A child's age and developmental level affect the manifestations of disturbed conduct and influence the child's likelihood to meet the diagnostic criteria for a conduct disorder as opposed to childhood antisocial behavior. Therefore, a child of 5 or 6 years of age is not likely to meet the criteria for three antisocial symptoms—for example, physical confrontations, the use of weapons, and forcing someone into sexual activity—but a single symptom, such as initiating fights, is common in children 5 to 6 years of age. The term *juvenile delinquent* is defined by the legal system as a youth who has violated the law in some way, but the term does not imply that the youth meets the criteria for a mental disorder.

Epidemiology

Estimates of antisocial behavior range from 5 to 15 percent of the general population and somewhat less among children and adolescents. Reports have documented a higher frequency of antisocial behaviors in urban settings than in rural areas. In one report, the risk of coming into contact with the police for antisocial behavior was estimated to be 20 percent for teenage boys and 4 percent for teenage girls.

Etiology

Antisocial behaviors can occur in the context of a mental disorder or in its absence. Antisocial behavior is multidetermined and occurs most frequently in children or adolescents with many risk factors. Among the most common risk factors are harsh and physically abusive parenting, parental criminality, and a child's tendency toward impulsive and hyperactive behavior. Protective factors can attenuate the risk of antisocial behaviors by exerting an independent influence on strengthening core aspects of functioning and thereby decreasing risk. Protective factors can include high intelligence, an easy or self-directed temperament, high levels of social skill, competence in school or in other domains of artistic or athletic skill, and, finally, a strong bond with at least one parent. Additional associated features of children and adolescents with antisocial behavior are low IQ, academic failure, and low levels of adult supervision.

Psychologic Factors. If they have been poorly parented, children experience emotional deprivation, which leads to low self-esteem and unconscious anger. When children are not given any limits, their consciences are deficient because they have not internalized parental prohibitions that account for superego formation. Therefore, they have so-called *superego lacunae*, which allow them to commit antisocial acts without guilt. At times, such children's antisocial behavior is a vicarious source of pleasure and gratification for parents who act out their own forbidden wishes and impulses through their children. A consistent finding in persons who perform repeated acts of violent behavior is a history of physical abuse.

Diagnosis and Clinical Features

The DSM-IV-TR contains the following statement about child or adolescent antisocial behavior:

> This category can be used when the focus of clinical attention is antisocial behavior in a child or adolescent that is not due to a mental disorder (e.g., Conduct Disorder or an Impulse-Control Disorder). Examples include isolated antisocial acts of children or adolescents (not a pattern of antisocial behavior).

The childhood behaviors most associated with antisocial behavior are theft, incorrigibility, arrests, school problems, impulsiveness, promiscuity, oppositional behavior, lying, suicide attempts, substance abuse, truancy, running away, associating with undesirable persons, and staying out late at night. The more symptoms present in childhood, the greater is the probability of adult antisocial behavior; however, the presence of many symptoms also indicates the development of other mental disorders in adult life.

Differential Diagnosis

Substance-related disorders (including alcohol, cannabis, and cocaine use disorders), bipolar I disorder, and schizophrenia in childhood often manifest themselves as antisocial behavior.

A 9-year-old child was arrested by police for breaking into a local hardware store. He was accompanied by two friends. The three had ridden their bikes in a suburban neighborhood until after dark and engaged in a play of "cops and robbers," taking turns in pursuing and being pursued. To make the game more lifelike, one of the three suggested that they actually break into this store, whose owner was a somewhat gruff and intimidating man. The three decided that such an adventure would be quite exciting and proceeded to smash in the glass door with a brick. Shortly after the glass broke, the police arrived and arrested them. Parents were called to come and to collect their children. None of the three had any previous contact with the police or any social service agency. Although they previously engaged in some mischief in the neighborhood, such as throwing toilet paper on people's houses and egging cars, none of the three had any serious infractions of societal rules, and none of the three boys had any more of these events cluster in the past few months. One of them had a history of ADHD and some learning difficulties at school, whereas the other two boys had no particular risk factors for the persistence of antisocial behavior. The antisocial activities of the child with ADHD progressed to the point of fulfilling conduct disorder criteria in early adolescence. Much of his future acting out consisted of drug-related offenses, that is, the use and sales of drugs, stealing, and other covert delinquent activities. The two boys without risks proceeded to develop through a normative, turbulent, and lively adolescence without any further legal involvement. (Courtesy of Hans Steiner, M.D., and Niranjan Karnik, M.D., Ph.D.)

Treatment

Antisocial behavior does not specifically represent a corresponding psychiatric disorder; therefore, a comprehensive psychiatric assessment and the context in which the antisocial behavior emerged must be conducted to delineate the place of the antisocial behavior with respect to any comorbid psychopathology.

Disturbances of conduct frequently accompany the onset of various other psychiatric disorders. The first step in determining the appropriate treatment for a child or an adolescent who is manifesting antisocial behavior is to evaluate the need to treat any coexisting mental disorder, such as bipolar I disorder, a psychotic disorder, or a depressive disorder, that may be contributing to the antisocial behavior. The treatment of antisocial behavior usually involves behavioral management, which is most effective when the patient is in a controlled environment in a structured day or residential setting. In less severe situations, the child's family members are able to manage the symptoms in collaboration with the clinician by using a cooperative behavioral program.

In some cases, special educational settings are necessary to provide the essential monitoring and feedback needed to diminish the undesired behaviors. In some cases, even regular school classroom teachers can help to modify antisocial behavior in the classroom. Rewards for prosocial behaviors and positive reinforcement for the control of unwanted behaviors have merit.

Medications generally are not used in patients with rare or occasional antisocial behaviors, especially when no comorbid psychiatric disorders exist. Medications have been used with some success when repetitive episodes of explosive behavior, aggression, or violent outbursts ensue. Lithium (Eskalith), divalproex (Depakote), and atypical antipsychotics such as risperidone (Risperdal), olanzapine (Zyprexa), quetiapine (Seroquel), ziprasidone (Geodon), or aripiprazole (Abilify) may reduce explosive behavior and rage outbursts. For young children who are sensitive to the extrapyramidal side effects of antipsychotics, chlorpromazine (Thorazine), despite its sedating properties, may be better tolerated and more efficacious in managing acute aggression. The use of diphenhydramine (Benadryl) or lorazepam (Ativan) may be helpful as adjunctive medications in the short-term control of aggressive behavior. When symptoms of ADHD, such as hyperactivity and impulsivity, are contributing factors, short- or long-acting methylphenidate agents (Ritalin, Concerta) or short- or long-acting amphetamine and amphetamine salts (Adderall, Adderall XR) may help to reduce impulsivity and decrease aggression.

It is more difficult to treat children and adolescents who exhibit long-term patterns of antisocial behavior, particularly covert behaviors, such as stealing and lying. Group therapy in the context of residential treatment centers has been used for these behaviors, and cognitive problem-solving approaches are potentially helpful.

IDENTITY PROBLEM

The conceptualization of identity encompasses cognitive, psychodynamic, psychosexual, neurobiologic, and cultural development. The developmentalist Erik Erikson proposed, in writings collected in his book *Identity and the Life Cycle*, that the central task of adolescence is to achieve a sense of selfsameness and continuity in time. The normative developmental process for an adolescent was conceptualized by Erikson as an adolescent crisis of identity. The transition between a childhood identity and the process of accepting a more mature sense of self is the resolution of the "crisis." The notion of an identity crisis in adolescence gained widespread attention among clinicians and the popular media during the late 1960s and early 1970s when many adolescents displayed rejection of mainstream cultural values and ideas and demonstrated alternate lifestyles. The concept of *identity disorder* as a psychiatric diagnosis was embraced in the 1980s when the DSM-III characterized it as a disorder usually first evident in childhood. It was meant to include adolescents who presented with "severe subjective distress regarding uncertainty about a variety of issues relating to identity" to the point where they became impaired. According to the DSM-IV-TR, identity problem refers to uncertainty about issues such as goals, career choice, friendships, sexual behavior, moral values, and group loyalties. An identity problem can cause severe distress for a young person and can lead a person to seek psychotherapy or guidance. Identity problem, however, is not recognized as a mental disorder in the DSM-IV-TR. It sometimes manifests in the context of such mental disorders as mood disorders, psychotic disorders, and borderline personality disorder.

Epidemiology

No reliable information is available regarding predisposing factors, familial pattern, sex ratio, or prevalence, but problems with identity formation seem to be a result of life in modern society. Today, children and adolescents often experience great instability in family life, problems with identity formation, conflicts between adolescent peer values and the values of parents and society, and exposure through the media and education to various moral, behavioral, and lifestyle possibilities.

Etiology

The causes of identity problems often are multifactorial and include the pressures of a highly dysfunctional family and the influences of coexisting mental disorders. In general, adolescents with major depressive disorder, psychotic disorders, and other mental disorders report feeling alienated from family members and experience some turmoil. Children who have had difficulty mastering expected developmental tasks all along are likely to have difficulty with the pressure to establish a well-defined identity during adolescence. Erikson used the term *identity versus role diffusion* to describe the developmental and psychosocial tasks challenging adolescents to incorporate past experiences and present goals into a coherent sense of self.

Diagnosis and Clinical Features

The DSM-IV-TR contains the following statement about identity problem:

> This category can be used when the focus of clinical attention is uncertainty about multiple issues relating to identity such as long-term goals, career choice, friendship patterns, sexual orientation and behavior, moral values, and group loyalties.

The essential features of identity problem seem to revolve around the question, "Who am I?" Conflicts are experienced as irreconcilable aspects of the self that the adolescent cannot integrate into a coherent identity. As Erikson described identity problem, youth manifests severe doubting and an inability to make decisions, a sense of isolation, inner emptiness, a growing inability to relate to others, disturbed sexual functioning, a distorted time perspective, a sense of urgency, and the assumption of a negative identity. The associated features frequently include marked discrepancy between the adolescent's self-perception and the views that others have of the adolescent; moderate anxiety and depression that are usually related to inner preoccupation rather than external realities; and self-doubt and uncertainty about the future, with either difficulty making choices or impulsive experiments in an attempt to establish an independent identity. Some persons with identity problem join cult-like groups.

Differential Diagnosis

Identity problem must be differentiated from a mental disorder (e.g., borderline personality disorder, schizophreniform disorder, schizophrenia, or a mood disorder). At times, what initially seems to be an identity problem may be the prodromal manifestations of one of these disorders. Intense but normal conflicts associated with maturing, such as adolescent turmoil and midlife crisis, may be confusing, but they usually are not associated with marked deterioration in school, vocational or social functioning, or severe subjective distress. Considerable evidence indicates that adolescent turmoil often is not a phase that is outgrown but an indication of true psychopathology.

Course and Prognosis

The onset of identity problem most frequently occurs in late adolescence as teenagers separate from the nuclear family and attempt to establish an independent identity and value system. The onset usually is characterized by a gradual increase in anxiety, depression, regressive phenomena (e.g., loss of interest in friends, school, and activities), irritability, sleep difficulties, and changes in eating habits. The course usually is relatively brief as developmental lags respond to support, acceptance, and the provision of a psychosocial moratorium.

Extensive prolongation of adolescence with continued identity problem can lead to the chronic state of role diffusion, which may indicate a disturbance of early developmental stages and the presence of borderline personality disorder, a mood disorder, or schizophrenia. An identity problem usually resolves by the mid-20s. If it persists, the person with the identity problem may be unable to make career commitments or lasting attachments.

Cory, an 8-year-old girl, was adopted in Taiwan at 10 months of age by a white Midwestern couple. As she grew, her vulnerability to separations became increasingly more pronounced. Even the possibility that her adoptive mother would leave her for the day triggered what appeared to be dramatic disruptions in Cory's reality contact, as well as outbursts of rage and misbehavior in school. She pleaded with her mother to care for the many aches and pains that plagued her. If her mother stayed with her, they could both enjoy the girl's favorite game—the mother playing the part of an Asian queen, with Cory as her beloved princess. Yet, the girl's demands, including the requirements of "royalty," were so exhausting that, at times, the mother would seek relief at her own mother's home in a nearby town.

Such "abandonment" would more than perturb the idyllic fantasy of the queen and her princess. Without the love, protection, and presence of the queen, Cory herself changed, turning into a "Chinese bitch." Later, in therapy, she discussed how a vivid fantasy would come to her at times of separation. In this fantasy, a witch, a vicious vixen of mixed Caucasian and Asian features, taunted Cory and threatened to drag her down into a bottomless pit.

Cory hated this witch nearly as much as she hated the "Chinese bitch" she herself became. She hated, in particular, the rage and anguish that overwhelmed her. To punish the "bitch," she would hit herself and poke at her skin until it bled.

By the time she reached adolescence, Cory's self-mutilating behavior was firmly established. She responded to frustration, separations, or perceived threats of abandonment by cutting herself or burning herself with cigarette lighters. Eventually, she was able to verbalize the multiple functions that self-injury served for her. It forced others to respond to her instead of ignoring her; it allowed her to "stick it" to others without having to take responsibility for her aggression; it produced in her feelings that countered the sense of deadness and emptiness that came on her when she felt desperate; and, last, but certainly not least, it created for her the illusion that she could control hope and healing, as she could literally see the healing taking place in her skin after she had wounded it, rather than waiting for someone else to hurt her or depending on others to provide her with a sense of hope. (Courtesy of Efrain Bleiberg, M.D.)

Treatment

Considerable consensus exists among clinicians, in the absence of an evidence base, that adolescents experiencing identity problems may respond to brief psychosocial intervention. Individual psychotherapy directed toward encouraging growth and development usually is considered the therapy of choice. Adolescents with identity problems often feel developmentally unprepared to deal with the increasing demands for social, emotional, and sexual independence. Issues of separation and individuation from their families can be challenging and overwhelming. Treatment is aimed at helping these adolescents to develop a sense of competence and mastery about necessary social and vocational choices. A therapist's empathic acknowledgment of an adolescent's struggle can be helpful in the process.

19

Psychiatric Treatment

▲ 19.1 Individual Psychotherapy

Individual psychotherapy for children and adolescents can take many forms, including short- and long-term approaches within a variety of conceptual frameworks, such as cognitive-behavioral, behavioral, psychodynamic, supportive, interpersonal, and "eclectic" mixtures of these techniques. In recent years, randomized clinical trials have provided data to support the efficacy of cognitive-behavioral interventions for a wide range of childhood psychiatric disorders, including obsessive-compulsive disorder (OCD), anxiety disorders, and depressive disorders. The initial goal of any psychotherapeutic strategy is to establish a working relationship with the child or adolescent. In general, successful individual psychotherapeutic interventions with children also require establishing a therapeutic rapport with parents. To approach a child therapeutically requires a sense of the normal development of a child of a given age, as well as an understanding of the context in which particular symptoms emerged. Individual psychotherapy with children focuses on improving children's adaptive skills and diminishing specific symptomatology. Treatment reflects an understanding of children's developmental levels and shows cultural sensitivity toward families and environments in which children live. Most children do not seek psychiatric treatment; they are taken to a psychotherapist because of a disturbance noted by a family member, a schoolteacher, or a pediatrician. Children often believe that they are being taken for treatment because of their *misbehavior* or as a punishment for *wrongdoing*.

Children and adolescents are the most accurate informants of their own thoughts, feelings, moods, and perceptual experiences; external behavior problems are often identified by others, yet children's internal experiences may be largely unknown. Children often can describe their feelings in a particular situation but cannot execute therapeutic changes without an advocate's help. Thus, child psychotherapists function as advocates for their child patients in interactions with schools, legal agencies, and community organizations. Child psychotherapists may be called on to make recommendations that affect various aspects of children's lives.

THEORIES AND TECHNIQUES

Emotional, social, and academic issues relating to children of varying ages and developmental levels can be addressed by clinicians using a working knowledge of diverse psychotherapeutic techniques and their applications in childhood. Psychodynamic approaches are generally mixed with supportive components and behavioral management techniques to build a comprehensive treatment plan for a child. Individual psychotherapy with a child frequently takes place in conjunction with family therapy, group therapy, and, when indicated, psychopharmacology. Several theoretical systems underlie psychotherapeutic approaches with children, including psychoanalytic theories, behavioral theories, family systems theories, and developmental theories.

Psychoanalytic Theories

In classic psychoanalytic theory, exploratory psychotherapy applies to patients of all ages by reversing the evolution of psychopathologic processes. A principal difference noted with advancing age is a sharpening distinction between psychogenetic and psychodynamic factors. The younger the child, the more are the genetic and dynamic forces intertwined. The development of these pathologic processes generally is believed to begin with experiences that have proved to be particularly significant to children and to have affected them adversely. Although in one sense the experiences were real, in another sense, they may have been misinterpreted or imagined. In any event, to children, these were traumatic experiences that caused unconscious complexes. Being inaccessible to conscious awareness, the unconscious elements readily escape rational adaptive maneuvers and are subject to pathologic misuse of adaptive and defensive mechanisms. The result is the development of conflicts leading to distressing symptoms, character attitudes, or patterns of behavior that constitute the emotional disturbance.

The psychoanalytic view of emotional disturbances in children has increasingly assumed a developmental orientation. Thus, the maladaptive defensive functioning is directed against conflicts between impulses that characterize a specific developmental phase and environmental influences or a child's internalized representations of the environment. In this framework, disorders result from environmental interference with maturational timetables or conflicts with the environment engendered by developmental progress. The result is difficulty in achieving or resolving developmental tasks and fulfilling capacities that are specific to later phases of development. These developmental stages can be expressed in various ways, from Anna Freud's lines of development to Erik Erikson's concept of sequential psychosocial capacities.

The goal of therapy is to help children to develop good conflict-resolution skills so they can function at their appropriate developmental levels. Therapy may again be necessary as children face the challenges of subsequent developmental periods.

Psychoanalytic psychotherapy, a modified form of psychotherapy, is expressive and exploratory and endeavors to reverse the evolution of emotional disturbance through reenacting and desensitizing traumatic events by freely expressing thoughts and feelings in an interview-play situation. Ultimately, therapists help patients to understand the warded-off feelings, fears, and wishes that have beset them.

Whereas the psychoanalytic psychotherapeutic approach seeks improvement by exposure and resolution of buried conflicts, suppressive-supportive-educative psychotherapy works in the opposite fashion by aiming to facilitate repression. Therapists, capitalizing on patients' desire to please, encourage them to substitute new adaptive and defensive mechanisms. In this therapy, clinicians use interpretations minimally; instead, they emphasize suggestion, persuasion, exhortation, operant reinforcement, counseling, education, direction, advice, abreaction, environmental manipulation, intellectual review, gratification of the patient's current dependent needs, and similar techniques.

Behavioral Theories

All behavior, whether adaptive or maladaptive, is a consequence of the same basic principles of behavior acquisition and maintenance. Behavior is either learned or unlearned. What renders behavior abnormal or disturbed is its social significance. Although theories and their derivative therapeutic intervention techniques have become increasingly complex over the years, all learning can be subsumed in two global basic mechanisms. One is classic *respondent conditioning*, akin to Ivan Pavlov's famous experiments, and the second is *operant instrumental learning*, which is associated with B. F. Skinner, although it is basic to both Edward Thorndike's law of effect, which is about the influence of reinforcing consequences of behavior, and Sigmund Freud's pain-pleasure principle. Both of these basic mechanisms assign the highest priority to the immediate precipitants of behavior and deemphasize remote underlying causal determinants that are important in the psychoanalytic tradition.

The respondent conditioning theory asserts that only two types of abnormal behavior exist: behavioral deficits that result from a failure to learn and deviant maladaptive behavior that is a consequence of learning inappropriate things. Such concepts have always been an implicit part of the rationale underlying all child psychotherapy. Intervention strategies derive much of their success, particularly with children, from rewarding previously unnoticed good behavior, thereby highlighting it, and making it occur more frequently than in the past.

Family Systems Theories

Although families have long been an interest of child psychotherapists, the understanding of transactional family processes has been greatly enhanced by conceptual contributions from cybernetics, systems theory, communications theory, object relations theory, social role theory, ethology, and ecology. The bedrock premise entails the idea of a family functioning as a self-regulating, open system that possesses its own unique history and structure. This structure is constantly evolving as a consequence of dynamic interaction between the family's mutually interdependent systems and persons who share a complementarity of needs. From this conceptual foundation, a wealth of ideas has emerged under rubrics such as family development, life cycle, homeostasis, functions, identity, values, goals, congruence, symmetry, myths, and rules; roles such as spokesperson, symptoms bearer, scapegoat, affect barometer, pet, persecutor, victim, arbitrator, distractor, saboteur, rescuer, breadwinner, disciplinarian, and nurturer; structure, such as boundaries, splits, pairings, alliances, coalitions, enmeshed, disengaged; and concepts such as double bind, scapegoating, pseudomutuality, and mystification. Increasingly, appreciation of the family system sometimes explains why a minute therapeutic input at a critical junction may result in far-reaching changes, whereas in other situations, huge amounts of therapeutic effort seem to be absorbed with minimal evidence of change.

Developmental Theories

Underlying child psychotherapy is the assumption that, in the absence of unusual interference, children mature in basically orderly, predictable ways that can be codified in a variety of interrelated psychosociobiologic sequential systematizations. The central, overriding role of a developmental frame of reference in child psychotherapy distinguishes it from adult psychotherapy. A therapist's orientation should entail more than knowledge of age-appropriate behavior derived from such studies as Arnold Gesell's description of the morphology of behavior. It should encompass more than psychosexual development with ego psychologic and sociocultural amendments, exemplified by Erikson's epigenetic schema. It extends beyond familiarity with Jean Piaget's sequence of intellectual evolution as a basis for knowing the level of abstraction at which children of various ages may be expected to function or for assessing their capacities for moral orientation.

TYPES OF PSYCHOTHERAPIES

Developing a psychotherapeutic intervention for a particular child includes evaluation of the child's age, developmental level, type of problem, and communication style. Whichever style or combination of techniques a therapist chooses to use in psychotherapy, the relationship between child and therapist is a critical element. The relationship itself often is the primary, if not the sole, ingredient in psychotherapy. The therapist provides a safe space in which to listen, empathize, and solve problems with the child.

John, a bright 14-year-old, was treated with brief (25 sessions) psychotherapy. The initial complaint was that his grades had dropped during the academic year; he had withdrawn from sports, was anhedonic, had difficulty relating to his peers, and whined a lot. His parents divorced when John was 7 years old. He had two younger sisters, ages 12 and 9. John "hated" his father; therefore, he missed many visitations with him, pretending that he was sick or too busy to see him. His sisters kept close contact with the father. His mother had a live-in boyfriend who moved in the year that John became symptomatic. John also "hated" the boyfriend. He felt miserable and reproached everyone in his environment. During the first two therapy sessions, two issues to be addressed were delineated: John feeling rejected by his father and mother (who had found another man) and his issues with rivalry. During the following treatment sessions, an empathetic and supportive therapist helped John acquire insight into his feelings through interpretation of his defenses, transferential manifestations, and clarifications. John and the therapist discussed strategies and activities to be carried out during the treatment period to alleviate his discomfort. By session 16, John had reestablished regular contact with his father and was able to tolerate his mother's boyfriend. The termination phase included the integration of what had been discussed, learned, and practiced, and gave John the ability to understand his internal conflicts and find more appropriate ways of managing them. His rivalry issues had diminished, as he was also able to share his father with his sisters. His biological parents and his mother's boyfriend were seen in parallel. The sessions consisted of psychoeducational approaches concerning John's developmental level of functioning and the way he perceived and experienced his environment. His parents were helped to recognize and handle John's problems, as well their own conflicts, and strategies were proposed for facilitating John's development. At termination, it was agreed that John would return to see the therapist for one follow-up session every 3 months in the first year and every 6 months in the following 2 years. At the 2-year follow-up, it was apparent that John had improved academically and had resumed his outside activities, such as sports. He remained sensitive to rejection, but he was able to use the skills he had learned to manage those feelings. (Courtesy of Euthymia D. Hibbs, Ph.D.)

Cognitive-behavioral therapy (CBT) is an amalgam of behavioral therapy and cognitive psychology. It emphasizes how children may use thinking processes and cognitive modalities to reframe, restructure, and solve problems. A child's distortions are addressed by generating alternative ways of dealing with problematic situations. Cognitive-behavioral strategies have been shown in multiple studies to be effective in the treatment of child and adolescent mood disorders, OCD, and anxiety disorders. A recent study compared a family-focused CBT—the Building Confidence Program—with traditional child-focused CBT with minimal family involvement for children with anxiety disorders. Both interventions included coping skills training and in vivo exposure, but the family CBT intervention also included parent communication training. Compared with the child-focused CBT, family CBT was associated with greater improvement on independent evaluators' ratings and parent reports of child anxiety but not on children's self-reports of improvement. Family-focused CBT has also been used with promising success in the treatment of pediatric bipolar disorder.

One of the limiting factors in providing CBT to children with OCD, anxiety disorders, and depressive disorders is the lack of sufficient numbers of trained child and adolescent cognitive-behavioral therapists. A recent study addressed the issue of the feasibility of combining a CBT via clinic-plus-Internet condition. Children who received the clinic-plus-Internet condition showed significantly greater reductions in anxiety from pre- to posttreatment condition and maintained gains for a period of 12 months compared with children who received no active treatment but were on a wait-list condition. The Internet treatment was acceptable to families, and dropout rate was minimal.

A recent study of CBT in conjunction with an attachment-based family therapy (ABFT) used in adolescents with anxiety disorders and their families showed significant improvements using individual CBT along with a family therapy condition. Participants followed at 6 to 9 months after the treatment showed significant decreases in anxiety and depressive symptoms. Cognitive behavior therapy has been shown in multiple randomized clinical trials to demonstrate efficacy in the treatment of anxiety disorders in children and adolescents. Using a variety of components, including behavioral exposure, cognitive restructuring, and psychoeducation, CBT has been shown to be adaptable to a variety of formats, including individual, family, and group treatment.

Michael was a 16-year-old boy from an intact middle-class family enrolled in the 11th grade of a public school. He sought evaluation and treatment for a long-standing history of shyness and anxiety in social situations. Evaluation revealed social phobia as the primary disorder. Michael was motivated for treatment and reported that he wished to feel more comfortable with other people and in social situations with peers. Consequently, Michael was treated with cognitive-behavioral group treatment for adolescents with social phobia, a 16-session course of treatment combining education, cognitive restructuring, behavioral exposure, relapse prevention, and four sessions of parent involvement. As treatment progressed, Michael increased his visibility at school-sponsored social events such that he caught the attention of a female classmate and was asked to attend the prom with her. The therapists designed several prom exposures whereby the various things that could happen at a dance or on a date were presented to Michael, including being offered alcohol or drugs, having a good time dancing, being left alone or ignored by his date, having an argument with the date, and having other girls ask him to dance. As it turned out, Michael's date did, in fact, ignore him and leave him at the dance. Michael, prepared for this less-than-desired outcome by the group experience, asked other girls to dance and interacted with other peers. He considered the evening a success and subsequently went on to other social events with friends made at the prom. In this case study, the importance of exposing youth to the range of potential outcomes for a given social situation was crucial to Michael's trust in the therapy and therapists and a belief in the credibility of treatment. Moreover, he was appropriately prepared through behavioral exposure and practice to handle what could have been an awkward and discouraging situation. (Courtesy of Anne Marie Albano, Ph.D.)

Freddy was a 3-year-old boy from an intact lower-income family, referred by his preschool teacher because of selective mutism. Freddy was the product of a normal, full-term pregnancy and vaginal delivery and attained all developmental milestones either as expected or early. However, temperamentally, he was a shy baby and toddler and reticent to explore surroundings on his own or to stay with adults other than his parents. Freddy spoke in full sentences and spontaneously up until 3 months before the referral, when he ceased speaking to anyone, including his parents. According to his parents, Freddy was left with a 16-year-old cousin for babysitting, but the cousin left the child alone in the apartment. Freddy let himself out of the apartment and was found wandering the street by the police. Subsequently, Freddy was taken into protective custody and spent a night in a foster placement, until his parents were able to rectify the situation with the authorities. Freddy stopped speaking from the moment of being taken by the police. He did not speak to his parents, but he did cry on their reunion. After his return home, Freddy did not speak to his parents for the first week, but then began asking for things and responding to his parents with simple one- or two-word sentences. He refused to speak to anyone else, however.

Freddy had begun preschool shortly before the incident and was speaking then but stopped after the incident. Although he was observed constantly, he was never "caught" speaking to peers. He was described as an overly obedient and pleasant child who smiled and played with others and followed requests without problem, but just stared at a speaker and offered no reply or nonverbal communication. During evaluation, it was revealed that Freddy enjoyed eating Froot Loops in a favorite cup as a treat. Treatment was designed to provide incentive for speaking through the delivery of a contingent reinforcer of high value, the Froot Loops. Hence, Froot Loops became available only in the preschool and the therapist's office and, temporarily, were not available in his home. The therapist enacted a process of graduated shaping of communication behaviors—first nonverbal and then vocal noises—and trained the preschool teacher to do the same. Froot Loop boxes were kept in full view of Freddy at all times during the initial phase of treatment and, when he was "caught" gazing at the box, the therapist or teacher would prompt Freddy for acknowledgment that he wanted the treat. Pointing, looking, and nodding in their direction resulted in receiving four Froot Loops. Next, Freddy was asked to make a sound or ask for the Froot Loop to receive the reward. This step was accomplished as he grunted and eventually said, "Loop." Finally, prompts to ask for the Froot Loops in a sentence were enacted, and Freddy complied with this demand. This phase of treatment took 2 days at the preschool and 2 hours of therapy to accomplish. Eventually, the boxes of Froot Loops were removed from the environments, but the teacher kept the cereal with her to deliver four Loops whenever Freddy made sounds or spoke in school. This shaping procedure took an additional 3 days to result in Freddy speaking to the teacher and peers, albeit in short sentences. The treat was faded—that is, delivered on a variable ratio schedule of every three to eight times that he spoke, to promote further speaking and decrease the association with the treat. By the end of the second week of training, Freddy was speaking at the rate and level that he had before the incident. His parents were instructed to provide the treat in the home as was usual. Moreover, they were cautioned to allow or prompt Freddy to speak for himself in social situations (e.g., order his own food at a restaurant, say hello to others, make his own requests before providing a treat) as a way of relapse prevention. (Courtesy of Anne Marie Albano, Ph.D.)

Maryanne was a 12-year-old girl with a family history of anxiety and mood disorders. Her parents brought her to treatment because of recurrent obsessions involving contamination and germs, with corresponding compulsions whereby she had her parents check her food and washed her hands repeatedly to the point of their becoming raw and bleeding. Evaluation revealed a fear that, unless her parents checked her food for bugs or germs, the meal was contaminated. Hence, her parents had to physically pull apart her food and examine it to her satisfaction, which could take upward of 1 hour for each meal. This caused much distress and discord between Maryanne and her family. In addition, Maryanne washed her hands constantly—after opening a door, reading a book, using a pencil, or touching any object that she deemed dirty. The process of exposure and response prevention was used whereby a hierarchy of her obsessions and compulsions was constructed, from the least upsetting (checking food prepared by her mother) to the most upsetting (touching something that was wet or slimy and then touching her mouth). Systematically, the therapist had Maryanne first engage in imaginary exposure to a scene (e.g., you take a bite of hamburger and something tastes gritty to you and you realize that your mom did not check the burger) until her anxiety dropped to minimal levels. This usually occurred after 25 minutes. Next, the scene was enacted in vivo, whereby foods were introduced with "contaminants" in them (e.g., putting pieces of uncooked rice into the burger to mimic "grit"), and Maryanne ate the food without having her parents check. As treatment progressed, Maryanne learned that her feared consequence of becoming sick was not likely to occur. Similarly, washing rituals were addressed by having her touch items with various substances coating them and then touching her face and mouth. Treatment occurred over a 14-session program with her parents taught to assist her with these exposures in the home. The parents were also instructed to refrain from engaging in her rituals. Relapse prevention plans were enacted to expand her range of food choices and situational contexts (cafeterias, food stands, restaurants) for exposure. By the end of treatment, Maryanne was eating without the need for checking and with minimal to no anxiety. Moreover, she was engaging in a wide range of activity without the need to wash after touching various objects. (Courtesy of Anne Marie Albano, Ph.D.)

Remedial, educational, and patterning psychotherapy is focused on teaching new attitudes and patterns of behavior to children who persist in using immature and inefficient patterns that are often presumed to be caused by a maturational lag. Supportive psychotherapy is particularly helpful in enabling a well-adjusted youngster to cope with emotional turmoil engendered by a crisis. It also is used with disturbed youngsters whose less-than-adequate ego functioning may be seriously disrupted by an expressive-exploratory mode or by other forms of therapeutic intervention.

At the beginning of most psychotherapy, regardless of a patient's age and the nature of the therapeutic interventions, the principal therapeutic elements perceived by patients tend to be supportive as a consequence of therapists' universal efforts to be reliably and sensitively responsive. In fact, some therapy may never proceed beyond the supportive level, whereas other therapy develops an expressive-exploratory or behavioral modification flavor on top of the supportive foundation.

Preschool-age children are sometimes treated through the parents, a process called *filial therapy*. Therapists using the strategy should be alert to the possibility that apparently successful filial treatment can obscure a significant diagnosis because patients are not treated directly. The first case of filial therapy was that of Little Hans, reported by Freud in 1905. Hans was a 5-year-old phobic child who was treated by his father under Freud's supervision.

Whereas historically psychotherapy had its roots in psychodynamic theories, evidence has shown that cognitive-behavioral therapeutic techniques are efficacious in the treatment of anxiety disorders and mood disorders in youth. Children generally are unaware of these unreal dangers, their fear of them, and the psychologic defenses they use to avoid both the danger and the fear. With the awareness that is facilitated, patients can evaluate the usefulness of their defensive maneuvers and can relinquish unnecessary maneuvers that constitute the symptoms of their emotional disturbance.

A 10-year-old girl was seen in twice-weekly psychodynamic psychotherapy. As the child left her sessions, her mother would ask each time, "How is she doing?" The therapist made a separate appointment with the parents to discuss these concerns further, while also exploring how the child felt about this meeting. The girl had concerns about "what they are going to say about me," but acceded with support and understanding from the therapist. After discussion with the parents, it was agreed that the therapist would meet with the parents once every month to discuss the child's progress and current functioning, provide support and guidance to the parents, and monitor the parents' anxiety. Once this plan was initiated, the mother's anxiety seemed to lessen, and she no longer waited expectantly after the sessions with her daughter. (Courtesy of David L. Kaye, M.D.)

A 6-year-old boy was brought for treatment because of long-standing severe aggression and destructiveness. In addition to an evaluation for medication, the child was seen in twice-weekly psychoanalytically oriented psychotherapy. The beginning sessions were marked by the repeated need to set limits and contain the child's aggressive behaviors. Two months into treatment, he began to pump himself up, roar, and announce that he was "the Incredible Hulk." He would then proceed to stomp around the play therapy room, attempting to destroy the toys. The therapist then said, "You know you can't really *be* the Hulk. You can *pretend* that you are the Hulk, and then maybe we can play this together." After a number of similar exchanges, the child gradually and increasingly became able to play the part without becoming it. (Courtesy of David L. Kaye, M.D.)

Child psychoanalysis—an intensive, uncommon form of psychoanalytic psychotherapy—works on unconscious resistance and defenses during three to four sessions a week. Under these circumstances, therapists anticipate unconscious resistance and allow transference manifestations to mature to a full transference neurosis, through which neurotic conflicts are resolved. Interpretations of dynamically relevant conflicts are emphasized in psychoanalytic descriptions, and elements that are predominant in other types of psychotherapies are not overlooked. Indeed, in all psychotherapy, children should derive support from the consistently understanding and accepting relationship with their therapists. Remedial educational guidance is provided when necessary.

Probably the most vivid examples of the integration of psychodynamic and behavioral approaches, although they are not always explicitly conceptualized as such, appear in the milieu of child and adolescent psychiatric therapy in inpatient, residential, and day treatment facilities. Behavioral change is initiated in these settings, and its repercussions are explored concurrently in individual psychotherapeutic sessions, so that the action in one arena and the information stemming from it augment and illuminate what occurs in the other arena.

DIFFERENCES BETWEEN CHILDREN AND ADULTS

Logic suggests that psychotherapy with children, who generally are more flexible than adults and have simpler defenses and other mental mechanisms, should consume less time than comparable treatment of adults. Experience usually does not confirm this expectation because children usually lack some elements that contribute to successful treatment. A child, for example, typically does not seek help. As a consequence, one of a therapist's first tasks is to stimulate a child's motivation for treatment. Children commonly begin therapy involuntarily, often without the benefit of true parental support. Although parents may want their children to be helped or changed, the desire often is generated by frustrated anger toward the children. Typically, the anger is accompanied by relative insensitivity to what therapists perceive as the children's need and the basis for a therapeutic alliance. Therefore, whereas adult patients frequently perceive advantages in getting well, children may envision therapeutic change as nothing more than conforming to a disagreeable reality, an attitude that heightens the likelihood of their perceiving a therapist as the parent's punitive agent. This is hardly the most fertile soil in which to nurture a therapeutic alliance.

Children have a limited capacity for self-observation, with the notable exception of some obsessive children who resemble adults in this ability. Such obsessive children, however, usually isolate the vital emotional components. In exploratory-interpretative psychotherapies, the development of a capacity for ego splitting—that is, simultaneous emotional involvement and self-observation—is most helpful. Only by identifying with a trusted adult and in alliance with this adult can children approach such an ideal. A therapist's gender and the relatively superficial aspects of the therapist's demeanor may be important elements in the development of a trusting relationship with a child.

Recognition of the importance of play constituted a major forward stride in these efforts.

PLAYROOM

The structure, design, and furnishing of the playroom are important. Some therapists maintain that the toys should be few, simple, and carefully selected to facilitate the communication of fantasy. Other therapists suggest that a wide variety of playthings should be available to increase the range of feelings that children can express. These contrasting recommendations have been attributed to differences in therapeutic methods. Some therapists tend to avoid interpretation, even of conscious ideas, whereas others recommend the interpretation of unconscious content directly and quickly.

Therapists tend to change their preferences in equipment as they accumulate experience and develop confidence in their abilities. Although special equipment—such as genital dolls, amputation dolls, and see-through anatomically complete (except for genitalia) models—has been used in therapy, many therapists have observed that the unusual nature of such items risks making children wary and suspicious of a therapist's motives. Until dolls available to children in their own homes include genitalia, the psychologic content that special dolls are designed to elicit may be more available at the appropriate time with conventional dolls.

Although the choices of play materials vary among therapists, the following equipment can constitute a well-balanced playroom or play area: multigenerational families of flexible but sturdy dolls of various races; additional dolls representing special roles and feelings, such as police officer, doctor, and soldier; dollhouse furnishings with or without a dollhouse; toy animals; puppets; paper, crayons, paint, and blunt-ended scissors; a sponge-like ball; clay or something comparable; tools such as rubber hammers, rubber knives, and guns; building blocks, cars, trucks, and airplanes; and eating utensils. The toys should enable children to communicate through play. Therapists should avoid toys and materials that are fragile or break easily, that can result in physical injury to a child, or that can increase a child's guilt.

INITIAL APPROACH

Various approaches are associated with each therapist's individual style and perception of children's needs, from approaches in which a therapist endeavors to direct children's thought content and activity (release therapy, some behavior therapy, and certain educational patterning techniques) to exploratory methods in which a therapist endeavors to follow children's leads. Although children determine the focus, therapists structure the situation. Encouraging children to say whatever they wish and to play freely, as in exploratory psychotherapy, establishes a definite structure. Therapists create an atmosphere in which they get to know all about a child—the good side as well as the bad side, as children would put it. A therapist may communicate to a child that the child's response elicits neither anger nor pleasure but only understanding from the therapist. Such an assertion does not imply that therapists have no emotions, but it assures the young patient that the therapist's personal feelings and standards are subordinate to understanding the youngster.

THERAPEUTIC INTERVENTIONS

Psychotherapy with children and adolescents generally is more directed and active than it often is with adults. Children usually cannot synthesize histories of their own lives, but they are excellent reporters of their current internal states. Even with adolescents, a therapist often takes an active role, is somewhat less open-ended than with adults, and offers more direction and advocacy than with adults. A child or adolescent therapist often makes exclamations and expresses confrontations in which attention is directed to data of which patients are cognizant. A therapist may use interpretations designed to expand patients' awareness of themselves by making explicit the elements that have previously been expressed implicitly in the patients' thoughts, feelings, and behavior. Beyond interpretation, therapists may educatively offer new information to which patients have not been exposed previously. At the most active end of the continuum are advising, counseling, and directing, which are designed to help patients to adopt a course of action or a conscious attitude.

Nurturing and maintaining a therapeutic alliance may require educating children about the process of therapy. Another educational intervention may entail assigning labels to affects that have not been part of a youngster's experience. Rarely does therapy have to compensate for a real absence of education about acceptable decorum and playing games. Children usually are in therapy not because they have never been exposed to educational efforts, but because repeated educational efforts have failed. Therefore, therapy generally need not include additional teaching efforts, despite the frequent temptation to offer them.

The temptation for therapists to offer themselves as a model for identification may also stem from helpful educational attitudes toward children. Although this may sometimes be an appropriate therapeutic strategy, therapists should not lose sight of the pitfalls of this apparently innocuous maneuver.

PARENTS

Psychotherapy with children requires parental involvement, which does not necessarily reflect parental culpability for a youngster's emotional difficulties but is a reality of a child's dependent state.

Parents are involved in child psychotherapy to varying degrees. For preschool-age children, the entire therapeutic effort may be directed toward the parents, without any direct treatment of the child. At the other extreme, children can be treated in psychotherapy without any parental involvement beyond the payment of fees and perhaps transporting the child to the therapy sessions. Most practitioners, however, prefer to maintain an informative alliance with parents to obtain additional information about the child.

Probably the most frequent parental arrangements are those developed in child guidance clinics—that is, parent guidance focused on the child or the parent–child interaction and therapy for the parents' individual needs concurrent with the child's therapy. Parents may be seen by their child's therapist or by someone else. Recently, increasing efforts have been made to shift the focus from the child as the primary patient to the child as the family's emissary to the clinic. In such family therapy, all or selected members of the family are treated simultaneously as a family group. Although the preferences of specific clinics and practitioners for either an individual or a family therapeutic approach may be unavoidable, the final decision regarding which therapeutic strategy or combination to use should be derived from the clinical assessment.

CONFIDENTIALITY

The issue of confidentiality takes on greater meaning as children grow older. Very young children are unlikely to be as concerned about this issue as are adolescents. Confidentiality usually is preserved unless a child is believed to be in danger or to be a danger to someone else. In other situations, a child's permission usually is sought before a specific issue is raised with parents. Advantages exist to creating an atmosphere in which children can feel that all words and actions are viewed by therapists as simultaneously both serious and tentative. In other words, children's communications do not bind therapists to a commitment; nevertheless, they are too important to be communicated to a third party without a patient's permission. Although such an attitude may be implied, sometimes therapists should explicitly discuss confidentiality with children. Most of what children do and say in psychotherapy is common knowledge to the parents.

The therapist should try to enlist parents' cooperation in respecting the privacy of children's therapeutic sessions. The respect is not always readily honored because parents are naturally curious about what occurs, and they may be threatened by a therapist's apparently privileged position.

Routinely reporting to a child the essence of communications with third parties about the child underscores the therapist's reliability and respect for the child's autonomy. In certain treatments, the report can be combined with soliciting the child's guesses about these transactions. A therapist also may find it fruitful to invite children, particularly older children, to participate in discussions about them with third parties.

> A 13-year-old boy was noted by his parents to be extremely worried about contracting germs from his surroundings. He insisted on washing his hands more than 25 times a day and would often spend more than an hour a day making sure that his body and hands were clean and "free of contamination." After evaluation, the diagnosis of OCD was made, and the boy and his parents opted for CBT. The therapist started by helping the boy to rank his fears on a scale of 1 to 10, with 10 assigned to objects that he believed were most germ-laden, and 1 assigned to those objects that were of little or no concern. The boy was then taught both relaxation techniques and how to engage in thought interruption, and he used these techniques in a step-wise fashion to overcome first the more benign elements on his list, followed by the most severe. Eventually, he was able to modify his behavior by combining his understanding of what worried him most with his capacity to master and eventually overcome his fears. (Courtesy of Eugene V. Beresin, M.D., and Steven C. Schlozman, M.D.)

INDICATIONS

Psychotherapy usually is indicated for children with emotional disorders that seem to be sufficiently permanent to impede maturational and developmental forces. Psychotherapy also may be indicated when a child's development is not impeded but is inducing reactions in the environment that are considered pathogenic. Such disharmonies ordinarily are dealt with by the child with parental assistance; however, when these efforts are persistently inadequate, psychotherapeutic interventions may be indicated.

Psychotherapy should be limited to instances in which positive indicators point to its potential usefulness. For a child to benefit from psychotherapy, the home situation must provide a certain amount of nurturance, stability, and motivation for therapy. A child must have adequate cognitive resources to participate in the process and profit from it. Psychotherapy must be judged with common sense. If a psychotherapy situation is not effective, it is important to determine whether the therapist and patient are poorly matched, whether the type of psychotherapy is inappropriate to the nature of the problems, and whether the child is cognitively inappropriate for the treatment.

▲ 19.2 Group Psychotherapy

Group formats have been demonstrated to be useful in randomized clinical trials using cognitive-behavioral techniques to treat childhood anxiety disorders. Groups have been used for a wide range of clinical situations, including aggressive adolescents requiring anger management training, children who need social skills improvement, survivors of childhood sexual abuse and other traumatic events such as the September 11 World Trade Center attacks, adolescents with social phobia and obsessive compulsive disorder (OCD), children with psychotic disorders, adolescents with substance abuse, and children and adolescents with learning disorders. A recent study formed a psychotherapy group for adolescent survivors of homicide victims. Group therapy can be done with children of all ages, using developmentally appropriate formats. Group therapy can be structured to address a variety of communication skills, including issues of interpersonal competence, peer relationships, and social skills. Group psychotherapy can be modified to suit groups of children of various ages and can focus on behavioral, educational, and social skills and psychodynamic issues. The mode in which the group functions depends on children's developmental levels, intelligence, and problems to be addressed. In behaviorally and cognitive-behavioral groups, the group leader is a directive, active participant who facilitates prosocial interactions and desired behaviors. In groups using psychodynamic approaches, the leader may monitor interpersonal interactions less actively than in behavior therapy groups.

Gathering children and adolescents into groups may lead to greater psychologic impact than treating them individually. A number of factors, described by Irving Yalom, may contribute to the effectiveness of groups. These factors include the following theoretical components:

Hope: Hope may be generated by gathering with others who are experiencing similar difficulties and by observing others actively mastering the problems.

Universality: Children and adolescents with psychiatric disorders often feel isolated and alienated from peers. Working together in groups may diffuse the isolation and help children and adolescents to view their disorder as only a small part of their overall identity.

Imparting information: Children and adolescents are familiar with a format of gaining new information in a group setting, such as in school. The group therapy format provides an opportunity to reinforce learning when the child or adolescent "helps" or demonstrates what he or she has learned to peers.

Altruism: Helping other peers in a group setting by supporting them and identifying with their struggles can improve children's or adolescents' self-esteem and help them to gain a sense of mastery over their own issues.

Improved Social Skills: Group therapy is a safe format in which children and adolescents with poor social skills can improve their interpersonal and communication abilities under the supervision of a leader and with peers who also benefit from the practice scenarios.

Groups can be highly effective modalities to provide peer feedback and support to children who are either socially isolated or unaware of their effects on their peers. Groups with very young children generally are highly structured by the leader and use imagination and play to foster socially acceptable peer relationships and positive behavior. Therapists must be keenly aware of the level of children's attention span and the need for consistency and limit setting. Leaders of preschool-age groups can model supportive adult behavior in meaningful ways for children who have been deprived or neglected. School-age children's groups can be single sex or include both boys and girls. School-age children are more sophisticated in verbalizing their feelings than preschoolers, but they also benefit from structured therapeutic games. Children of school age need frequent reminders about rules, and they are quick to point out infractions of the rules to each other. Interpersonal skills can be addressed nicely in group settings with school-age children.

Same-sex groups are often used among early adolescents. Physiologic changes in early adolescence and the new demands of high school lead to stress that may be ameliorated when groups of same-age peers compare and share. With older adolescents, groups more often include both boys and girls. Even with older adolescents, the leader often uses structure and direct intervention to maximize the therapeutic value of the group. Adolescents who are feeling dejected or alienated may find a special sense of belonging in a therapy group.

Johnny was a high-functioning, 14-year-old boy diagnosed with autistic disorder. He had been in individual and family therapy for several months before he was considered ready for group therapy. Johnny was an awkward-looking adolescent who looked and acted younger than his chronologic age. His academic level was above average, but his social development was very limited. A supercilious, hypermoralistic attitude of more recent development contributed considerably to his social isolation, particularly after starting 7th grade. He was assigned to an established group of early adolescents with a mixture of clinical conditions, meeting once weekly for 75 minutes. Initially, Johnny limited his participation to monosyllabic answers to direct questions, then he would go back to reading a book on the history of Napoleon, his favorite subject and object of fascination. Group members chose to ignore him after a while. Over a period of several weeks, his interest in the book seemed to abate. Johnny brought it, but it remained unopened on his lap. He would make an occasional remark, mostly to criticize another group member for his "vulgarity." The group laughed at his remarks, but scapegoating could be avoided. They seemed to respect his "differentness." Two months later, Peter, a very shy schizoid 13-year-old boy joined the group. After a few sessions Johnny developed an unexpected interest in Peter and sat by him and encouraged him to interact with the group. Soon Johnny was not bringing a book any longer and was more actively involved with group members. He responded to social cues in a more age-typical and appropriate manner, and although he continued having morbid preoccupations with power and a fascination with Napoleon, the intensity was considerably diminished. Johnny's growing interest in people was clinically evident. Group therapy was used in combination with individual and family therapy and psychotropic medication over 18 months. Although the group experience was only one component of the treatment plan, it became a most significant tool to help Johnny with his interpersonal deficits. (Courtesy of Alberto C. Serrano, M.D.)

PRESCHOOL-AGE AND EARLY SCHOOL-AGE GROUPS

Work with a preschool-age group usually is structured by a therapist through the use of a particular technique, such as puppets or artwork, or is couched in terms of a permissive play atmosphere. In therapy with puppets, children project their fantasies onto the puppets in a way not unlike ordinary play. The main value lies in the cathexis afforded children, especially if they show difficulty expressing their feelings. Here, the group aids the child less by interaction with other members than by action with the puppets.

In play group therapy, the emphasis rests on children's interactional qualities with each other and with the therapist in the permissive playroom setting. The therapist should allow children to produce fantasies verbally and in play but also use active restraint when children undergo excessive tension. The toys are the traditional ones used in individual play therapy. The children use the toys to act out aggressive impulses and relive their home difficulties with group members and with the therapist. The children selected for group treatment have a common social hunger and need to be like their peers and be accepted by them. Selected children usually include those with phobias, effeminate boys, shy and withdrawn children, and children with disruptive behavior disorders.

Modifications of these criteria have been used in group psychotherapy for autistic children, parent group therapy, and art therapy. A modification of group psychotherapy has been used for toddlers with physical disabilities who show speech and language delays. The experience of twice-weekly group activities involves mothers and children in a mutual teaching and learning setting. This experience has proved effective for mothers, who received supportive psychotherapy in the group experience; their formerly hidden fantasies about their children emerged and were dealt with therapeutically.

SCHOOL-AGE GROUPS

Activity group psychotherapy is based on the idea that poor, divergent experiences have led to deficits in children's appropriate personality development; therefore, corrective experiences in a therapeutically conditioned environment modify them. Because some latency-age children have deep disturbances involving fears, high anxiety levels, and guilt, a modification of activity-interview group psychotherapy has evolved. The format uses interview techniques, verbal explanations of fantasies, group play, work, and other communications. In this type of group psychotherapy, children verbalize in a problem-oriented manner, with the awareness that the problems brought them together and the group aims to change them. They report dreams, fantasies, daydreams, and traumatic and unpleasant experiences. Open discussion includes both the experiences and the group behavior.

Therapists vary in their use of time, cotherapists, food, and materials. Most groups meet after school for at least 1 hour, although other group leaders prefer a 90-minute session. Some therapists serve food during the last 10 minutes; others prefer serving times when the children are together for talking. Food, however, does not become a major feature and is never central to the group's activities.

PUBERTAL AND ADOLESCENT GROUPS

Group therapy methods similar to those used in younger-age groups can be modified to apply to pubertal children, who are often grouped monosexually. Their problems resemble those of late latency-age children, but they (especially the girls) are also beginning to feel the effects and pressures of early adolescence. Groups offer help during a transitional period; they seem to satisfy the social appetite of preadolescents, who compensate for feelings of inferiority and self-doubt by forming groups. This therapy takes advantage of the influence of the socialization process during these years. Because pubertal children experience difficulties in conceptualizing, pubertal therapy groups tend to use play, drawing, psychodrama, and other nonverbal modes of expression. The therapist's role is active and directive.

Activity group psychotherapy has been the recommended group therapy for pubertal children who do not have significantly disturbed personality patterns. The children, usually of the same sex and in groups of not more than eight, freely engage in activities in a setting especially designed and planned for its physical and environmental characteristics. Samuel Slavson, a pioneer in group psychotherapy, pictured the group as a substitute family in which the passive, neutral therapist becomes the surrogate for parents. The therapist assumes various roles, mostly in a nonverbal manner, as each child interacts with the therapist and other group members. Currently, however, therapists tend to see the group as a form of peer group, with its attendant socializing processes, rather than a reenactment of the family.

Late adolescents, 16 years of age and older, often may be included in groups of adults. Group therapy has been useful in the treatment of substance-related disorders. Combined therapy (the use of group and individual therapy) also has been used successfully with adolescents.

OTHER GROUP SITUATIONS

Groups are also helpful in more focused treatments, such as specific social skills training for children with attention-deficit/hyperactivity disorder (ADHD) or cognitive-behavioral group interventions for depressed children and for children with bereavement problems or eating disorders. In these more specialized groups, the issues are more specific, and actual tasks (as in social skills groups) can be practiced within the group. Some residential and day treatment units use group psychotherapy techniques. Group psychotherapy in schools for underachievers and children from low socioeconomic levels has relied on reinforcement and on modeling theory in addition to traditional techniques and has been supplemented by parent groups.

In controlled conditions, residential treatment units have been used for specific studies in group psychotherapy, such as behavioral contracting. Behavioral contracting with reward-punishment reinforcement provides positive reinforcements among preadolescent boys with severe concerns in basic trust, low self-esteem, and dependence conflicts. Somewhat akin to formal residential treatment units are social group work homes. For children who undergo many psychologic assaults before placement, supportive group psychotherapy offers ventilation and catharsis, but more often it succeeds in letting children become aware of the enjoyment of sharing activities and developing skills.

Public schools—also a structured environment, although not usually considered the best site for group psychotherapy—have been used by several workers. Group psychotherapy as group counseling readily lends itself to school settings. One such group used gender- and problem-homogeneous selection for groups of six to eight students who met once a week during school hours over 2 to 3 years.

INDICATIONS

Many indications exist for the use of group psychotherapy as a treatment modality. Some indications are situational; a therapist may work in a reformatory setting, in which group psychotherapy seems to reach adolescents better than individual treatment does. Another indication is time economics: More patients can be reached in a given time by the use of groups than by individual therapy. Group therapy best helps a child at a given age and developmental stage and with a given type of problem. In young age groups, children's social hunger and their potential need for peer acceptance help to determine their suitability for group therapy. Criteria for unsuitability are controversial and have been loosened progressively.

PARENT GROUPS

In group psychotherapy, as in most treatment procedures for children, parental difficulties can present obstacles. Sometimes, uncooperative parents refuse to bring a child or to participate in their own therapy. The extreme of this situation reveals itself when severely disturbed parents use a child as their channel of communication to work out their own needs. In such circumstances, a child is in the unfortunate position of receiving positive group experiences that seem to create havoc at home.

Parent groups, therefore, can be a valuable aid to group psychotherapy for their children. A recent study showed that a cognitive-behavioral group intervention for parents can successfully teach them how to use therapeutic interventions with their anxiety-disordered children. Parents of children in therapy often have difficulty understanding their children's ailments, discerning the line of demarcation between normal and pathologic behavior, relating to the medical establishment, and coping with feelings of guilt. Parent groups assist in these areas and help members to formulate guidelines for action.

▲ 19.3 Residential, Day, and Hospital Treatment

National trends in treatment and delivery systems for children and adolescents with psychiatric disorders indicate a significant decline in the availability of child and adolescent inpatient beds. Given that there are just fewer than 10 million children and adolescents with psychiatric disorders, questions arise as to the most effective ways of providing them with psychiatric care. Given the paucity of psychiatric inpatient units for children and adolescents, those children with severe psychiatric conditions may turn to residential treatment centers and various types of intensive outpatient programs or partial hospital treatment programs.

Residential treatment centers and facilities are appropriate settings for children and adolescents with mental disorders who require a highly structured and supervised setting for a substantial time. Such settings have the advantage of providing a stable, consistent environment with a high level of psychiatric monitoring but one that is less intensive than a hospital. Children and adolescents with serious psychiatric disturbances often end up in residential facilities because of difficulties in managing their own psychiatric problems and because of family situations in which appropriate supervision and parenting are impossible. Residential settings offer many treatments, including behavioral management, psychotherapy, medication, special education, and the therapeutic milieu itself. Children and adolescents who benefit from residential settings have a wide variety of psychiatric problems and commonly have difficulty with impulse control and structuring their own time. Many residents of such programs also have families with serious psychiatric, financial, and parenting difficulties. Given the multitude of treatment modalities available for children and adolescents with psychiatric disorders, including cognitive-behavioral and interpersonal individual therapies, social skills and cognitive-behavioral group therapies, family education and therapy, psychopharmacology, special educational services, and therapeutic recreational therapies, residential facilities are even more critical in providing the setting in which to conduct the evidence-based research for these interventions.

Partial hospitalization has been used more frequently with the advent of managed care as an alternative to hospitalization to provide short-term crisis stabilization or as a step-down from inpatient treatment for children and adolescents with psychiatric disorders. Day treatment programs, sometimes used interchangeably with the term *partial hospitalization*, are designed to serve the needs of children and adolescents with severe disorders who require interventions focused on improved level of function but who do not meet criteria of medical necessity to be in the hospital. A variety of intensive outpatient programming constitutes a day treatment program. One of the key ingredients of a day treatment program is the provision of a therapeutic day that optimally includes an educational component. Day treatment programs are excellent alternatives for children and adolescents who require more intensive support, monitoring, and supervision than is available in the community but who can live successfully at home if they receive the proper level of intervention. In most cases, children and adolescents who attend day hospital programs have serious mental disorders and might warrant psychiatric hospitalization without the program's support. Family therapy, group and individual psychotherapy, psychopharmacology, behavioral management programs, and special education are integral parts of these programs.

Tammy, age 13, was first seen in a pediatric emergency department on a Saturday morning by a psychiatry resident who determined that, although she had continued suicidal ideation, she did not have a specific plan and could be treated without hospitalization. Over the weekend, the resident contacted Tammy and her family twice by phone and arranged for her to be admitted to a partial hospital program on Monday morning. During her first few days in the program, she was monitored closely by the staff, and her suicide potential was evaluated at the end of each day by the medical director. During the first week, her suicidal ideation resolved in response to the support and structure of the program. At the end of her second week in the partial hospital program, she was stabilized, started on antidepressant medication, and transitioned to outpatient family and group therapy after stated commitments to follow-up by the patient and her parents. The use of partial hospitalization prevented a psychiatric inpatient admission for this acutely symptomatic adolescent. (Courtesy of Laurel J. Kiser, Ph.D., M.B.A., Jerry Heston M.D., and David Pruitt, M.D.)

During a hospitalization for a life-threatening suicide attempt, Jamie's family's managed care company decertified his admission, saying he was no longer at acute risk for suicide. Because of continued serious depressive symptoms and chronic family dysfunction, he was determined to be inappropriate for routine outpatient management. He was admitted to a day program with a strong family systems orientation. Over the course of his 8-week treatment, he was able to develop a therapeutic alliance with his individual therapist, and significant family restructuring was accomplished. The consulting child and adolescent psychiatrist was able to manage Jamie's medication and regularly monitor his suicide potential. At the end of 8 weeks, his depressive symptoms were decreased to the extent that he could transition to outpatient therapy and return to school successfully. This use of the ambulatory behavioral continuum allowed for prompt discharge from the hospital with continued consolidation of progress in a highly structured system. (Courtesy of Laurel J. Kiser, Ph.D., M.B.A., Jerry Heston M.D., and David Pruitt, M.D.)

Eric was a 7-year-old boy referred to a rural community mental health center for services. Eric presented with a family history of schizophrenia, extreme irritability, labile mood, noncompliance, tantrums, and physical violence toward his peers and adults. He had received multiple school suspensions and was at risk for expulsion. On intake to services, the clinician recommended participation in a newly established day treatment program housed at Eric's elementary school. The clinician also recommended individual therapy, family therapy, case management, psychiatric evaluation, and nursing services.

During Eric's 6-month participation in the day treatment program, his academic program was infused with daily mental health services in the classroom setting. His daily goals included increasing compliance, decreasing anger outbursts, and decreasing physical aggression. He was able to improve peer relations while receiving immediate feedback and direct instruction on social skills by a master's-level clinician, teacher, and teacher's assistant. Each of the adult staff was able to consistently apply behavior management principles in their domain areas. Eric's parents actively participated in parent conferences, as well as in family therapy sessions. After initial reluctance, they agreed to schedule a psychiatric evaluation, after which Eric was further stabilized on medication. Eric was gradually transitioned to a regular classroom setting, where he is being maintained successfully. He continues with outpatient services. (Courtesy of Laurel J. Kiser, Ph.D., M.B.A., Jerry Heston, M.D., and David Pruitt, M.D.)

HOSPITALIZATION

Psychiatric hospitalization is needed when a child or adolescent exhibits dangerous behavior, is contemplating suicide, or is experiencing an exacerbation of a psychotic disorder or another serious mental disorder. Safety, stabilization, and effective treatment are the goals of hospitalization. Recently, the length of stay for child and adolescent psychiatric patients has decreased because of financial pressures and increased availability of day treatment programs. Psychiatric hospitalization may be some children's first opportunity to experience a stable, safe environment. Hospitals often are the most appropriate places to start use of new medications, and they provide an around-the-clock setting in which to observe a child's behavior. Children may show remission of some symptoms by virtue of their removal from a stressful or abusive environment. After a child has been observed for several weeks, the best treatment and disposition may become clear.

RESIDENTIAL TREATMENT

More than 20,000 emotionally disturbed children are in residential treatment centers in the United States, and this number is increasing. Deteriorating social conditions, particularly in cities, often make it impossible for a child with a serious mental disorder to live at home. In these cases, residential treatment centers serve a real need. They provide a structured living environment in which children may form strong attachments to, and receive commitments from, staff members. The purpose of the center is to provide treatment and special education for children and their families.

Staff and Setting

Staffing patterns include various combinations of child-care workers, teachers, social workers, psychiatrists, pediatricians, nurses, and psychologists; therefore, residential treatment can be very expensive. The Joint Commission on the Mental Health of Children made the following structural and setting recommendations:

> In addition to space for therapy programs, there should be facilities for a first-rate school and a rich evening activity program, and there should be ample space for play, both indoors and out. Facilities should be small, seldom exceeding 60 patients in capacity with a limit of 100 patients, and they should make provisions for children to live in small groups. The centers should be located near the families they serve and should be readily accessible by public transportation. They should be located for ready access to special medical and educational services and to various community resources, including consultants. The centers should be open institutions whenever possible; locked buildings, wards, or rooms should be required only rarely. In designing residential programs, the guiding principle should be that children should be removed from their normal life settings the least possible distance in space, in time, and in the psychologic texture of the experience.

Indications

Most children who are referred for residential treatment have had multiple evaluations by professionals, such as school psychologists, outpatient psychotherapists, juvenile court officials, or state welfare agency staff. Attempts at outpatient treatment and foster home placement usually precede residential treatment. Sometimes, the severity of a child's problems or the inability of a family to provide for the child's needs prohibits sending a child home. Many children sent to residential treatment centers have disruptive behavior problems in addition to other problems, including mood disorders and psychotic disorders. In some cases, serious psychosocial problems, such as physical or sexual abuse, neglect, indigence, or homelessness, necessitate out-of-home placement. The age range of the children varies among institutions, but most children are between 5 and 15 years of age. Boys are referred more frequently than girls.

An initial review of data enables the intake staff to determine whether a particular child is likely to benefit from the treatment program; often, for every child accepted for admission, three are rejected. The next step usually is interviews with the child and the parents by various staff members, such as a therapist, a group-living worker, and a teacher. Psychologic testing and neurologic examinations are given, when indicated, if they have not already been performed. The child and parents should be prepared for these interviews.

Group Living

Most of a child's time in a residential treatment setting is spent in group living. The group-living staff consists of child-care workers who offer a structured environment that forms a therapeutic milieu; the environment places boundaries and limitations on the children. Tasks are defined within the limits of children's abilities; incentives, such as additional privileges, encourage them to progress rather than regress. In milieu therapy, the environment is structured, limits are set, and a therapeutic atmosphere is maintained.

The children often select one or more staff members with whom to form a relationship; through this relationship, they express, consciously and unconsciously, many of their feelings about their parents. The child-care staff should be trained to recognize such transference reactions and to respond to them in a way that differs from the children's expectations, which are based on their previous or even current relationships with their parents.

To maintain consistency and balance, the group-living staff members must communicate freely and regularly with each other and with the other professional and administrative staff members of the residential setting, particularly the children's teachers and therapists. The child-care staff members must recognize any tendencies toward becoming the good (or bad) parent in response to a child's splitting behavior. This tendency may be manifest as a pattern of blaming other staff members for a child's disruptive behavior. Similarly, the child-care staff must recognize and avoid such individual and group countertransference reactions as sadomasochistic and punitive behavior toward a child.

The structured setting should offer a corrective emotional experience and opportunities for facilitating and improving children's adaptive behavior, particularly when such problems as speech and language deficits, intellectual retardation, inadequate peer relationships, bed wetting, poor feeding habits, and attention deficits are present. Some attention deficits are the basis of a child's poor academic performance and unsocialized behavior, including temper tantrums, fighting, and withdrawal.

Behavior modification principles also have been used, particularly in group work with children. Behavior therapy is part of a residential center's total therapeutic effort.

Education

Children in residential treatment frequently have severe learning disorders, disruptive behavior, and attention-deficit disorders such as attention-deficit/hyperactivity disorder (ADHD). Usually, the children cannot function in a regular community school and consequently need a special on-grounds school. A major goal of the on-grounds school is to motivate children to learn. The educational process in residential treatment is complex; Table 19.3–1 shows some of its components.

Therapy

Most residential facilities use a basic behavior modification program to set guidelines and to give the residents a concrete sense of how to earn privileges. These behavioral programs range in detail and intensity. Some programs operate with level systems that are associated with privileges and responsibilities. Some programs use a token economy system in which residents earn points for appropriate behavior and for meeting specific goals. Most programs include basic tasks of living as well as specific therapeutic goals for the residents.

Psychotherapy offered in these programs generally is supportive and oriented toward reunion with the family when possible. Insight-oriented psychotherapy is included when it can be used by a resident.

Table 19.3–1
Education Process in Residential Treatment

Preentry Assessment	Intervention Program Planning		Evaluation and Reevaluation	Educational Placement
Nature of emotional conflict	Educational skill development	Anxiety reduction program	Weekly staff meetings	Regular school
	Remedial reading	Supportive adult relationships	Interdisciplinary meetings and conferences	Special class
Nature of learning difficulties	Basic skill development	Stable, trusted models	Daily teacher reports	Private school
	Perceptual motor and impulse-control teaching	Life-space interviewing	Psychologic testing Continuous criterion testing	State institution
	Arts and crafts skills	Individual psychotherapy	Semiannual educational testing	
	Music skills	Removal from classroom area	Semiannual total staff evaluation	
	Total group project	Guidance room standardized		
	Academic skills built on six instructional cycles of 25 days in which assessment diagnosis, individual objectives and prescription, and new objectives or alternatives are planned	Quiet room safety in unit		

Courtesy of Melvin Lewis, M.B., B.S., F.R.C. Psych., D.C.H.

Parents

Concomitant work with parents is essential. Children usually have a strong tie to at least one parent, no matter how disturbed the parent may be. Sometimes, a child idealizes the parent, who repeatedly fails the child. At other times, the parent has an ambivalent or unrealistic expectation that the child will return home. In some instances, the parent must be helped to enable the child to live in another setting when it is in the child's best interest. Most residential treatment centers offer individual or group therapy for parents, couples or marital therapy, and, in some cases, conjoint family therapy.

DAY TREATMENT

The concept of daily comprehensive therapeutic experiences that do not require removing children from their homes or families derived partly from experiences with a therapeutic nursery school. Day hospital programs for children were then developed, and the number of programs continues to grow. The main advantages of day treatment are that children remain with their families and the families can be more involved in than they are in residential or hospital treatment. Day treatment also is much less expensive than residential treatment. At the same time, the risks of day treatment are a child's social isolation and confinement to a narrow band of social contacts in the program's disturbed peer population.

Indications

The primary indication for day treatment is the need for a more structured, intensive, and specialized treatment program than can be provided on an outpatient basis. At the same time, the home in which the child is living should be able to provide an environment that is at least not destructive to the child's development. Children who are likely to benefit from day treatment may have a wide range of diagnoses, including autistic disorder, conduct disorder, ADHD, and mental retardation. Exclusion symptoms include behavior that is likely to be destructive to the children themselves or to others under the treatment conditions. Therefore, some children who threaten to run away, set fires, attempt suicide, hurt others, or significantly disrupt the lives of their families while they are at home may not be suitable for day treatment.

Programs

The same ingredients that lead to a successful residential treatment program apply to day treatment. These ingredients include clear administrative leadership, team collaboration, open communication, and an understanding of children's behavior. Indeed, having a single agency offer both residential and day treatment has advantages.

A major function of child-care staff in day treatment for psychiatrically disturbed children is to provide positive experiences and a structure that enables the children and their families to internalize controls and function better than in the past regarding themselves and the outside world. Again, the methods used are essentially similar to those in full residential treatment programs.

Because the ages, needs, and range of diagnoses of children who may benefit from some form of day treatment vary, many day treatment programs have been developed. Some programs specialize in special educational and structured environmental needs of children with mental retardation. Others offer special therapeutic efforts required to treat children with autism and schizophrenia. Still other programs provide the total spectrum of treatment usually found in full residential treatment, of which they may be a part. Children may move from one part of the program to another and may be in residential treatment or day treatment according to their needs. The school program always is a major component of day treatment, and psychiatric treatment varies according to a child's needs and diagnosis.

Results

Recently, attempts have been made to analyze the treatment outcome of day treatment and partial hospitalization. Many different dimensions exist to analyzing overall benefits of such programs. Assessment of level of improvement in clinical status, academic progress, peer relationships, community interactions (legal difficulties), and family relationships are some pertinent areas to measure. In a recent follow-up 1 year after discharge from a partial hospital program, comparison of patients at admission and 1 year postdischarge showed statistically significant improvement in clinical symptoms on each subscale of the Child Behavior Checklist, except for sexual problems. These improvements were in mood symptoms, somatic complaints, attention problems, thought problems, delinquent behavior, and aggressive behavior. The assessment of long-term effectiveness of day treatment is fraught with difficulties, from the point of view of a child's maintenance of gains, a therapist's view of psychologic gains, or cost-to-benefit ratios.

At the same time, the advantage of day treatment has encouraged further development of programs. Moreover, the lessons learned from day treatment programs have moved mental health disciplines toward having services follow children rather than perpetuating discontinuities of care. The experiences of day treatment for psychiatric conditions of children and adolescents have also encouraged pediatric hospitals and departments to adopt a model that promotes continuity of care for the medical treatment of children with chronic physical illnesses.

▲ 19.4 Biological Therapies

PHARMACOTHERAPY

Over the last decade, there has been a fundamental shift in the research arena of pediatric psychopharmacology. Placebo-controlled trials have been undertaken to ascertain short-term efficacy for a great number of psychotropic drugs: fluoxetine (Prozac), sertraline (Zoloft), paroxetine (Paxil), escitalopram (Lexapro), nefazodone, quetiapine (Seroquel), olanzapine (Zyprexa), risperidone (Risperdal), mirtazapine (Remeron), and venlafaxine (Effexor). Published data support the efficacy and safety of fluoxetine, sertraline, and escitalopram for the treatment of depression in children and adolescents. Fluoxetine, however, is the only U.S. Food and Drug Administration (FDA)–approved selective serotonin reuptake inhibitor (SSRI) for treating major depressive disorder (MDD) in children younger then 7 years of age. Several SSRIs have been shown to be beneficial in the treatment of childhood obsessive-compulsive disorders (OCDs), including paroxetine, sertraline, fluoxetine, and fluvoxamine.

Long-acting stimulant medications, such as methylphenidate preparations (Concerta), methylphenidate transdermal patch (Daytrana), and amphetamine and amphetamine salt preparations (Adderall XR), permit a once-a-day treatment strategy that is accepted as a first-line treatment for attention-deficit/hyperactivity disorder (ADHD). Other novel nonstimulant agents include atomoxetine (Strattera), which is also approved to treat adult ADHD.

Perhaps the most significant contributions in the last decade have been the publicly funded research studies comparing combinations of pharmacologic interventions with psychosocial treatments alone and in combination for several childhood disorders, including OCD and MDDs. Both the Pediatric OCD Treatment Study (POTS) (2004) and the Treatment for Adolescents with Depression Study (TADS) (2004) found cognitive-behavioral psychotherapy in combination with SSRI medications to have advantages over either treatment alone for the treatment of childhood anxiety disorders.

Another area of progress is in testing medication efficacy and safety in younger age groups. For example, the Preschooler with ADHD Treatment Study (PATS) was the first multisite study of preschool children with ADHD treated with a parent training component combined with methylphenidate. Another large study is the Treatment of Early Onset Schizophrenia Spectrum Disorders (TEOSS) trial in children and adolescents (8 to 19 years of age). This is a multisite trial comparing the effects of atypical antipsychotics (risperidone and olanzapine) to the conventional antipsychotic molindone (Moban).

The use of serotonin-dopamine antagonists (SDAs) has become the norm and has largely replaced the conventional antipsychotics. This is due to its improved side-effect profile with regard to neuromotor side effects and its broader efficacy. At the same time the use of SDAs has been associated with greater weight gain and hence higher risk of obesity, diabetes, and dyslipidemia, which can increase the risk of cardiovascular morbidity and mortality. Children and adolescents exposed to these medications require close monitoring and assessment.

In 2004, the FDA released a statement on the recommendation of the Psychopharmacologic Drugs and Pediatric Advisory Committees of a black box warning relating to an increased risk for suicidality in pediatric patients for all antidepressant medications—including SSRIs—but not contraindicating their use. Several reviews since then, however, have concluded that the data do not indicate a significant increase in the risk of suicide or serious suicide attempt after starting treatment with antidepressant drugs. Rather than a worsening effect, antidepressant use was associated with the protective effect against new-onset and ongoing suicidal ideation. One study showed that the rates of suicide attempts in patients treated with an antidepressant were one third of those observed for patients not treated with an antidepressant. A strongly worded editorial in the *Journal of the American Psychiatric Association* (July 2007) was concluded, "It is much more likely that suicidal behavior leads to treatment than that treatment leads to suicidal behavior." There is pressure on the FDA to remove the black box warning, and if the evidence continues to mount, it is likely that this will happen. In the meantime, psychiatrists should not withhold antidepressant medication in suicidal children or adolescents. At the same time, they must remain vigilant and monitor their suicidal patients closely, regardless of the medication prescribed.

Therapeutic Considerations

An evaluation for psychopharmacotherapy must first include an assessment of a child's psychopathology and physical condition to rule out any predisposition for side effects (Table 19.4–1). An assessment of the child's caregivers focuses on their ability to provide a safe, consistent environment in which a clinician can conduct a drug trial. The physician must consider the risk-to-benefit ratio and must explain it to the patient, if he or she is old enough, and to the child's caregivers and others (e.g., child welfare workers) who may be involved in the decision to medicate.

The clinician must obtain baseline ratings before medicating. Behavioral rating scales help to objectify the child's response to medication. The physician generally starts at a low dose and titrates upward on the basis of the child's response and the appearance of adverse effects. Optimal drug trials cannot be rushed (e.g., by insurance-imposed, inadequately short hospital stays or by infrequent outpatient visits), nor can drug trials be prolonged by the physician's insufficient contact with the patient and the caregivers. The success of drug trials often hinges on the physician's daily accessibility.

Childhood Pharmacokinetics

Compared with adults, children have greater hepatic capacity, more glomerular filtration, and less fatty tissue. Thus, stimulants,

Table 19.4–1
Diagnostic Processes of Biological Therapy

1. Diagnostic evaluation
2. Symptom measurement
3. Risk–benefit ratio analysis
4. Periodic reevaluation
5. Termination and tapered drug withdrawal

antipsychotics, and tricyclic drugs are eliminated more rapidly by children than by adults; lithium (Eskalith) may also be eliminated more rapidly, and children may be less able to store drugs in their fat. Because of children's quick elimination, the half-lives of many medications may be shorter in children than in adults.

Little evidence indicates that clinicians can predict a child's blood level from the dose or a treatment response from the plasma level. Relatively low serum levels of haloperidol (Haldol) seem to be adequate to treat Tourette's disorder in children. No correlation is seen between the methylphenidate (Ritalin) serum level and a child's response. The data are incomplete and conflicting about major depressive disorder and serum levels of tricyclic drugs. Serum level is related to response for tricyclic drugs in the treatment of enuresis.

With lithium therapy, a ratio of lithium concentration in saliva to that in serum can be established for a child by averaging three to four individual ratios. The average ratio can then be used to convert subsequent saliva levels to serum levels and thus avoid some venipuncture in children who are stressed by blood tests. As with serum levels, regular clinical monitoring for adverse effects is necessary. Table 19.4–2 lists representative drugs and their indications, doses, adverse reactions, and monitoring requirements.

Indications

Attention-Deficit/Hyperactivity Disorder. Pharmacotherapy remains the primary treatment for ADHD in children, adolescents, and adults. Multiple studies support the efficacy of stimulant medications for ADHD. Practice is leaning toward more use of once-a-day, long-acting preparations of stimulants such as methylphenidate, amphetamine and amphetamine salts, and dexmethylphenidate (Focalin LA). The most frequently researched and used stimulant is methylphenidate. Dextroamphetamine (Dexedrine) has comparable efficacy and, unlike methylphenidate, is approved by the FDA for children 3 years of age and older; the starting age for methylphenidate is 6 years. Adderall combines dextroamphetamine and amphetamine salts. The extended-release preparations, such as Concerta and Adderall XR, have the advantage of covering symptoms throughout the school day without the necessity of taking another dose, as well as a more continuous delivery of medication. A prodrug of amphetamine, lisdexamfetamine (Vynase), was recently approved for once-daily dosing. Stimulants reduce hyperactivity, inattentiveness, aggressiveness, and impulsivity in about 75 percent of children with ADHD. The dose-related adverse effects of stimulants are listed in Table 19.4–3.

The Daytrana patch has been approved by the FDA in the treatment of ADHD in children of age 6 to 12 years. Daytrana comes in patches that can deliver 15, 20, and 30 mg when worn for 9 hours per day. The medication begins to have its effects on the target symptoms of ADHD approximately 2 hours after the patch is placed and continues to deliver medication throughout the wear time. Given that its active ingredient is methylphenidate, the side effects are generally the same as those for methylphenidate, except for the potential skin irritation that may emerge from wearing the patch. The patch should not be worn in the presence of a heating pad or electric blanket because heat increases the rate of methylphenidate delivery into the skin. Patients with glaucoma or known hypersensitivity to methylphenidate products should not begin treatment with Daytrana. Daytrana has the advantages of being able to deliver medication until the patch is removed and, for children who are unable to swallow pills, a unique administration option.

Atomoxetine is a new nonstimulant medication and is a selective serotonin-norepinephrine reuptake inhibitor (SNRI). It is the first nonstimulant approved by the FDA for the treatment of ADHD in children, adolescents, and adults. Atomoxetine is well absorbed after ingestion and reaches its maximal plasma concentration after about 1 to 2 hours. Common side effects of atomoxetine include abdominal discomfort, decreased appetite, weight loss, dizziness, sedation, and irritability. Rarely, minor increases in blood pressure and heart rate have been noted. Atomoxetine is metabolized by the cytochrome P450 (CYP) 2D6 hepatic enzyme system, and a fraction of the population (about 7 percent of whites and 2 percent of African-Americans) are poor metabolizers, which may increase the plasma half-life by about fivefold. When combined with other medications that inhibit CYP 2D6, such as fluoxetine and paroxetine, diminished metabolism of atomoxetine can occur, and the dose may need to be decreased. Atomoxetine is generally initiated at 0.5 mg per kg given once per day and increased to a therapeutic dose ranging between 1.4 and 1.8 mg per kg either in one dose or in two divided doses. Some studies suggest that it may be effective in treating comorbid anxiety, chronic tic disorders, and tic symptoms in the subset with Tourette's syndrome. It has less abuse potential, does not produce euphoria, and may be particularly useful in ADHD with substance abuse disorder.

Other non–FDA-approved treatments for ADHD are antidepressants, including tricyclics (imipramine [Tofranil] and desipramine [Norpramin, Pertofane]). Bupropion (Wellbutrin) and venlafaxine have also been reported to be useful in patients with ADHD. There is limited data regarding the efficacy of modafinil (Provigil) and clonidine (Catapres).

The dietary management of hyperactivity has historically received public attention, but controlled studies have not substantiated its benefit.

Antipsychotics are not indicated in the treatment of ADHD, unless accompanied by psychosis, given the risks of sedation and tardive dyskinesia. ADHD often precedes and coexists with tic disorders.

Autistic Disorder. Until recently no specific pharmacotherapy was approved for the core symptoms of autistic disorder; these include impulsivity and inattention, compulsive and ritualistic behaviors, irritability, temper outbursts with or without

Table 19.4–2
Common Psychoactive Drugs in Childhood and Adolescence

Drug	Indications	Dosing Regimen	Adverse Reactions and Monitoring
Antipsychotics (also known as *major tranquilizers* or *neuroleptics*) Divided into (1) high potency, low dose (e.g., haloperidol [Haldol], pimozide [Orap], trifluoperazine [Stelazine], thiothixene [Navane]), (2) low potency, high dose (more sedating; e.g., chlorpromazine [Thorazine]), and (3) atypicals (e.g., risperidone [Risperdal], olanzapine [Zyprexa], quetiapine [Seroquel], and clozapine [Clozaril])	Psychoses; agitated self-injurious behaviors in MR, PDDs, CD, and Tourette's disorder: haloperidol and pimozide Clozapine: refractory schizophrenia in adolescence	All can be given in two to four divided doses or combined into one dose after gradual build-up Haloperidol: child, 0.5–6 mg/day; adolescent, 0.5–16 mg/day Clozapine: dose not determined in children; <600 mg/day in adolescents Risperidone: 1–3 mg/day Olanzapine: 2.5–10 mg/day Quetiapine: 25–500 mg/day	Sedation, weight gain, hypotension, lowered seizure threshold, constipation, extrapyramidal symptoms, jaundice, agranulocytosis, dystonic reaction, tardive dyskinesia Hyperprolactinemia with atypicals except quetiapine Monitor blood pressure, CBC count, LFTs, and prolactin if indicated; with thioridazine, pigmentary retinopathy is rare but dictates ceiling of 800 mg in adults and proportionally lower in children; with clozapine, weekly WBC counts for development of agranulocytosis and EEG monitoring because of lowering of seizure threshold
Stimulants			
Dextroamphetamine (Dexedrine) and amphetamine-dextroamphetamine (Adderall): FDA approved for children 3 years and older Methylphenidate (Ritalin, Concerta) and pemoline (Cylert): FDA approved for children 6 years and older	In ADHD for hyperactivity, impulsivity, and inattentiveness Narcolepsy	Dextroamphetamine and methylphenidate are generally given at 8 AM and noon Dextroamphetamine: about half the dose of methylphenidate Methylphenidate: 10–60 mg/day or up to about 0.5 mg/kg per dose Adderall: about half the dose of methylphenidate	Insomnia, anorexia, weight loss (possibly growth delay), rebound hyperactivity, headache, tachycardia, precipitation or exacerbation of tic disorders With pemoline, monitor LFTs because hepatotoxicity and liver failure are possible
Daytrana patch	ADHD	15, 20, 30 mg Wear for 9 hrs/day	Skin irritation
Nonstimulants			
Atomoxetine (Straterra)	ADHD	Begin with 0.5 mg/kg, up to 1.8 mg/kg	Abdominal pain, loss of appetite
Mood stabilizers			
Lithium: considered an antimanic drug; also has antiaggression properties	Studies support use in MR and CD for aggressive and self-injurious behaviors; can be used for same in PDD; also indicated for early-onset bipolar disorder	600–2,100 mg in two or three divided doses; keep blood levels to 0.4–1.2 mEq/L	Nausea, vomiting, polyuria, headache, tremor, weight gain, hypothyroidism Experience with adults suggests renal function monitoring
Divalproex (Depakote)	Bipolar disorder, aggression	Up to about 20 mg/kg per day; therapeutic blood level range appears to be 50–100 μg/mL	Monitor CBC count and LFTs for possible blood dyscrasias and hepatotoxicity Nausea, vomiting, sedation, hair loss, weight gain, possibly polycystic ovaries
Carbamazepine (Tegretol): an anticonvulsant	Aggression or dyscontrol in MR or CD Bipolar disorder	Start with 10 mg/kg per day, can build to 20–30 mg/kg per day; therapeutic blood-level range appears to be 4–12 mg/day	Drowsiness, nausea, rash, vertigo, irritability; monitor CBC count and LFTs for possible blood dyscrasias and hepatotoxicity; must obtain blood concentrations

(continued)

Table 19.4–2 (Continued)

Drug	Indications	Dosing Regimen	Adverse Reactions and Monitoring
Antidepressants			
Tricyclic antidepressants: imipramine (Tofranil), nortriptyline (Pamelor), clomipramine (Anafranil)	Major depressive disorder, separation anxiety disorder, bulimia nervosa, enuresis; sometimes used in ADHD, sleepwalking disorder, and sleep terror disorder Clomipramine is effective in childhood OCD and sometimes in PDD	Imipramine: start with divided doses totaling about 1.5 mg/kg per day; can build up to not more than 5 mg/kg per day; eventually combine in one dose, usually 50–100 mg before sleep Clomipramine: start at 50 mg/day; can raise to not more than 3 mg/kg per day or 200 mg/day	Dry mouth, constipation, tachycardia, arrhythmia
Selective serotonin reuptake inhibitors: fluoxetine (Prozac), sertraline (Zoloft), fluvoxamine (Luvox), paroxetine (Paxil), citalopram (Celexa)	OCD; may be useful in major depressive disorder, anorexia nervosa, bulimia nervosa, repetitive behaviors in MR or PDD	Less than adult doses	Nausea, headache, nervousness, insomnia, dry mouth, diarrhea, drowsiness, disinhibition
Bupropion (Wellbutrin)	ADHD	Start low and titrate up to between 100 and 250 mg/day	Disinhibition, insomnia, dry mouth, gastrointestinal problems, tremor, seizures
Anxiolytics			
Benzodiazepines			
Clonazepam (Klonopin)	Panic disorder, generalized anxiety disorder	0.5–2.0 mg/day	Drowsiness, disinhibition
Alprazolam (Xanax)	Separation anxiety disorder	Up to 1.5 mg/day	Drowsiness, disinhibition
Buspirone (BuSpar)	Various anxiety disorders	15–90 mg/day	Dizziness, upset stomach
α_2-Adrenergic receptor agonists			
Clonidine (Catapres)	ADHD, Tourette's disorder, aggression	Up to 0.4 mg/day	Bradycardia, arrhythmia, hypertension, withdrawal hypotension
Guanfacine (Tenex)	ADHD	0.5–3.0 mg/day	Same as with clonidine plus headache, stomachache
β-Adrenergic receptor antagonist (beta blocker)			
Propranolol (Inderal)	Explosive aggression	Start at 20–30 mg/day and titrate	Monitor for bradycardia, hypotension, bronchoconstriction Contraindicated in asthma and diabetes
Other agents			
Naltrexone (ReVia)	Hyperactivity or self-injurious behavior in autism or MR	0.5–1.0 mg/kg per day	Drowsiness, vomiting, anorexia, headache, nasal congestion, hyponatremic seizures
Desmopressin (DDAVP)	Nocturnal enuresis	20–40 μg intranasally	Headache, nasal congestion, hyponatremic seizures (rare)

ADHD, attention-deficit/hyperactivity disorder; CBC, complete blood count; CD, conduct disorder; EEG, electroencephalogram; FDA, U.S. Food and Drug Administration; LFT, liver function test; MR, mental retardation; OCD, obsessive-compulsive disorder; PDD, pervasive development disorder; WBC, white blood cell.

Table 19.4–3 Common Dose-Related Side Effects of Stimulants

Insomnia
Decreased appetite
Irritability or nervousness
Weight loss

self-injurious behaviors, and anxiety symptoms. In October 2006, the FDA approved the use of risperidone for treating irritability in children and adolescents (5 to 16 years of age) with autism. Other pharmacologic agents used in the treatment of autistic disorder are atypical antipsychotics, such as olanzapine and aripiprazole. Both risperidone and olanzapine are associated with weight increase and hence require lifestyle management. Some studies have suggested the use of metformin (Fortamet,

Glucophage, Riomet) in children and adolescents for weight stabilization. Clinicians should be aware of the rare adverse effect of lactic acidosis associated with metformin and need to inform the patient and the caregivers. Other medications used in managing behavioral control of autistic disorder include the α_2-adrenergic agonists clonidine and guanfacine (Tenex). Both have been shown to reduce irritability, hyperactivity, and oppositional behavior.

In the past, haloperidol was used with varying degrees of success in reducing temper tantrums, aggression, stereotypies, self-injurious behavior, and hyperactivity. Haloperidol is now chosen much less frequently compared with the atypical antipsychotic agents because of its increased risks of extrapyramidal symptoms and withdrawal dyskinesia. SSRIs, including fluoxetine and citalopram, have been studied in autistic disorder because of the association between the compulsive behaviors in OCD and stereotypic behaviors common in children with autism. Clomipramine (Anafranil) and fluoxetine have shown promise in ending stereotypies and other behaviors in autistic children and adults. The opioid antagonists naloxone (Narcan) and naltrexone have not proved effective in diminishing self-injurious behavior in children with autistic disorder. A variety of agents, including β-adrenergic receptor antagonists (beta blockers), lithium, and anticonvulsants are used in clinical practice to ameliorate the multiple symptoms seen in children with pervasive developmental disorder (PDD). Stimulants are often tried to reduce hyperactivity and inattentiveness in children with autism.

Atomoxetine has shown improvement in children with PDD. Atypical and to a limited extent typical antipsychotics are effective in treating the aggression, irritability, and self-injurious behavior associated with PDD.

Conduct Disorder. The explosive and assaultive behaviors associated with some forms of conduct disorder continue to be treated with pharmacotherapy. Atypical antipsychotics, such as risperidone, olanzapine, quetiapine, and aripiprazole (Abilify), cause behavioral improvement with fewer long-term adverse effects. Lithium has been shown in multiple investigations to reduce aggression in conduct disorder, and propranolol (Inderal) has been chosen in open trials as an agent to control aggression, although no evidence supports its use in children and adolescents. Carbamazepine (Tegretol) has not been shown to be effective in controlling aggression in child and adolescent conduct disorders.

When conduct disorder is associated with ADHD, a trial of a stimulant is indicated; stimulants are faster acting than atypical antipsychotics or mood-stabilizing agents used in clinical practice to control dangerously aggressive behaviors.

The management of severe aggression, disruptive behavior, and ADHD remains a challenge. Combinations of antipsychotics with mood-stabilizing agents or stimulants are sometimes used in treatment-resistant cases, although few studies attest to the efficacy or safety of drug combinations. Atypical antipsychotic medications—SDAs—such as risperidone, olanzapine, clozapine (Clozaril), ziprasidone (Geodon), and aripiprazole, have enabled a wider range of treatment-resistant patients to benefit from neuroleptic treatment. SDAs produce less risk of extrapyramidal adverse effects and less potential for the development of tardive dyskinesia. Nevertheless, all antipsychotics pose some risk of extrapyramidal adverse effects and tardive dyskinesia. One challenge in obtaining optimal pharmacologic treatment for children is to decrease maladaptive behaviors and promote productive academic functioning. To this end, clinicians must consider adverse medication effects that result in cognitive "dulling." Certain pharmacologic agents used in pediatric populations are associated with a specific disorder or with target symptoms that appear in several disorders. For example, haloperidol was shown in studies to be effective in the treatment of Tourette's disorder, but it has also been used to control severe aggression.

Tourette's Disorder. The high-potency antipsychotics haloperidol and pimozide (Orap) still have the greatest body of evidence as effective medications for Tourette's disorder, although they also have considerable drawbacks. Pimozide prolongs the QT interval and thus requires electrocardiographic (ECG) monitoring. Clonidine, a presynaptic α-adrenergic blocking agent, is less effective than either of the aforementioned antipsychotics but has the advantage of avoiding the risk for tardive dyskinesia; sedation is a frequent side effect of clonidine.

Tic disorders often coexist with ADHD in children and adolescents. Stimulant use is controversial; it can precipitate tics and should be avoided in these patients, although recent studies indicate that the prohibition may not be totally warranted. Clonidine reduces tics in both ADHD and comorbid cases. A small study supports the use of nortriptyline (Pamelor).

Enuresis. Before initiating psychopharmacotherapy for treating enuresis, clinicians must consider the merits of waiting for a possible spontaneous remission and of using behavioral techniques; bell-and-pad conditioning (a bell awakens the child when the mattress becomes wet), perhaps the most elaborate behavioral treatment, seems to be more successful than medication.

Desmopressin (DDAVP) is effective in about 50 percent of patients and has largely replaced the use of imipramine, a tricyclic antidepressant, because of its increased safety profile. Improvement ranges from complete cessation of wetting to continued wetting but with less urine volume. Desmopressin has been used intranasally in doses of 10 to 40 mg per day. When it is used over months, nasal discomfort can occur, and water retention is potentially a problem. Patients who respond with full dryness should continue to take the medication for several months to prevent relapses. Desmopressin is available in oral tablets, and a controlled multicenter study found equal efficacy between intranasal and oral administration of desmopressin in the treatment of enuresis. A dose of 400 mg of oral desmopressin was associated with greater effectiveness than 200 mg.

Separation Anxiety Disorder, Generalized Anxiety Disorder, and Social Phobia. A substantial evidence base exists for the efficacy of SSRI medications in the treatment of separation anxiety, generalized anxiety disorder, and social phobia in children and adolescents. Randomized clinical trials have confirmed efficacy of fluoxetine, fluvoxamine, sertraline, and paroxetine in the treatment of these anxiety disorders. Thus, SSRIs are recommended as first-line medications in the treatment of childhood anxiety. Separation anxiety disorder, generalized anxiety disorder, and social phobia are often studied together because they so commonly coexist. A given child with one of these anxiety disorders has a 60 percent chance of having a second one and a 30 percent chance of having all three. Several randomized clinical trials have provided data to support the use of sertraline, fluoxetine, and fluvoxamine. Alprazolam (Xanax) and clonazepam (Klonopin) have not been shown to be helpful in anxiety disorders. Cognitive-behavioral therapy (CBT) has been shown to be an effective intervention in childhood anxiety disorders.

Schizophrenia. The atypical antipsychotic agents represent a major advance in the pharmacologic treatment for schizophrenia in children and adolescents, as well as in adults. An Australian and U.S. study showed that atypical antipsychotics may be effective in treating the prodromal symptoms of schizophrenia and reducing the conversion rate to psychosis. Based on small sample size and attrition time, however, no conclusions can be drawn, and further studies are warranted. The atypical antipsychotic agents have largely replaced traditional antipsychotics because of their more favorable side-effect profiles, greater effectiveness for negative symptomatology, and mood-stabilizing effects. Although the atypical agents are generally recommended as first-line agents in the treatment of psychotic disorders in children and adolescents, only one published controlled National Institute of Mental Health (NIMH) trial has been conducted using an atypical agent in the treatment of schizophrenia for youth. The NIMH study for clozapine provided evidence of its superiority to haloperidol (clozapine mean dose of 176 mg per day) for treating positive and negative symptoms of schizophrenia in 21 youth. The serious drawbacks of clozapine, however, limit its use as a first-line agent for this disorder. In the NIMH trial, 5 patients developed significant neutropenia and 2 of them experienced seizures. Clozapine is chosen for treatment-resistant schizophrenia.

Open-label trials in schizophrenic youth have suggested the efficacy of other atypical antipsychotic agents such as olanzapine, risperidone, and quetiapine. Case reports have suggested that ziprasidone is effective. One of the main side effects of the atypical antipsychotic agents is significant weight gain. A newer atypical agent, aripiprazole, awaits clinical trials to confirm its potential as an efficacious and more weight-neutral agent for the treatment of childhood psychoses. Although conventional antipsychotics such as haloperidol, loxapine (Loxitane), and thioridazine (Mellaril) have been shown to be significantly superior to placebo in the treatment of psychosis in youths, given their side-effect profiles they are typically not chosen as first-line treatments. Schizophrenia with onset in late adolescence is treated as is adult-onset schizophrenia. As noted, atypical antipsychotics have been linked to obesity, particularly in children and adolescents. It is imperative to screen and educate patients, discuss the adverse reactions, and monitor for any metabolic abnormalities, including hyperglycemia and dyslipidemia. Other risk factors for diabetes include increasing age, race, genetic factors, lack of physical activity, and dietary factors.

As in adults, 50 percent of adolescents with schizophrenia have partial or poor response to treatment. Possible augmentation strategies include lithium, anticonvulsants, and, more recently, lamotrigine.

Mood Disorders. Randomized clinical trials have provided evidence for the efficacy and safety of fluoxetine, sertraline, and citalopram (Celexa) in the treatment of major depression in children and adolescents. The SSRIs are the drugs of choice in the pharmacologic treatment of depressive disorders in children and adolescents. Given the FDA placement of the black box warning in 2004 on all antidepressants used in children and adolescents because of the slightly increased risk of suicidal behaviors, it is imperative that close monitoring of suicidal ideation and behavior be followed by all clinicians who prescribe these medications. Tricyclic drugs have not been shown to be superior to placebo in double-blind, placebo-controlled studies of children and adolescents with major depressive disorder and have been largely replaced by the SSRIs in the treatment of childhood mood disorders. The SSRIs are favored because of their apparent efficacy, mild adverse-effect profile, and lower risk in overdose. Although most side effects of SSRIs are tolerable, recent anecdotal reports indicate occasional SSRI-induced apathy in children and adolescents treated with them.

Manic episodes in childhood and adolescence are treated as they are in adulthood. Use of lithium in treating adolescent mania has been supported in many open trials, and it is the only medication approved by the FDA for mania in adolescents (12 years and older). Divalproex is used frequently to treat bipolar disorder in children and adolescents. Few case reports and open-label studies of atypical antipsychotics support the effectiveness of these medications in pediatric bipolar disorder. Many double-blind and open-label studies of olanzapine, risperidone and quetiapine have demonstrated efficacy of these medications. Co-occurring conditions like ADHD, oppositional defiant disorder, conduct disorder, anxiety disorder, and substance abuse require combination of medications. It is not unusual to combine atypicals with valproic acid and lithium or SSRIs when significant anxiety is present. These situations require close monitoring for destabilization of mood symptoms and switch into mania.

Obsessive-Compulsive Disorder. The current literature provides evidence from randomized clinical trials of the efficacy and safety of fluoxetine, fluvoxamine, and sertraline as first-line agents for children and adolescents with OCD. CBT when

Table 19.4–4
Effects of Psychotropic Drugs on Cognitive Tests of Learning Functions[a]

			Test Function			
Drug Class	Continuous Performance Test (Attention)	Matching Familiar Figures (Impulsivity)	Paired Associates (Verbal Learning)	Porteus Maze (Planning Capacity)	Short-Term Memory[a]	WISC (Intelligence)
Stimulant	↑	↑	↑	↑	↑	↑
Antidepressant	↑	0	0	0	0	0
Antipsychotic	↑↓	0	↓	↓	↓	0

↑, improved; ↑↓, inconsistent; ↓, worse; 0, no effect. WISC, Wechsler Intelligence Scale for Children.
[a]Various tests, digit span, word recall, etc.
Adapted from Amar MG. Drugs, learning and the psychotherapies. In: Werry JS, ed. *Pediatric Psychopharmacology: The Use of Behavior Modifying Drugs in Children.* New York: Brunner/Mazel; 1978:356, with permission.

combined with sertraline results in the best outcome for children and adolescents with OCD compared with medication or therapy alone. Previously, clomipramine was proved to be effective in diminishing obsessions and compulsions in children and adolescents, but although clomipramine is often well tolerated, the SSRIs have a more favorable adverse-effect profile and appear to be as effective as clomipramine.

Eating Disorders. The treatment of anorexia nervosa does not focus primarily on pharmacologic interventions, but drugs can be important adjuncts in many cases. The SSRIs are not used uncommonly in this population; the target symptoms are obsessions and compulsions and high levels of anxiety and depressive symptoms. Cyproheptadine (Periactin) was used historically and reported to benefit some patients with anorexia, and antidepressants may benefit those with comorbid depressive disorders. The compromised metabolism of many patients with anorexia can put them at high risk for cardiac arrhythmias, however, if tricyclic drugs are administered.

Evidence from controlled studies indicates that high-dose SSRI treatment (fluoxetine at doses of approximately 60 mg per day) can reduce binge eating and purging in bulimia nervosa. Bupropion must be used with care in patients with bulimia nervosa because of the risk of seizures.

Mental Retardation. No pharmacotherapy exists that is specifically designed for mental retardation; however, children and adolescents with mental retardation are at higher risk for comorbid psychiatric disorders. The psychopharmacotherapy for youth with mental retardation most often addresses behavioral problems, especially aggression, and the coexistence of other mental disorders. For severe aggression, antipsychotics are most commonly used, and cognitive dulling can best be avoided with high-potency drugs or atypical antipsychotics. β-Adrenergic receptor antagonists have reduced aggression in uncontrolled studies of adults and children with mental retardation. Lithium and anticonvulsants such as carbamazepine may also be tried. Antipsychotics have the advantage of a fast onset of action and little need for laboratory monitoring of their adverse effects, but the use of other drugs eliminates the risk for tardive dyskinesia.

The endogenous opioid antagonists, such as naltrexone (ReVia), and the SSRIs, such as fluoxetine, have been prescribed in an attempt to diminish self-injurious behavior in patients with mental retardation. When ADHD coexists with mental retardation, methylphenidate often is effective.

Recently, attempts have been made to treat the behavioral problems associated with fragile X syndrome with folic acid supplements. Some prepubescent children experienced less active or less aggressive behavior and concentrated better when they took folic acid than they did before treatment.

Learning Disorders. No pharmacologic agent significantly improves any learning disorder, but many children with other mental disorders also have learning disorders, and many who have learning disorders also have behavioral problems. These associations and the importance of school and learning in children's lives raise questions about the cognitive effects of psychotropics. Table 19.4–4 summarizes the effects of drugs on cognitive tests of learning functions. In children with learning disorders who have attention problems, even in the absence of meeting the full criteria for ADHD, methylphenidate facilitates performance on several standard cognitive, psycholinguistic, memory, and vigilance tests but does not improve children's academic achievement ratings or teacher ratings. Cognitive impairment from psychotropic drugs, especially antipsychotics, may be an even greater problem for persons with mental retardation than for those with learning disorders.

Sleep Terror Disorder and Sleepwalking Disorder. Sleep terror disorder and sleepwalking disorder occur in the transition from deep delta-wave sleep (stages 3 and 4) to light sleep. Benzodiazepines and tricyclics are effective in these disorders. They work by reducing both delta-wave sleep and arousals between sleep stages. The medications should be used temporarily and only in severe cases because tolerance to the medications develops. Cessation of these medications can lead to severe rebound worsening of the disorders, and reducing delta sleep in children may have deleterious effects; thus, behavioral approaches are preferred for these disorders.

Patients with early-onset panic disorder and panic attacks have benefited from clonazepam in several open trials.

Adverse Effects and Complications

Antidepressants. Adverse effects related to antidepressants have diminished significantly since SSRI antidepressants were widely accepted as first-line treatments for depressive disorders in children and adolescents. Tricyclics are rarely recommended because of the significant risks of dangerous adverse effects. The adverse effects of tricyclics for children usually are similar to those for adults and result from the drugs' anticholinergic properties. The adverse effects include dry mouth, constipation, palpitations, tachycardia, loss of accommodation, and sweating. The most serious adverse effects are cardiovascular; in children, diastolic hypertension is more common, and postural hypotension occurs more rarely than in adults. ECG changes are most likely seen in children receiving high doses. Slowed cardiac conduction (PR interval greater than 0.20 second or QRS interval greater than 0.12 second) may necessitate lowering the dose. FDA guidelines limit doses to a maximum of 5 mg/kg a day. The drugs can be toxic in an overdose, and, in small children, ingestion of 200 to 400 mg can be fatal. When the dose is lowered too rapidly, withdrawal effects occur, mainly gastrointestinal symptoms—cramping, nausea, and vomiting—and sometimes apathy and weakness. Appropriate treatment is to taper the dose more slowly.

Antipsychotics. Historically, the best-studied antipsychotics given to pediatric age groups are chlorpromazine (Thorazine) and haloperidol. High-potency and low-potency antipsychotics are believed to differ in their adverse-effect profiles. The phenothiazine derivatives (chlorpromazine and thioridazine) have the most pronounced sedative and atropinic actions, whereas the high-potency antipsychotics are commonly believed to be associated with extrapyramidal reactions, such as Parkinsonian symptoms, akathisia, and acute dystonias. The risk of tardive dyskinesia in relation to antipsychotics leads to caution in the use of these drugs. Tardive dyskinesia, which is characterized by persistent abnormal involuntary movements of the tongue, face, mouth, or jaw and sometimes the extremities, is a known hazard when giving antipsychotics to patients of all age groups. No known treatment is effective. Tardive dyskinesia has not been reported in patients taking less than 375 to 400 g of chlorpromazine equivalents. Because nonpersistent choreiform movements of the extremities and trunk are common after abrupt discontinuation of antipsychotics, clinicians must distinguish these symptoms from persistent dyskinesia.

SDAs have generally replaced the conventional antipsychotics as first-line agents in the treatment of all psychotic disorders in children and adolescents. Some of the common adverse effects of atypical antipsychotics, including clozapine, olanzapine, and quetiapine, include sedation, dry mouth, increased appetite, and dizziness. Ziprasidone has been associated with prolonged QT interval, whereas aripiprazole can induce akathisia.

OTHER BIOLOGICAL THERAPIES

Electroconvulsive therapy (ECT) is rarely initiated in childhood and adolescence. In cases of catatonia, treatment-resistant mania, and severe depression, however, the suggestion is that it is efficacious.

Psychosurgery for severe and intransigent OCD is virtually absent from the literature in children and adolescents.

No controlled studies provide evidence that food allergies or sensitivities play a role in childhood mental disorders. Diets that eliminate food additives, colorings, and sugar are difficult to maintain and usually have no effect. Megavitamin therapy has not been shown to influence behavioral disorders (unless the child has a frank vitamin deficiency) and can cause serious adverse effects.

Significant advances have been made in scientific studies assessing the efficacy and safety of pharmacologic agents in the treatment of childhood psychiatric disorders, and, given the trend of increased use of psychotropic medications in the treatment of childhood disorders, future large multisite studies are needed to confirm optimal pharmacologic treatments and combinations of psychosocial and pharmacologic treatments.

▲ 19.5 Psychiatric Treatment of Adolescents

Psychiatric treatment is indicated for an adolescent in whom is found a disturbance of thought, affect, or behavior to the point that it disrupts normal functioning. For adolescents, this includes influences on eating, sleeping, and school function, as well as relationships with family and peers. A variety of serious psychiatric disorders, including schizophrenia, bipolar disorder, eating disorders, and substance abuse, typically have their onset during adolescence. In addition, the risk for completed suicide drastically increases in adolescence. Although some stress is virtually universal in adolescence, most teenagers without mental disorders can cope well with the environmental demands. Teenagers with preexisting mental disorders may experience exacerbations during adolescence and may become frustrated, alienated, and demoralized.

Clinicians and parents must be sensitive to adolescents' perceptions of themselves. A range of emotional maturity exists in a group of teenagers of the same age. Issues that are specific to adolescents are related to their new, evolving identities, the development of sexual activity, and their plans to meet future life goals.

DIAGNOSIS

Adolescents can be assessed in both their specific stage-appropriate functions and their general progress in accomplishing the tasks of adolescence. For almost all adolescents in today's culture, at least until their late teens, school performance and peer relationships are the primary barometers of healthy functioning. Intellectually normal adolescents who are not functioning satisfactorily academically or teens who are isolated from peers have significant psychologic problems whose nature and causes should be identified.

Questions to be asked regarding adolescents' stage-specific tasks are the following: What degree of separation from their parents have they achieved? What sort of identities are evolving? How do they perceive their past? Do they perceive themselves as responsible for their own development or only the passive recipients of their parents' influences? How do they perceive themselves with regard to the future, and how do they anticipate their future responsibilities for themselves and others? Can they think about the varying consequences of different ways of living? How do they express their sexual and affectionate interests? These tasks occupy all adolescents and normally are performed at varying times.

Adolescents' family and peer relationships must be evaluated. Do they perceive and accept both good and bad qualities in their parents? Do they see their peers and boyfriends or girlfriends as separate persons with needs and identities of their own, or do others exist only for the adolescents' own needs?

A respect for, and, if possible, some actual understanding of, an adolescent's subcultural and ethnic background are essential. For example, in some groups, depression is acceptable; in other groups, overt depression is a sign of weakness and is masked by antisocial acts, substance misuse, and self-destructive risks. A psychiatrist need not be of the same race or group identity as a given adolescent to treat him or her effectively. Respect and knowledgeable concern are human qualities and are not group restricted.

INTERVIEWS

Whenever circumstances permit, both an adolescent patient and his or her parents should be interviewed. Other family members also may be included, depending on their involvement in the teenager's life and difficulties. Clinicians should see the adolescent first, however; preferential treatment helps to avoid the appearance of being the parents' agent. In psychotherapy with an older adolescent, the therapist and the parents usually have little contact after the initial part of the therapy because ongoing contact inhibits the adolescent's willingness to open up.

Interview Techniques

All patients test and mistrust therapists, but adolescents often manifest these reactions crudely, intensely, provocatively, and for prolonged periods. Clinicians must establish themselves as trustworthy and helpful adults to promote a therapeutic alliance. They should encourage adolescents to tell their own stories, without interrupting to check discrepancies; such a tactic would seem like correcting the patient and expressing disbelief. Clinicians should ask patients for explanations and theories about what happened. Why did these behaviors or feelings occur? When did things change? What caused the identified problems to begin when they did?

Sessions with adolescents generally follow the adult model; the therapist sits across from the patient. In early adolescence, however, board games (e.g., checkers) may help to stimulate conversation in an otherwise quiet, anxious patient.

Language is crucial. Even when a teenager and a clinician come from the same socioeconomic group, their languages are seldom the same. Psychiatrists should use their own language, explain any specialized terms or concepts, and ask for an explanation of unfamiliar in-group jargon or slang. Many adolescents do not talk spontaneously about illicit substances and suicidal tendencies but do respond honestly to a therapist's questions. A therapist may need to ask specifically about each substance and the amount and frequency of its use.

The sexual histories and current sexual activities of adolescents are increasingly important pieces of information for adequate evaluation. The nature of adolescents' sexual behaviors often is a vignette of their whole personality structures and ego development, but a long time may elapse in therapy before adolescents begin to talk about their sexual behavior.

The parents of a 13-year-old boy noted that it was difficult for him to get up in the morning. He seemed as though he was not sleeping. When asked about his sleep, he was reluctant to answer and simply indicated that he was having "a little trouble" falling asleep at night. His parents began watching him and found that he was up until 2 or 3 AM. He was getting up out of bed numerous times. They also found that he took longer and longer time in the bathroom. In school, he often missed classes and was found in the bathroom. When confronted, he disclosed that he had developed a number of bedtime rituals that took longer and longer to complete because if he did them incorrectly, he had to repeat them. They included checking the locks on the windows and doors, placing objects in the "right" places on his dresser, and repeating a prayer 16 times. He also revealed that when in the bathroom, he had to wash his hands a certain way and dry them "just so," or he feared something terrible would happen. His psychiatric evaluation revealed significant obsessive-compulsive disorder (OCD) and social phobia. Treatment was initiated, including use of a selective serotonin reuptake inhibitor (SSRI), cognitive-behavioral therapy (CBT), and problem-solving family therapy. Over the course of 6 months, his OCD responded well to the combination of medications and CBT, and the family learned ways of helping him both at home and in school. (Courtesy of Eugene V. Beresin, M.D., and Steven C. Schlozman, M.D.)

A 14-year-old girl gymnast began increasing her daily exercise and restricting her diet. She had never achieved menses because of her low weight. She became fixated on the size of her thighs and belly and lost so much weight that her coach and pediatrician did not allow her to participate in athletics. She became increasingly terrified of getting fat and secretly exercised any chance she could. She was a perfectionist in academics as well as in gymnastics. Because of excessive weight loss, she was hospitalized, and the diagnosis of anorexia nervosa, nonpurging type, was established without comorbid disorders. After hospitalization with modest weight gain, an outpatient plan was initiated, including regular meetings with her pediatrician for monitoring of vital signs, weekly meetings with a nutritionist, weekly family therapy, and individual psychodynamic psychotherapy. In her psychotherapy, over the course of 2 years, she was able to understand that her perfectionism was a defense against low self-esteem, that she was very angry with her mother, who lived vicariously through her gymnastics and did not validate who she really was, and that she was, as an only child, the focus in her family, holding her parents' marriage together. Over time, she was able to understand the function of her anorexia as a way to avoid her maturation as a woman, as a dysfunctional means of developing some kind of identity, and as a passive-aggressive attack on her parents. With time, her weight increased, and she was able to resume her athletics and developed close friends. (Courtesy of Eugene V. Beresin, M.D., and Steven C. Schlozman, M.D.)

TREATMENT

Psychiatric treatment of an adolescent can occur in numerous venues and modalities. Treatment can focus on individual or group settings and can include interventions that are pharmacologic (when indicated), psychosocial, and from an environmental perspective. The best choices for treatment of psychiatric disorders in adolescents must take into account the characteristics of the individual adolescent and the family or social milieu. Adolescents' striving for autonomy may complicate problems of compliance with therapy and may result in the need for stabilization in inpatient settings, whereas this level of care may not be necessary at a different stage of life. Therefore, the following discussion is less a set of guidelines than a brief summary of what each treatment modality can or should offer.

Individual Psychotherapy

Individual psychosocial modalities with an evidence base for efficacy with adolescents include cognitive-behavioral treatments for psychiatric disorders, such as anxiety disorders, mood disorders, and OCD. Interpersonal therapy is a technique that has been applied to mood disorders in adolescents. Few adolescent patients are trusting or open without considerable time and testing, and it is helpful to anticipate the testing period by letting patients know that it is to be expected and is natural and healthy. Pointing out the likelihood of therapeutic problems—for instance, impatience and disappointment with the psychiatrist, the therapy, the time required, and the often intangible results—may help to keep problems under control. Therapeutic goals should be stated in terms that adolescents understand and value. Although they may not see the point in exercising self-control, enduring dysphoric emotions, or forgoing impulsive gratification, they may value feeling more confident than in the past and gaining more control over their lives and the events that affect them.

Typical adolescent patients need a real relationship with a therapist they can perceive as a real person. The therapist becomes another parent because adolescents still need appropriate parenting or reparenting. Thus, a professional who is impersonal and anonymous is a less useful model than one who can accept and respond rationally to an angry challenge or confrontation without fear or false conciliation—one that can impose limits and controls when adolescents cannot, can admit mistakes and ignorance, and can openly express the gamut of human emotions. Adolescents perceive as indifference or collusion a failure to take a stand about self-damaging and self-destructive behavior or to respond actively to manipulative and dishonest behavior.

Countertransference reactions can be intense in psychotherapeutic work with adolescents, and therapists must be aware of them. An adolescent often expresses hostile feelings toward adults, such as parents and teachers. A therapist may react with over identification with the adolescent or with the parents. Such reactions are determined, at least in part, by the therapist's experiences during his or her adolescence or, when applicable, the therapist's experiences as a parent.

Individual outpatient therapy is appropriate for adolescents whose problems are manifest in conflicted emotions and nondangerous behavior, who are not too disorganized to be maintained outside a structured setting, and whose families or other living environments are not sufficiently disturbed to negate the influence of therapy. Such therapy characteristically focuses on intrapsychic conflicts and inhibitions; on the meanings of emotions, attitudes, and behavior; and on the influence of the past and the present. Antianxiety agents can be considered in adolescents whose anxiety may be high at certain times during psychotherapy, but adolescents' potential for abusing these drugs must be weighed carefully.

Psychopharmacotherapy and Combined Therapy

Randomized clinical trials have provided evidence of the superiority of CBT in combination with SSRI medication in the treatment of mood disorders, OCD, and, most likely, anxiety disorders in adolescents.

Attention-deficit/hyperactivity disorder (ADHD) in adolescents has not been studied systematically with regard to the effectiveness of treating it by combination therapy with CBT. In the Multimodal Treatment Study of Children with ADHD (MTA), psychosocial interventions did not add to the efficacy of the stimulant treatments for the core symptoms of ADHD. Other outcome measures of psychosocial improvements are needed, however, in future studies of combination treatment. Psychostimulants, such as methylphenidate (Ritalin, Concerta), dextroamphetamine (Dexedrine), and amphetamine salts (Adderall, Adderall XR), however, have been found to be efficacious in adolescents in the treatment of ADHD.

Advances in drug development have widened the choice of medications with which to treat mood disorders (e.g., SSRIs) and schizophrenia (e.g., serotonin-dopamine antagonists [SDAs], including risperidone [Risperdal], olanzapine [Zyprexa], and clozapine [Clozaril]). Although these medications have been used to treat adolescent disorders, systematic research is required to determine the efficacy and safety profiles of these medications for treatment of adolescent psychopathology.

A comprehensive workup is needed before starting psychopharmacotherapy with adolescents, including a physical examination; blood tests to evaluate hematologic, kidney, liver, thyroid, and other physiologic functions; and an electrocardiogram (ECG) to measure cardiac function. Neurologic assessment with an electroencephalogram (EEG) is necessary if seizure disorder is suspected or if the medication is likely to lower the seizure threshold.

A 17-year-old girl complained of episodes of rapid heartbeat, sweating, trembling, and fears of going out alone to the shopping mall. She had entered her senior year in high school, was considering her choice of colleges, and was planning to take her college entrance examination. Her parents wanted her to maintain the family tradition and go to the college from which her mother graduated. Psychoanalytically oriented outpatient treatment and treatment with an SSRI were instituted to alleviate the panic disorder symptoms. The psychotherapy focused on the patient's conflicts with her parents, highlighting her chronic concern that she could not meet parental expectations and fears of her independence. Medication appeared to reduce symptoms of tachycardia, tremulousness, and preoccupation with lack of competence. Psychotherapy was maintained for 8 months during her last year in high school. (Courtesy of Cynthia R. Pfeffer, M.D.)

Group Psychotherapy

In many ways, group psychotherapy is a natural setting for adolescents. Most teenagers are more comfortable with peers than with adults. A group diminishes the sense of unequal power between the adult therapist and the adolescent patient. Participation varies, depending on an adolescent's readiness. Not all interpretations and confrontations should come from the parent-figure therapist; group members often are adept at noticing symptomatic behavior in each other, and adolescents may find it easier to hear and consider critical or challenging comments from their peers.

Group psychotherapy usually addresses interpersonal and current life issues. Some adolescents, however, are too fragile for group psychotherapy or have symptoms or social traits that are too likely to elicit peer group ridicule; they need individual therapy to attain sufficient ego strength to struggle with peer relationships. Conversely, other adolescents must resolve interpersonal issues in a group before they can tackle intrapsychic issues in the intensity of one-on-one therapy.

Family Therapy

Family therapy is the primary modality when adolescents' difficulties mainly reflect a dysfunctional family (e.g., teenagers with school refusal, runaways). The same may be true when developmental issues, such as adolescent sexuality and striving for autonomy, trigger family conflicts or when family pathology is severe, as in cases of incest and child abuse. In these instances, adolescents usually need individual therapy as well, but family therapy is mandatory if an adolescent is to remain in the home or return to it. Serious character pathology, such as that underlying antisocial and borderline personality disorders, often develops from highly pathogenic early parenting. Family therapy is strongly indicated whenever possible for such disorders, but most authorities consider it adjunctive to intensive individual psychotherapy when individual psychopathology has become so internalized that it persists regardless of the current family status.

Inpatient Treatment

Residential treatment schools often are preferable for long-term therapy, but hospitals are more suitable for emergencies, although some adolescent inpatient hospital units also provide educational, recreational, and occupational facilities for long-term patients. Adolescents whose families are too disturbed or incompetent, who are dangerous to themselves or others, who are out of control in ways that preclude further healthy development, or who are seriously disorganized require, at least temporarily, the external controls of a structured environment.

Long-term inpatient therapy is the treatment of choice for severe disorders that are considered wholly or largely psychogenic in origin, such as major ego deficits that are caused by early massive deprivation and that respond poorly or not at all to medication. Severe borderline personality disorder, for example, regardless of the behavioral symptoms, requires a full-time corrective environment in which regression is possible and safe and in which ego development can take place. Psychotic disorders in adolescence often require hospitalization, but psychotic adolescents often respond to appropriate medication so that therapy usually is feasible in an outpatient setting, except during exacerbation. Adolescent patients with schizophrenia who exhibit a long-term deteriorating course may require hospitalization periodically.

Day Hospitals

In day hospitals, which have become increasingly popular, adolescents spend the day in class, individual and group psychotherapy, and other programs but they go home in the evenings. Day hospitals are less expensive than full hospitalization and usually are preferred by patients.

CLINICAL PROBLEMS

Atypical Puberty

Pubertal changes that occur 2.5 years earlier or later than the average age are within the normal range. Body image is so important to adolescents, however, that extremes of the norm may be distressing to some either because markedly early maturation subjects them to social and sexual pressures for which they are unready or because late maturation makes them feel inferior and excludes them from some peer activities. Medical reassurance, even if based on examination and testing to rule out pathophysiology, may not suffice. An adolescent's distress may show as sexual or delinquent acting out, withdrawal, or problems at school that are sufficiently serious to warrant therapeutic intervention. Therapy also may be prompted by similar disturbances in some adolescents who fail to achieve peer-valued stereotypes of physical development despite normal pubertal physiology.

Substance-Related Disorders

Some experimentation with psychoactive substances is almost ubiquitous among adolescents, especially if this category of behavior includes alcohol use. Most adolescents, however, do not become abusers, particularly of prescription drugs and illegal substances. Any regular substance abuse represents disturbance. Substance abuse sometimes is self-medication against depression or schizophrenic deterioration, and sometimes it signals a character disorder in teenagers whose ego deficits render them unequal to the stresses of puberty and the tasks of adolescence. Some substances, including cocaine, have a physiologically reinforcing action that acts independently of preexisting psychopathology. When substance abuse covers an underlying illness or is a maladaptive response to current stresses or disturbed family dynamics, treatment of the underlying cause may diminish the substance use; in most cases of significant abuse, however, the drug-taking behavior typically requires intervention. Substance abuse treatments typically include a 12-step program with behavioral monitoring to accomplish sobriety, as well as the ability to verbalize regarding the motivations for substance use. These philosophies are adapted to inpatient, intensive outpatient, and once-a-week outpatient treatment.

Suicide

Suicide is the second-leading cause of death among adolescents. Many hospital admissions of adolescents result from suicidal ideation or behavior. Among adolescents who are not psychotic, the highest suicidal risks occur in those who have a history of parental suicide, who are unable to form stable attachments, who display impulsive behavior, and who abuse alcohol or other substances. Many adolescents who complete suicide have backgrounds that include longstanding family conflict and social problems since early childhood and the escalation of subjective distress under the pressure of a sudden perceived conflict or loss. Early childhood loss of parents also can increase the risk of depression in adolescence. Adolescents who are susceptible to rapid and extreme mood swings and a history of impulsive behavior are at greater risk of responding to despair with impulsive suicide attempts. Alcohol and other substances are known added risks for suicidal behavior in adolescents with suicidal ideations. The developmentally predictable "omnipotent" attitudes of adolescents may cloud the immediate sense of the permanence of death and result in impulsive self-destructive behavior.

During a psychiatric evaluation of an adolescent with suicidal thoughts, plans and past attempts must be discussed directly when the concern arises and information is not volunteered. Recurring suicidal thoughts should be taken seriously, and a clinician must evaluate the possibility of imminent clinical danger requiring inpatient hospitalization versus an adolescent's ability to engage in an agreement or contract mandating that he or she will seek help before engaging in self-destructive behavior. Adolescents typically are honest in their refusal of such agreements, and, in such cases, hospitalization is indicated. Hospitalization of a suicidal adolescent by a clinician is an act of serious, protective concern.

20

Special Areas of Interest

▲ 20.1 Forensic Issues

Forensic child and adolescent psychiatry is a subspecialty of the branch of psychiatry involving the relationships between psychiatry and the law. Board certification in forensic psychiatry is based on a 1-year fellowship that is not specifically geared to children and adolescents; however, many programs offer exposure to child and adolescent cases. Traditionally, forensic child and adolescent psychiatrists have dealt largely with custody evaluation and recommendations and with the ramifications of child abuse and neglect. Child and adolescent psychiatrists are increasingly being sought out by patients and attorneys for evaluations and expert opinions related to child sexual and physical abuse and criminal behaviors perpetrated by minors and for evaluation of the relations between traumatic life events and the emergence of psychiatric symptoms in children and adolescents. As more youth enter the juvenile justice system, an increasing need exists for forensic psychiatrists with expertise in evaluation and treatment for detainees and committed youths. The American Academy of Child and Adolescent Psychiatry (AACAP) developed Practice Parameters for the Forensic Evaluation of Children and Adolescents Who May Have Been Physically or Sexually Abused for custody evaluations and for children with posttraumatic stress disorder (PTSD). Throughout the development of medicine, ethical principles have alluded to moral obligations as a guide for acceptable physician behavior, for example, the Hippocratic oath. During the last few decades, however, more complex ethical and moral dilemmas have arisen with the greater sophistication of medical technology. For example, a patient may be kept alive for long periods while in a coma, or a pregnant woman's life may be saved by aborting her fetus.

Society's view of children and their rights evolved dramatically during the 20th century. The institution of a juvenile court system about 100 years ago was an acknowledgment that children must be protected and provided for differently than adults. In 1980, the AACAP published a code of ethics that was developed to publicly endorse the ethical standards relating to this discipline. The code is based on the assumption that children are vulnerable and unable to take adequate care of themselves; as they mature, however, their capacity to make judgments of, and choices about, their well-being develop. The code has several caveats: From the standpoint of child and adolescent psychiatrists, issues of consent, confidentiality, and professional responsibility must be seen in the context of overlapping and potentially conflicting rights of children, parents, and society.

Confidentiality, or intensive trust, refers to the relationship between two persons with respect to the "entrustment of secrets." Until the 1970s, little attention was paid to issues of confidentiality pertaining to minors. In 1980, among the items in the AACAP Code of Ethics, six principles were related to confidentiality. Breaches and limits of confidentiality can be obtained in cases of child abuse or maltreatment or for purposes of appropriate education. Although unnecessary with a child or adolescent, consent for disclosure should be obtained when possible. In 1979, the American Psychiatric Association (APA) stated that a child of 12 years of age could give consent for disclosure of confidential information, and, with the exception of safety issues, a minor's consent is required for disclosure of information to others, including the child's parents. According to the AACAP Code of Ethics, the consent of a minor is not required for disclosure of confidential information. Specific ages for consent are not addressed in the code. Child and adolescent psychiatrists often face the dilemma of weighing the potential benefits and possible harm in sharing information obtained confidentially from a child with the child's parents. Although the smoothest transition occurs when the child and the physician agree that certain information can be shared, in many situations that border on "dangerousness to the child or others," the child or adolescent does not agree to share the information with a parent or another responsible adult. Among adolescents, these secrets that are sometimes shared with a psychiatrist may involve drug or alcohol use, unsafe sex practices, or a thrill-seeking act that places the adolescent in danger. A psychiatrist may choose to work with the child or adolescent toward agreeing to share confidential information when it is determined by the treating psychiatrist that the probable outcome would be beneficial. The initial treatment contract, however, limits confidentiality to situations of "danger" to the child or others.

Other arenas that can pose confidentiality dilemmas include educational and scientific settings, research activities, and third-party agencies. Professional settings, such as annual psychiatric conventions, often include individual case presentations. In the context of a clinical symposium, doctors should realize that confidentiality means more than changing or dropping a patient's name; other information in a case study may pose a threat to a patient's privacy. Research projects sometimes are impeded by laws designed to protect the privacy of children and their families. In some cases, long-term follow-up studies may no longer be legal because of a time limitation on a written consent for study. Third-party payers are requiring more and more confidential information before they consider reimbursement of psychiatric services. Information disclosed to insurance companies often is shared with many reviewers in the company, which also places it in danger of being merged into a data base in a computer system that is neither highly restricted nor confidential.

In general, there is no way to simplify the many difficult, complex confidentiality issues that may emerge in treating children and adolescents. Child and adolescent psychiatrists function as advocates for their patients and must always remain aware of minors' vulnerabilities and the importance of maintaining trust in the treatment relationship.

CHILD CUSTODY

Child custody evaluations by child and adolescent psychiatrists may be initiated by divorcing parents who cannot come to an agreement regarding custody of their children or can be requested by an attorney. Attorneys are most likely to seek child custody evaluations when allegations are made of parental incompetence or issues of alleged physical or sexual abuse arise. Comprehensive custody evaluations by mental health professionals may play a significant role in successful negotiations of custody by parents without the necessity of proceeding to a trial.

The evolution of child custody decision making has been influenced by increasing awareness and recognition of the rights of children and women, as well as by a broadening perspective on the developmental and psychologic needs of the children involved. Historically, children were considered to be their fathers' property. At the beginning of the 20th century, the "tender years" doctrine became the standard for determining child custody. According to this doctrine, the relationship between mother and infant, later generalized to mother and child, is responsible for the optimal emotional development of the child; the doctrine thus supported custody decisions in the mother's favor in most cases. With this doctrine as its guide, psychologic issues in developing children became an acceptable dimension to consider in the determination of custody. In controversial and unclear cases, psychologic expert testimony began to be accepted as a valuable part of child custody decision making.

The "best interest of the child" standard replaced the "tender years" doctrine and expanded considerations of the optimal parent to include assessing issues of emotional climate, safety, and educational and social opportunities for the child. The "best interest of the child" grew from the movement to support legislation about the rights of children in the areas of compulsory education, child labor laws, and child abuse and neglect protection laws. Therefore, although "best interest" standards have broadened the dimensions considered in evaluating which parent is best able to serve the best interest of the child, how to measure these qualities in a parent remains vague. In view of the lack of clarity regarding what specific qualities in a parent best correspond to the interest of the child, child and adolescent psychiatrists have increasingly been asked to help make decisions by defining relevant psychologic conditions in parents and in the relationships between parents and children.

Psychiatric evaluators may be asked to give an opinion about child custody at various points during the separation and divorce process. Sometimes, a psychiatric evaluation is requested by the parents before any legal action occurs. When the parents and an evaluator can agree on custody decisions before the legal process, a court is likely to go along with these decisions rather than launch an additional investigation. A psychiatric evaluation may be ordered by the court or by the attorneys representing the feuding parents. In such cases, an evaluator is faced with two disgruntled parents who often are consumed by their mutual conflict to the point that neither is willing to compromise, even in the child's interest. The advantage in such cases, however, is that evaluators represent the court and can act as advocate for the child without the same pressures faced by an evaluator hired by only one parent. A psychiatric evaluation also may be initiated by a guardian *ad litem,* an attorney who is appointed by the court to represent the child. Psychiatric evaluators also may be requested to give an opinion about custody during a mediation process. Mediation is a legal process that usually involves one attorney and one evaluator. Because mediation can occur outside the judicial system, some families may prefer it accepting it to going through a trial. In addition to custody, psychiatric evaluators often are asked to give opinions about visitation.

In undertaking a custody evaluation, an evaluator is expected to determine the best interests of the child while keeping in mind the standard elements that the court considers. These considerations include the wishes of the parents and the child; relationships with significant others in the child's life; the child's adjustment to the current home, school, and community; the psychiatric and physical health of all parties; and the level of conflict and potential danger to the child under the care of either parent. A psychiatric evaluator must maintain his or her role as an advocate for the best interest of the child and is not to consider the fairest outcome for parents. The psychiatric evaluator conducts a series of interviews, often including at least one separate interview with each parent and the child alone and one interview with the child and both parents. The evaluator may obtain a written waiver of confidentiality from all parties because he or she may have to make disclosures to opposing attorneys and in court before the judge. The evaluator uses direct questioning as well as observations of the relationships between the child and each parent. The age and developmental needs of the child are considered in making a judgment regarding which parent may better serve the child's interests. As part of the psychiatric assessment of the child custody evaluation, the evaluator determines the need for psychiatric treatment of any of the parties involved.

The child custody evaluation generally is provided in a written report. This document is not confidential and can be used in court. The report contains a description of the relationship between the child and parents, the capabilities of the parents, and, finally, the custody recommendations. In view of data supporting the importance of continuing a relationship with both parents in most cases, it is recommended that joint custody be considered before other options. When sufficient cooperation exists to negotiate for joint custody, the best interests of the child often are served. Joint custody may not be the best option for a child when the relationship of the child with either parent is jeopardized and undermined by the other. The next-most-frequent choice when joint custody is not advisable is full custody by one parent with visitation rights for the other parent. The parent awarded full custody should be able to support the visitations and relationship with the noncustodial parent. In custody disputes involving a biological parent and a nonbiological parent, the biological parent generally has the right to custody unless he or she is shown to be unable to provide for the child. After the custody evaluation has been submitted in writing, the results must be communicated to the parents, the child, and possibly their respective attorneys. The evaluator may be called on to testify in court, and the parties can use the custody evaluation to mediate other areas of their dispute.

Many complications can occur in an ongoing bitter dispute between divorcing or divorced parents. Both true and false allegations of psychiatric illness, drug or alcohol abuse, or sexual or physical abuse are not uncommon during custody battles. The evaluator must be prepared to verify any allegations and to carefully discuss their effects on custody and visitation. Evidence suggests that markedly elevated numbers of unfounded allegations of child sexual abuse occur during the course of custody disputes.

Joey, age 8 years, has been in a therapeutic foster home for 2 years, having been removed from his home along with his younger sister (who was subsequently returned home) owing to profound neglect, as well as abuse. Although he is receiving appropriate services, he remains volatile, with extensive developmental problems; and typically becomes more aggressive and regressed after weekly supervised visits with his family. Joey's guardian *ad litem* requests that Dr. Jacobs perform a forensic evaluation to determine whether visits should continue. She reviews extensive records, evaluates each parent, obtains history from them and the foster parent, and then observes a visit. Joey's little sister totally dominates the visit, and the parents are at a loss to control her aggressive and hyperactive behavior. Joey is passive and not very engaged with either parent. According to the visitation supervisor, this is a fairly typical visit. When Dr. Jacobs meets individually with Joey, Joey expresses concerns that his sister is still being abused at home, and his need to check on her seems to be the only reason he wants to continue the visits. Dr. Jacobs tells Joey that both parents are getting help and doing better with their parenting, but he remains unconvinced. Joey evidences a positive relationship with his foster father and, in contrast, has little to say about his parents. Dr. Jacobs recommends a psychiatric evaluation of the sister, but Joey's parents do not follow through with one. She further recommends cutting visits back to monthly, but Joey's anxiety and aggressive behavior persist around these limited visits. It also becomes apparent that the parents are not up to the demands of caring for two special-needs children. She recommends ceasing efforts at parental reunification but maintaining some contact between Joey and his sister. (Courtesy of Diane H. Schetky, M.D.)

JUVENILE OFFENDERS

The creation of a separate juvenile court system in the United States first occurred by statute in the state of Illinois in the late 1800s. Its mandate was to rehabilitate rather than to punish. Despite the protective intentions of the legal system, children and adolescents involved in the juvenile justice system are at high risk for multiple psychiatric disorders and suicidal thoughts and behavior. A recent survey of 991 youth at an initial juvenile justice intake revealed high levels of suicidal ideation, with recent attempts more common in females, youth with major depression or substance use disorders, and those who were violent offenders. The omission of various constitutional safeguards, such as the rights to counsel, confrontation, and cross-examination of an accuser, eventually led to criticism and disillusionment with this system. Juvenile offenders of small and significant crimes often were sent to state-run residential programs that were criticized for being overcrowded, neglectful, and frankly abusive. Despite the strong sentiment to increase due process protection for juveniles rather than pretrial, trial, and sentencing, the juvenile court system includes intake, adjudication, and disposition. The intake is a determination of whether probable cause exists that the youth committed a crime. A youth who confesses may be diverted from the court system altogether at this time, and appropriate plans for rehabilitation can be made in a community setting. For more serious crimes or when juveniles deny perpetrating a crime, the process continues. Juveniles must be represented by counsel, and an attorney is provided if the family cannot afford to provide its own.

Unlike in adult court, in juvenile court guilt or innocence is determined by a judge, not a jury. The case is argued by a prosecuting attorney and a defense attorney, and the judge is bound by the same standards as in adult court; that is, a judgment of delinquency requires proof beyond a reasonable doubt. When the charge is substantiated and the judgment is for delinquency, the juvenile is an "adjudicated delinquent." Disposition must next be determined. Dispositions include a wide range of options, from placement in youth correctional facilities, to placement in residential treatment settings, to psychiatric hospitalizations for further evaluation. *Delinquent acts* refer to ordinary crimes committed by juveniles; *status offenses* refer to behaviors that would not be criminal if perpetrated by adults, such as truancy, running away, or drinking alcohol. Sometimes, youths who are believed to have committed a serious crime are turned over (receive a waiver) to adult criminal court.

A psychiatrist may be asked to evaluate a juvenile to make recommendations about appropriate diversion plans. Psychiatric evaluation can be sought for adjudicated delinquents to determine whether treatment for a psychiatric illness would work to prevent future delinquent acts and, if so, in what setting. Psychiatric evaluations also may be requested when the court is considering a waiver to adult court. In some states, such decisions are based, in part, on the youth's psychiatric history and current mental status.

MENTAL HEALTH NEEDS OF YOUTH IN THE JUVENILE JUSTICE SYSTEM

Youth in the juvenile justice system are at extremely high risk for psychiatric disturbance, and unmet mental health needs have reached such high proportions that they are of public health concern. Adolescents in juvenile justice residential facilities not only have higher rates of psychiatric disorders, including depression, substance use, and suicidal behavior, but they are also significantly more likely to have been victims of physical and sexual abuse, educational failure, and family conflict. Few studies have documented the needs of juveniles in residential facilities and the medical and psychiatric care available. A recent study collected data from the U.S. Department of Justice censuses of all public and private juvenile justice facilities in the United States. The Juvenile Residential Facilities Census (JRFC) and the Census of Juveniles in Residential Placement (CJRP) investigated data on death rates of youth under the age of 21 years who had been charged with, or adjudicated for, an offense and were housed in the facility because of the offense. In the 2-year period covered by the 2000 and 2002 statistics, a total of 62 deaths of youth occurred. The leading cause of death was suicide (20 cases), followed by accidents (17 cases), illness (14 cases), and homicides by nonresidents (6 cases). No deaths resulted from acquired immunodeficiency syndrome (AIDS), homicide by another resident, or an injury that occurred before placement. The risk for death of youth in juvenile justice facilities was found to be 8 percent higher than the death rate for the general population of adolescents aged 15 to 19 years. Above all, the risk for suicide is clearly increased in the juvenile justice facility compared with the general population, indicating a significant need for increased mental health evaluation and treatment in this population.

ADVERSE LIFE EVENTS AND PSYCHIATRIC SYMPTOMS

Child and adolescent psychiatrists are frequently sought out to evaluate children or adolescents who have been exposed to a traumatic or adverse life event and are exhibiting a variety of psychiatric symptoms. The child and adolescent psychiatrist may be asked to determine whether a child or adolescent is experiencing posttraumatic stress disorder or whether a given set of symptoms is likely to have been caused by exposure to the adverse life event. A recent report by William Bernet and David Corwin detailed an evidence-based approach to estimating present and future damages from a traumatic event such as, for example, sexual abuse. In such as case this requires the child and adolescent psychiatrist to carefully interview the patient and family, as well as review the literature on the aspects of childhood sexual abuse that would help to render an opinion based on individual and systematic approaches to similar situations. Thus, the first question asked is whether the child was injured by the sexual abuse. Given the clinical case history of the child in question, intrusive painful memories, depressed mood, suicidal ideation, poorly controlled rage, and substance abuse after the sexual abuse are reasonable indicators of harm. The question of whether the child who has been sexually abused is at increased risk of future psychiatric problems can be reasonably ascertained by reviewing the literature on children who were sexually abused, which shows them to have rates of psychiatric disorders two to three times higher than would otherwise be expected. Regarding the efficacy of treatment, the psychiatrist should be able to extrapolate from the literature that such a child would likely be better off with a psychosocial intervention after abuse than with none. Thus, the principles of evidenced-base approaches to forensic evaluations can increase the validity and usefulness of the recommendations.

Another common request to a child and adolescent psychiatrist is to render an expert opinion regarding whether, for example, a child diagnosed with autistic disorder is likely to have been at greater risk for the disorder because of a particular treatment given to the mother during pregnancy. It is much easier for a child and adolescent psychiatrist to verify the presence of a psychiatric disorder in a child than to determine its exact cause. Evaluations requiring a psychiatrist to make a judgment identifying a single cause of a complex psychiatric disorder are generally difficult or impossible because of the lack of data linking psychiatric disorders to single causes.

> Dr. Abibi is called by a defense attorney to review discovery material in a case that alleges permanent harm and suffering in 6-year-old Tony, who is alleged to have been sexually abused at age 3 in his day care center. Dr. Green, the forensic expert for the plaintiff, has evaluated the child and performed psychologic testing of him and concluded that the boy's conduct problems are all related to the alleged abuse, which the child has difficulty recalling. His early history on the boy is cursory, however, and he has little information about the mother, who is a single parent, and did not review medical records. In her thorough review of discovery material, Dr. Abibi learns that Tony has witnessed extensive domestic violence and his mother's rape, shown signs of hyperactivity since age 2, and has exhibited much anxiety related to his mother's safety and several separations from

her at times when she was unable to care for him owing to depression. Tony also has had delayed language development. Dr. Green, at the time of his deposition, was asked why he had not asked about these matters. He said he considered the mother's personal life a private matter and did not see its relevance to the litigation. Dr. Abibi, when deposed, points out that many other factors beside the alleged abuse might account for Tony's behavioral problems. (Courtesy of Diane H. Schetky, M.D.)

▲ 20.2 Adoption and Foster Care

As many as 500,000 to 700,000 children are in foster care each year in the United States. Foster care caseloads more than doubled in the last two decades. In recent years, child abuse and neglect and abandonment, often in conjunction with parental substance abuse and psychiatric illness, have emerged as significant reasons for placement. Foster care is intended to be temporary out-of-home care provided by the welfare system for children and adolescents whose immediate families are unable to care for them. Given the severity of the vulnerable parents, however, care is often needed for many months and years. In 1997, President Clinton signed the Adoption and Safe Families Act (PL-105-89), a law designed to improve provisions for child safety, to decrease the length of time that a child remains in foster care without long-term planning and to limit the amount of time in which a biological parent has to undergo rehabilitation to 12 months. An additional law, PL-99-272, allocated federal funds to assist adolescents and young adults 16 to 21 years of age who leave foster care in transitioning to independent living.

EPIDEMIOLOGY AND DEMOGRAPHICS OF FOSTER CARE

Minority children are overrepresented in the foster care population. Approximately 38 percent are African-Americans, more than three times the representation in the general population. Whites make up approximately 48 percent, and Hispanics make up almost 15 percent. Of foster children, 55 to 69 percent are girls, and 83.4 percent enter foster care at a mean age of 3 years. Children placed in care as infants are more likely to stay in care. Those younger than 5 years of age comprise the fastest growing segment of the foster care population. Studies reveal that as many as 62 percent of foster children had prenatal drug exposure. A 1989 Department of Health and Human Services (HHS) study revealed that 30 to 50 percent of all drug-exposed children entered foster care; among African-Americans, parental drug use precipitated almost 80 percent of foster care placements. Parental drug use is positively correlated with maltreatment, with approximately 89 percent of maltreatment cases involving drug abuse. In one California study, 89 percent of maltreated infants tested positive for drugs at birth; cocaine was the drug identified in 85 percent of those who were positive for drug use.

Needs of Foster Care Children

Children entering foster care have enormous mental health needs; more than 80 percent of them have developmental, emotional, or behavioral problems. Growth abnormalities (including failure to thrive), neurologic abnormalities, neuromuscular disorders, language disorders, cognitive delays, and asthma are prevalent. Their health care needs cost six to ten times as much as matched non–foster care peers. Among foster care children 0 to 5 years of age, approximately 25 percent are seriously emotionally damaged. Attachment disorders are increasingly diagnosed. Foster care children use the full range of mental health services: outpatient, acute inpatient, day treatment, partial hospitalization, and residential treatment. Adolescents in foster care are at increased risk for substance abuse, teenage pregnancies, and sexually transmitted diseases, including infection with human immunodeficiency virus (HIV). With public health care increasingly adopting a managed health care system, which is designed to limit care, grave concern exists that the provision and delivery of services to this medically and psychiatrically vulnerable population can be seriously compromised.

Kinship Care for Foster Children

More states are recognizing kinship care as an alternative placement option and are authorizing licensing and reimbursement to kinship caregivers, who are generally women (mostly maternal grandmothers), of low income, of low education, and of minority status. Nationwide, approximately 23 percent of African-American children are in foster kinship care. It is unknown just how many children are in informal kinship care within the African-American population, which has had a long cultural tradition of taking in children of family members who are unable to care for their offspring. The few studies available indicate that outcomes, although mixed, are somewhat more positive than for those children in nonkinship care. Children reportedly receive more positive regard from caregivers in kinship care, and a consistent outcome, when it works, is that it provides more stability than nonrelative foster care. Most foster children have consistently said that they would rather be with a family member than stay in the system. When foster children feel embraced by their families of origin and the latter can provide appropriate nurturance and access to good therapeutic services, the foster children's sense of identity and belonging is less disrupted. As best as can be determined, however, no demonstrable difference is seen in the need for mental health, medical, and special educational services for these children. Research on kinship care is ongoing and should be providing increasingly reliable data. Initial data from Robert B. Clyman and associates on outcomes from kinship care are not favorable but should be interpreted cautiously and within the context of that particular research design.

THERAPEUTIC FOSTER CARE

Therapeutic foster care (TFC) has emerged as a cost-effective alternative to the more restrictive *residential treatment center* (RTC). Therapeutic effectiveness is mixed. TFC is designed to provide nurturing family-based care with specialized treatment interventions from an interdisciplinary treatment team. Therapeutic foster parents are supposed to be the agents of therapeutic change, functioning as *extenders* of the clinical treatment team. Because of the children's special needs, therapeutic foster parents must have more extensive training, receive a higher reimbursement, and receive more intensive monitoring, supervision, and support from the foster care agency. Although the concept of TFC is promising, good outcome data do not show consistent success. Several models exist, but implementation that shows fidelity to empirically tested models is often spotty. Some models, although efficacious in the research setting, have proved too expensive and complicated to implement in the real-world setting. The concept of professional therapeutic parents, who are actually paid competitive full-time wages to care for special-needs foster children, has been gaining increasing interest and definitely holds some promise as an alternative to current prevailing practice. Clinical practice demonstrates that, when adequate and appropriate intensive in-home services with good case management can be provided in a well-managed foster care setting, children can show significant gains.

Cultural Competence

Anna McPhatter defined *cultural competence* as the ability to use knowledge and cultural awareness to design psychosocial interventions that support and sustain healthy client–system functioning within a cultural context that is meaningful to the client. Because U.S. society is still significantly encumbered by racial conflicts, some children have been denied placement with families of a different race, and they have ended up in long-term foster care rather than in a permanent adoption placement. The Association of Black Social Workers is on record as opposing transracial placement of African-American children. In 1978, the Indian Child Welfare Act (PL 95-608) transferred to tribal courts the power to make placement decisions about Native American children to reverse the practice of placement in non–Native American homes. Adoption studies have shown that it is not inherently harmful for children to be cross-racially adopted. Congress passed the Multiethnic Placement Act of 1994 to facilitate transracial adoptions while maintaining the language of cultural awareness in placement decisions. The need for cultural sensitivity and respect and a capacity to facilitate a foster child's cultural development and identity are well acknowledged. These issues must be addressed in training providers of foster care services. Although it is common practice to include *cultural competence* as a requirement in the implementation of child welfare programs, no rigorous research has identified the essential variables that make for success in cultural competency.

PSYCHOLOGIC ISSUES IN FOSTER CARE CHILDREN

Foster care children are overrepresented in psychiatric populations. Among those who return home, 40 percent reenter the foster care system. These children struggle with issues of abandonment, neglect, rejection, and physical, emotional, and sexual maltreatment. The child's age, home environment, and the specific reasons for going into placement affect the emotional issues that he or she must handle. Early abandonment and neglect can lead to anaclitic depression. Attachment issues are prevalent in this young population because they have not had an opportunity to form secure attachments with consistent nurturing figures in early life.

Foster children are often unprepared for separations, which can be abrupt and repeated in the current foster care climate. Early separation from the primary caretaker is considered a major trauma for the child and sets the stage for a vulnerability to subsequent trauma. Children who bounce from foster home to foster home have their capacity to form enduring emotional attachments compromised; trust becomes a lifelong challenge. Defense mechanisms tend to be primitive, that is, denial, splitting, projection, and introjection. Characterologic problems are common in adulthood. Not surprisingly, children who have never had their narcissistic needs appropriately met may become unempathetic adults with pathologic narcissism, which is associated with criminality.

Children who have experienced traumatic physical and sexual abuse often become mistrustful, hypervigilant, aggressive, impulsive, oppositional, and avoidant as they attempt to negotiate a world that they experience as threatening, hostile, and uncaring. When children are raised in a psychosocial environment of trauma, aggression, and lack of empathy from adults, the psychologic seeds are sown for later violence against the self and others. The range of psychopathology of foster care children covers several psychiatric diagnostic categories. Attention-deficit/hyperactivity disorder (ADHD), attachment disorders, oppositional defiant disorder, conduct disorders, impulse-control disorders, posttraumatic stress disorder (PTSD), dissociative disorders, mood and anxiety disorders, sleep disorders, and developmental disorders are among those that are frequently diagnosed. A pervasive problem is one of dysregulation of behavior, emotions and affect, attention, and sleep. Review of the empirical data on the effect of maltreatment on the neurobiology of the developing brain shows that stress hormones play an important role in adaptation and coping, and that these capacities are compromised in varying degrees of severity in abused and neglected children. The data also show that, because of the developmental plasticity of the brain, if appropriate early intervention can be done, hope exists for remediation and repair at the neurobiologic level.

A boy was placed in care because of maternal drug involvement. When seen for a psychiatric evaluation, it was noted that all of his primary teeth were full of dental caries. The foster mother was asked about dental care, and she responded that the dentist had said that he would wait until the teeth had fallen out, because they were his first set of teeth and did not require intervention. This response aroused suspicion about neglect as being the cause of the behavioral (encopresis and smearing) and emotional problems with which this youngster presented. A neglect report was made and the investigation revealed that the boy was not only neglected, but was also being physically abused in that foster care placement. Subsequent to removal and placement with a good foster family, this boy has shown considerable emotional stabilization, does well academically and socially, and is now being adopted by that family. (Courtesy of Marilyn B. Benoit, M.D., Steven L. Nickman, M.D., and Alvin Rosenfeld, M.D.)

FAMILY PRESERVATION

Family preservation came under increasing scrutiny in the last decade. Estimates on the percentage of children who are reportedly reunited vary from 66 to 90 percent. Philosophically, family reunification appears to be the right thing to do, yet approximately 40 percent of reunified children reenter out-of-home care. The field needs discriminating criteria that would identify psychosocial profiles of families that could best benefit from family preservation services. In 1996, the Child Welfare League of America (CWLA) acknowledged the failure of family preservation efforts and requested that child welfare policy makers rethink the current use of intensive family preservation. Recent research has validated poor outcomes with family preservation. It is hoped that the Adoption and Safe Families Act of 1997 (PL 105-89) will give child welfare agencies the opportunity to step back from the myopic view of family preservation and to consider seriously the needs of the child as the major priority. The American Academy of Child and Adolescent Psychiatry (AACAP) and the CWLA jointly launched a national effort to address the mental health needs of children in foster care. This effort is supported by a broad-based coalition of agencies that are all stakeholders in foster care. The coalition proposes that the foster care system be child focused but inclusive of the biological and foster families in intervention planning on the child's behalf if families are to be preserved. Another area of concern regarding improving family preservation is that of substance abuse as a major contributing factor to family dysfunction. The data are clear that this is the major contributor to children's going into care. The high incidence of comorbid mental illness in a biological parent makes rehabilitation a challenging endeavor that requires more comprehensive interventions than are currently provided.

One case of a 7-year-old boy who was in foster care for 2 years is illustrative of why some family preservation efforts fail. When he was returned to his biological mother, she was in a new marriage with a new baby. Her husband was new to parenting. The family was financially strapped and lived under harsh conditions. The mother did the required parenting course for resuming custody of her child, but no supports were put in place to assist this young couple financially or with any family therapy, psychoeducation, or case management interventions. Frequent and increasingly urgent calls to the child welfare family reunification services were of no avail. The outcome for this youngster was that he was reabused and had to reenter the foster care system.

This outcome represents a failure of the system, but also translates into a fractured and debilitated family, with everyone internalizing a profound sense of failure and impotence. (Courtesy of Marilyn B. Benoit, M.D., Steven L. Nickman, M.D., and Alvin Rosenfeld, M.D.)

FOSTER CARE OUTCOMES AND RESEARCH INITIATIVES

The overall quality of outcome studies is poor. Some patterns, however, recur across studies. Several studies reveal that 15 to 39 percent of the homeless are foster care graduates, who are also overrepresented among adult substance abusers and clients in the criminal justice system. It is likely that the reasons that initially precipitated the child's foster care placement contributed to the negative adult outcomes. Studies indicate that children entering care who have been victimized, who have substance-abusing parents or parents with major mental illness or high criminality or both, and who come from homes with a high degree of domestic violence are at greater risk of having poor outcomes. Research on early maltreatment indicates that the influence of maltreatment on brain development can be profound over the life span. Developmental disabilities occur in more than 50 percent of the foster care population. Children returned to their families of origin typically have fared worse than those who have remained in long-term placement.

Several studies reported findings indicating that multiple placements and poor parental involvement consistently lead to negative outcomes. Federal mandate under PL 96-272 requires states to maintain a tracking system for children in foster care. New reporting systems—the Adoption and Foster Care Analysis and Reporting System (AFCARS) and the Statewide Automated Child Welfare Information System (SACWIS)—are available nationwide. States are being monitored for compliance with their use, and continued federal funds are contingent on the implementation of these information systems. Because foster care placement is the result of psychosocial environmental failure, fixing the existing system requires more than good information systems. Integration of sound, theory-driven, child-focused, family-centered services, collaboratively funded by multiple governmental agencies, is essential. Through the use of longitudinal, research-based performance measures, reliable data are emerging. The National Institute of Mental Health (NIMH) has funded research focusing on foster care children and youth. Some examples of such research initiatives include using preventive interventions for foster care youths to reduce problem behaviors and improve prosocial development, tailoring services to foster infants' needs, improving casework and collaboration across agencies, and examining the use of mental health services by youths leaving care. The complexity of the impact of ever-changing psychosocial variables makes this type of research challenging. Nonetheless, this research must be done if welfare funding is to be spent doing the right thing for needy children and their families. In 2004, in a groundbreaking study, the Pew Commission on Children in Foster Care made sweeping recommendations to overhaul the system, stating that "children deserve more from our child welfare system."

HISTORY OF ADOPTION

Adoption has existed in different forms throughout history. In ancient Babylonia, it provided for the transmission of property or artisan's skills, whereas in the Roman Empire, it was often used to elevate the status of an adult protégé. In some Pacific islands, adoption of young children formed part of an exchange system between related clans. Concerns expressed by adopted persons about not knowing their roots are as ancient as they are contemporary. Euripides' *Ion* contains a touching dialogue between a woman in search of the child she had given up years before and a young priest of Apollo, who does not know that he is the woman's son and says that the only mother he knows is Apollo's priestess.

In the 19th century, the newly established social work profession took on the task of adoption placement, facilitated by legislation that enabled children to become legal members of families, although, in some cases, the child was not entitled to an inheritance. Because of concerns about the possibility of children having undesirable inherited traits, they were kept and observed in hospitals for as long as 1 year to ensure suitability. With a change in focus to addressing the needs of children as a priority, infant placements are now encouraged to take place as soon as possible to promote secure attachment.

After World War II, European children were placed in the United States, and, after the Korean War, Korean children were placed in U.S. homes. Continuing transracial and transcultural (domestic and international) adoptive placements have raised some controversy, having opponents and proponents of the practice.

Historically, *closed adoptions* were common practice. That was done to ensure the sealed identities of birth and adoptive parents and was believed to be in the best interests of adopted children. That practice is now considered flawed, and contemporary, although still controversial, thinking is that most adoptees should grow up knowing of their adoptive status, as well as the identities of their birth parents. Adoptees and many birth parents and adoptive parents increasingly have shared interests in legislation that affects the open or closed status of birth records and the placement of children in families. The phrase *adoption triad* has come to stand for these shared interests, represented by the American Adoption Congress and other organizations. In addition, other organizations represent each of these three groups, and those organizations often have divergent agendas. Since the 1980s, adoption practice has been profoundly affected by federal legislation.

EPIDEMIOLOGY OF ADOPTION

From 1.5 to 2.0 percent of children grow up in nonrelated adoptive placements, whereas another 1.5 percent are adopted by relatives or stepparents. Figures from the National Adoption Information Clearinghouse (NAIC) indicate that, in 1992, 127,441 adoptions were finalized in the United States. Of these, 42 percent were by stepparents or relatives, and 58 percent were unrelated adoptions. Of the unrelated adoptions, 27 percent were conducted by public agencies (i.e., adoptions from the foster care system); 8 percent were from other countries, with the largest number coming from Korea; and 64 percent were arranged by a private agency or were independent adoptions, in approximately equal numbers. The number of completed adoptions from the U.S. foster care system does not give a full picture of the numbers of waiting children—primarily, minority children in the public child welfare system. The NAIC estimated that, as of March 1998, approximately 500,000 children were in foster care in the United States. Of these, 110,000 (just more than 20 percent) were eligible for adoption. Some were legally free for adoption and waiting in not-yet-legalized adoptive homes, whereas others were waiting to be placed in adoptive families. Other children not yet legally free for adoption lived in preadoptive foster placements, but most remained in traditional foster homes or residential facilities. The pattern of international adoptions by U.S. families varies with world events, such as wars, internal conflicts, and policy changes. A sense of this can be seen by comparing the rank-order list of countries sending the most children to the United States in 1991 and 2001: China ranked 17th in 1991 but first in 2001; Russia did not appear on the 1991 list but was second in 2001; whereas Colombia, in fourth place in 1991, descended to 12th place 10 years later.

TERNATIONAL ADOPTION

Each year more than 20,000 children are adopted from outside of the United States, and many of these are transracial adoptions. More than 17,000 children were adopted from Guatemala, for example, in the last two decades. In the Guatemalan adoptees, the mean age was 1.5 years, and the children had previously resided in orphanages, foster homes, or mixed-care settings. Investigation of the health records of children who were evaluated after arrival in the United States in an international adoption specialty clinic revealed that younger children at time of adoption had better growth, language development, cognitive skills, and activities of daily living than children who were older at time of adoption. Among children matched for age, gender, and time from adoption to evaluation, those who were previously living in foster care were observed to have higher cognitive scores and improved growth than children who had resided in orphanages. These findings support the priority of adoptive placement at younger ages and the benefits of foster care over orphanage care.

EARLY VERSUS LATE ADOPTION

Data suggest that adoption at an earlier age predicts better outcome than adoption in middle or late childhood. A recent prospective study examined factors related to successful outcome in public adoption of children ranging in age from 5 to 11 years. Prospective data were collected from domestic adoptions in the United Kingdom at 1- and 6-year follow-up for 108 adoptees who were placed primarily because of situations involving childhood abuse and neglect. Outcome was assessed by the disruption rate and measures of psychologic adaptation. At the adolescent follow-up, 23 percent of the adoption placements had been disrupted, 49 percent were continuing with positive adaptations, and 28 percent were ongoing but with significant conflicts. Four factors contributed independently to the risk of disruptions: older age at placement, report of being singled out and rejected by siblings, time in care, and greater degree of behavioral problems. Given that almost half of the placements were ongoing, later childhood age of adoption can be successful; however, the constellation of families and assessment of behavioral problems may determine the likelihood of positive outcome for adopted school-aged children.

BIRTH PARENTS: SEARCH AND REUNION

The increasing trend toward open adoption allows the opportunity for adoptees to more easily search and successfully find their birth parents. Many adoptive parents choose open adoptions so that they can experience a greater connection with the child if they have some relationship with the birth mother. Some adoptees want to develop an ongoing relationship with birth parents, but many who search are satisfied to meet birth parents without further correspondence. Outcomes of reunions with birth parents vary widely, and, in some cases, especially when the birth parents are well functioning and welcoming toward their child, the adoptee may experience a sense of relief and joy in knowing that their birth mother is no longer vulnerable.

▲ 20.3 Child Maltreatment and Abuse

Child and adolescent maltreatment and abuse is prevalent and its long-term consequences multiple. The estimated number of children maltreated in the United States each year is close to 1 million, and the annual number of deaths caused by abuse or neglect has been estimated to be nearly 1,500.

The National Longitudinal Study of Adolescent Health, a prospective study following a national sample of adolescents, recently investigated the prevalence, risk factors, and health consequences in adolescents who reported retrospective child maltreatment. The most common forms of maltreatment reported were being left home alone as a child, indicating potential supervision neglect (reported by 41.5 percent), physical assault (reported by 28.4 percent), physical neglect (reported by 11.8 percent), and sexual abuse (reported by 4.5 percent). Each type of maltreatment was associated with at least eight of the ten adolescent health risks examined, including self-report of depression, regular alcohol use, binge drinking, marijuana use, overweight status, generally "poor" health, inhalant use, and violent behaviors, including fighting and hurting others. Clearly, the effects of self-reported maltreatment had far-ranging and long-lasting associations with multiple detrimental consequences.

The identification, management, and treatment for child maltreatment require cooperative efforts among multiple professionals, including primary care physicians, emergency room staff, law enforcement, attorneys, social service staff, and mental health professionals. Perpetrators typically deny abuse or neglect, and maltreated children often fear disclosure of their abuse or neglect.

DEFINITIONS

DSM-IV-TR

The somewhat terse classification system provided by the text revision of the fourth edition of the *Diagnostic and Statistical Manual of Mental Disorders* (DSM-IV-TR) lists *physical abuse of child*, *sexual abuse of child*, and *neglect of child*. The three classifications appear in the chapter "Other Conditions That May Be a Focus of Clinical Attention" and in the section "Problems Related to Abuse or Neglect." These categories should be used when the focus of clinical attention is severe mistreatment of one individual by another. These conditions and problems are coded on Axis I.

The DSM-IV-TR does not include detailed definitions or criteria for diagnosis. Circumstances in which the focus of attention is on the perpetrator of child abuse or neglect or on the relational unit in which it occurs have one code. Three different codes cover situations in which the focus of attention is on the victim (for neglect of child, for physical abuse of child, or for sexual abuse of child).

Federal Law

The Child Abuse Prevention and Treatment Act was passed in 1974 and has been amended several times, most recently in 2003. In federal law, *child abuse* and *neglect* mean, as a minimum, any recent act or failure to act on the part of a parent or caretaker that results in death, serious physical or emotional harm, or sexual abuse or exploitation. It also includes an act or failure to act that presents an imminent risk of serious harm. In federal law, *sexual abuse* means the employment, use, persuasion, inducement, enticement, or coercion of any child to engage in or to assist any other person to engage in any sexually explicit conduct (or simulation of such conduct for the purpose of producing a visual depiction of such conduct) or the rape (and in cases of caretaker or interfamilial relationships, statutory rape), molestation, prostitution, or other forms of sexual exploitation of children or incest with children.

State Law

A large variety of legal definitions and guidelines exists at the state level. The legal definitions of terms related to the maltreatment of children vary from one jurisdiction to another, so clinicians should be aware of the definitions used in their locale. The following generic definitions are used in this section.

Neglect

Neglect, the most prevalent form of child maltreatment, is the failure to provide adequate care and protection for children. Children can be harmed by malicious or ignorant withholding of physical, emotional, and educational necessities. Neglect includes failure to feed children adequately and to protect them from danger. Physical neglect includes abandonment, expulsion from home, disruptive custodial care, inadequate supervision, and reckless disregard for a child's safety and welfare. Medical neglect includes refusal, delay, or failure to provide medical care. Educational neglect includes failure to enroll a child in school and allowing chronic truancy.

Physical Abuse

Physical abuse can be defined as any act that results in a nonaccidental physical injury, such as beating, punching, kicking, biting, burning, and poisoning. Some physical abuse is the result of unreasonably severe corporal punishment or unjustifiable punishment. Physical abuse can be organized by damage to the site of injury: skin and surface tissue, the head, internal organs, and skeletal system.

Emotional Abuse

Emotional or *psychologic abuse* occurs when a person conveys to children that they are worthless, flawed, unloved, unwanted, or endangered. The perpetrator may spurn, terrorize, ignore, isolate, or berate the child. Emotional abuse includes verbal assaults (e.g., belittling, screaming, threatening, blaming, or using sarcasm), exposing the child to domestic violence, overpressuring through excessively advanced expectations, and encouraging or instructing the child to engage in antisocial activities. The severity of emotional abuse depends on (1) whether the perpetrator actually intends to inflict harm on the child and (2) whether the abusive behaviors are likely to cause harm to the child. Some authors believe that the terms *emotional* or *psychologic abuse* should not be used and that *verbal abuse* more accurately describes the pathologic behavior of the caregiver.

Sexual Abuse

Sexual abuse of children refers to sexual behavior between a child and an adult or between two children when one of them is significantly older or uses coercion. The perpetrator and the victim may be of the same sex or the opposite sex. The sexual behaviors include touching breasts, buttocks, and genitals, whether the victim is dressed or undressed; exhibitionism; fellatio; cunnilingus; and penetration of the vagina or anus with sexual organs or objects. Sexual abuse can involve behavior over an extended time or a single incident. Developmental factors must be considered in assessing whether sexual activities between two children are abusive or normative. In addition to the forms of inappropriate sexual touching, *sexual abuse* also refers to sexual exploitation of children, for instance, conduct or activities related to pornography depicting minors and promoting or trafficking in prostitution of minors.

Ritual Abuse

Cult-based *ritual abuse*, which includes satanic ritual abuse, is physical, sexual, or psychologic abuse that involves bizarre or ceremonial activity that is religiously or spiritually motivated. Typically, multiple perpetrators abuse multiple victims over an extended period of time. Ritual abuse is a controversial concept; some professionals believed in the 1990s that ritual abuse was common, whereas others were skeptical about most allegations and descriptions of ritual abuse.

Perpetrators of Abuse

Some lack of consistency is seen in who may be defined as an *abuse perpetrator*. Usually, a person must be a parent or designated caregiver to be charged with neglect, physical abuse, or emotional abuse. Another adult (e.g., a stranger) who injures a child would be charged with battery, not with child abuse. On the other hand, a caretaker or any other person could be charged with child sexual abuse. State laws vary in this regard.

COMPARATIVE NOSOLOGY

Neither the first nor the second edition of the DSM (1968) mentioned child maltreatment. The Group for the Advancement of Psychiatry (1974) mentioned child maltreatment among the pathogenic factors of childhood mental disorders: "The deleterious effects . . . of open rejection or neglect, occasionally involving willful injury or inadequate feeding, are well documented." It did not, however, include child maltreatment in its proposed system of classification.

In the third edition of the DSM (DSM-III) (1980), the American Psychiatric Association Task Force on Nomenclature and Statistics introduced a chapter entitled "V Codes for Conditions Not Attributable to a Mental Disorder That Are a Focus of Attention or Treatment." The V Codes, which were modeled on the practice in the ninth edition of the *International Classification of Diseases*, Clinical Modification (ICD-9-CM), did not include specific categories for child maltreatment. It was intended, however, that child abuse would be coded as a *parent–child problem*, the category used "when a focus of attention or treatment is a parent–child problem that is apparently not due to a mental disorder of the individual (parent or child) who is being evaluated." The DSM-III specifically stated that "an example (of parent–child problem) is child abuse not attributable to a mental disorder of the parent." The emphasis on *parent–child problem* was apparently to identify the perpetrators of abuse, not the child victims of abuse.

The revised third edition of the DSM (DSM-III-R) (1987) provided a similar definition for *parent–child problem*: "This category can be used for either a parent or a child when the focus of attention or treatment is a parent–child problem that is apparently not due to a mental disorder of the person who is being evaluated." The example involving child abuse was replaced, however, by "conflict between a mentally healthy adolescent and her parents about her choice of friends."

In the fourth edition of the DSM (DSM-IV) (1994), the title of the chapter was changed to "Other Conditions That May Be a Focus of Clinical Attention." In addition, a specific section was introduced, "Problems Related to Abuse or Neglect," which included terms related to child maltreatment. The editors noted that this category was "included because of the clinical and public health significance of these conditions." For the first time, it was possible to diagnose clearly *physical abuse of child*, *sexual abuse of child*, and *neglect of child*. Furthermore, the DSM-IV made it possible to distinguish whether the person being evaluated is the perpetrator of abuse or the victim of abuse.

The terminology regarding child maltreatment in the DSM-IV-TR (2000) is the same as that in the DSM-IV. The DSM-IV and DSM-IV-TR terminology are the same as that in the tenth edition of the ICD (ICD-10); only the codes differ.

EPIDEMIOLOGY

Each year, the Children's Bureau, an agency within the Department of Health and Human Services, collects data on child maltreatment. The results are published in an annual document called *Child Maltreatment*. The agency estimated that, in 2002, approximately 3 million alleged victims were reported to child protective services. Of those reports, approximately 896,000 were substantiated; this represents 12.3 of every 1,000 children. The substantiated cases were distributed as follows: neglect, 60 percent; physical abuse, 20 percent; sexual abuse, 10 percent; and emotional abuse, 7 percent. The Children's Bureau estimated that 1,400 children died as the result of maltreatment in 2002. Approximately 41 percent of these deaths were children younger than 1 year of age.

The data were analyzed for patterns of maltreatment by the sex and age of victims. Rates of many types of maltreatment were similar for male and female children, but the sexual abuse rate for female children was higher than the sexual abuse rate for male children. According to the age distribution of victims of abuse, the group from 0 to 3 years of age had the highest victimization rate, and the rate of victimization declined as the age of the victims increased. For example, the rate for infants (0 to 3 years of age) was 16 per 1,000, whereas the rate for adolescents (16 to 17 years of age) was 6 per 1,000. Regarding the perpetrators of abuse, it was reported that, overall, 58 percent were female and 42 percent were male.

All of these figures are approximations because the actual number of cases of abuse is unclear. The reporting of abuse and the annual victimization rate increased during the 1980s and reached a high in 1993 (when the victimization rate was 15.2 per 1,000 children in the population). This increase resulted from greater public awareness and willingness to report child abuse, improvement in data collection techniques by individual states, and local economic conditions that placed a larger number of families under stress. The victimization rate fell after 1993 and reached a low in 1999 (when the victimization rate was 11.8 per 1,000 children).

ETIOLOGY

Physical Abuse

Although child abuse occurs at all socioeconomic levels, it is highly associated with poverty and psychosocial stress, especially financial stress. Child maltreatment is strongly correlated with less parental education, underemployment, poor housing, welfare reliance, and single parenting. Child abuse tends to occur in multiproblem families, that is, families characterized by domestic violence, social isolation, parental mental illness, and parental substance abuse, especially alcoholism. The probability of maltreatment may be increased by risk factors such as prematurity, mental retardation, and physical handicap. In addition, the risk of child abuse increases in families with many children.

Sexual Abuse

Social, cultural, physiologic, and psychologic factors all contribute to the breakdown of the incest taboo. Incestuous behavior has been associated with alcohol abuse, overcrowding, increased physical proximity, and rural isolation that prevents adequate extrafamilial contacts. Some communities may be more tolerant of incestuous behavior. Major mental disorders and intellectual deficiency have been described in some perpetrators of incest and sexual abuse.

DIAGNOSIS AND CLINICAL FEATURES

Abused children manifest a variety of emotional, behavioral, and somatic reactions. These psychologic symptoms are neither specific nor pathognomonic: The same symptoms can occur without any history of abuse. The psychologic symptoms manifested by abused children and the behaviors of abusive parents can be organized into clinical patterns. Although it may be helpful to note whether a particular case falls into one of these patterns, that in itself is not diagnostic of child abuse.

Physically Abused Children

In many cases, the physical examination and radiologic evaluation show evidence of repeated suspicious injuries. Abused children display behaviors that should arouse the suspicions of the health professional. For example, these children may be unusually fearful, docile, distrustful, and guarded. On the other hand, they may be disruptive and aggressive. They may be wary of physical contact and show no expectation of being comforted by adults, they may be on the alert for danger and continually size up the environment, and they may be afraid to go home.

The literature regarding the psychologic consequences of physical abuse and neglect indicates a wide range of effects: affect dysregulation, insecure and atypical attachment patterns, impaired peer relationships involving increased aggression or social withdrawal, and academic underachievement. Physically abused children exhibit a range of psychopathology, including depression, conduct disorder, attention-deficit/hyperactivity disorder (ADHD), oppositional defiant disorder, dissociation, and posttraumatic stress disorder (PTSD).

Physically Abusive Parents

Abusive parents typically delay seeking help for the injuries. The history given by the parents is implausible or incompatible with the physical findings. The parents blame a sibling or claim that the children injured themselves. The characteristics of abusive parents include a history of abuse in their own early lives, a lack of empathy for the child, unrealistic expectations of the child, and an impaired parent–child attachment, especially to babies who are defective in some way.

Carol, 4 years of age, had a change in her behavior at preschool approximately 3 months after the birth of her sister. Her teacher saw Carol push other children and hit a classmate with a wooden block, causing a laceration of the child's lip. When Carol's teacher took her aside to talk about her behavior, she noticed what seemed to be belt marks on Carol's abdomen and forehead. The teacher reported possible child abuse to protective services. Also, the family was referred for psychiatric evaluation.

Carol's baby sister was colicky and slept only for short periods of time throughout the day and night. She stopped crying only when her mother held her. Her mother, therefore, had little time for Carol, and Carol's father took over her care on evenings after day care and on weekends. He began to drink more than usual and became increasingly irritable. The parents argued over the mother's attention to the infant and the requirement that the father take care of Carol. Carol, who was a bright, curious, and talkative child, constantly asked questions and often asked to carry the baby. When refused, she would lie on the floor and have a tantrum. She also began to have difficulty falling asleep and awoke repeatedly during the night. Carol's father was unable to cope with her requests for attention and often told her to shut up and slapped her when she continued her demands. On many occasions, he responded to her tantrums or repeated questions by hitting her with his belt.

While protective services monitored the situation, Carol and her parents began a family therapy program that included parenting training and behavioral therapy for Carol, which was coordinated with the preschool. Carol's father attended Alcoholics Anonymous (AA) meetings and stopped drinking. He was able to control his anger at his daughter. Six months later, Carol's aggressive behavior ceased. She was doing well with peers, was sleeping through the night, and stopped having temper tantrums. (Courtesy of William Bernet, M.D.)

Sexually Abused Children

A variety of symptoms, behavioral changes, and diagnoses sometimes occur in sexually abused children: anxiety symptoms, dissociative reactions and hysterical symptoms, depression, disturbances in sexual behaviors, and somatic complaints.

Anxiety Symptoms. Anxiety symptoms include fearfulness, phobias, insomnia, nightmares that directly portray the abuse, somatic complaints, and PTSD.

Dissociative Reactions and Hysterical Symptoms. The child may exhibit periods of amnesia, daydreaming, trance-like states, hysterical seizures, and symptoms of dissociative identity disorder.

Depression. Depression may be manifested by low self-esteem and suicidal and self-mutilative behaviors.

Disturbances in Sexual Behaviors. Some sexual behaviors are particularly suggestive of abuse, such as masturbating with an object, imitating intercourse, and inserting objects into the vagina or anus. Sexually abused children may display sexually aggressive behavior toward others. Other sexual behaviors are less specific, such as showing genitals to other children and touching the genitals of others. A younger child may manifest age-inappropriate sexual knowledge. In contrast to these overly sexualized behaviors, the child may avoid sexual stimuli through phobias and inhibitions.

Somatic Complaints. Somatic complaints include enuresis, encopresis, anal and vaginal itching, anorexia, bulimia, obesity, headache, and stomachache.

These symptoms are not pathognomonic. Nonabused children may exhibit any of these symptoms and behaviors. For example, normal, nonabused children commonly exhibit sexual behaviors, such as masturbating, displaying their genitals, and trying to look at people who are undressing.

Approximately one third of sexually abused children have no apparent symptoms. Most adults who were abused as children have no significant abuse-related symptoms. On the other hand, the following factors tend to be associated with more severe symptoms in the victims of sexual abuse: greater frequency and duration of abuse, sexual abuse that involved force or penetration, and sexual abuse perpetrated by the child's father or stepfather. Other factors associated with poorer prognosis are the child's perception of being less believed, family dysfunction, and lack of maternal support. In addition, multiple investigatory interviews appear to increase symptoms.

Intrafamilial Sexual Abuse

Incest can be defined strictly as sexual relations between close blood relatives, that is, between a child and the father or mother, uncle or aunt, or sibling. Because of increased reporting, sibling incest is an area of growing concern. In its broader sense, incest includes sexual intercourse between a child and a stepparent or stepsibling. Although father–daughter incest is the most common form, incest can also involve father and son, mother and daughter, and mother and son.

Intrafamilial sexual abuse and other sexual abuse that occurs over a period of time are characterized by a particular pattern or sequence of steps. Victims of sexual abuse recount a gradual progression of boundary violations by the perpetrator, starting with tiny invasions and escalating to serious, overwhelming intrusions. Healthy, self-confident children rebuff the intrusions directly (via temper tantrums and verbal disagreements) or indirectly (through silence and distancing maneuvers) or by adopting any strategy that causes the offender to refrain.

Sexual abuse that occurs over a period of time evolves through five phases: engagement, sexual interaction, secrecy, disclosure, and suppression.

Engagement Phase. The perpetrator induces the child into a special relationship. For example, the daughter in father–daughter incest frequently may have had a close relationship with her father throughout her childhood and may be pleased at first when he approaches her sexually.

Sexual Interaction Phase. The sexual behaviors progress from less to more intrusive forms of abuse. As the behavior continues, the abused daughter becomes confused and frightened, because she never knows whether her father will be parental or sexual. If the victim tells her mother about the abuse, the mother may not be supportive. The mother often refuses to believe her daughter's reports or refuses to confront her husband with her suspicions. Because the father provides special attention to a particular daughter, her brothers and sisters may distance themselves from her.

Secrecy Phase. The perpetrator threatens the victim not to tell. The father, fearful that his daughter may expose their relationship and often jealously possessive of her, interferes with the girl's development of normal peer relationships.

Disclosure Phase. The abuse is discovered accidentally (when another person walks in the room and sees it), through the child's reporting it to a responsible adult, or when the child is brought for medical attention and an alert clinician asks the right questions.

Suppression Phase. The child often retracts the statements of the disclosure because of family pressure or because of the child's mental processes. That is, the child may perceive that violent or intrusive attention is synonymous with interest or affection. Many incest survivors rally around their perpetrators, seeking to capture any modicum of tenderness or interest. At times, affection for the perpetrator outweighs the facts of abuse, and children recant their statements about sexual assault, regardless of substantiated evidence of molestation.

> Financially comfortable parents lived in a pleasant, clean house in a nice neighborhood, but they had no friends. Their four teenagers never had visitors. One day, the oldest girl, 17 years of age, went to the police and told them that she had a baby at home and that her own father was the father of the baby. The girl said that her father had been having sexual relations with her for more than 4 years and that he was now doing the same with her younger sisters. The mother admitted knowing about the situation for years, but she had not reported it to the authorities for fear of losing her husband. (Courtesy of William Bernet, M.D.)

Extrafamilial Sexual Abuse

Of course, sexual abuse is not limited to incest. Children can be abducted and sexually abused by strangers. A perpetrator may observe a playground and may identify a child who is not closely supervised. A pedophile may molest this child and hundreds of other children before he or she is apprehended. For the child, this is usually a single, isolated experience.

On the other hand, children can be repeatedly abused by trusted adults, such as teachers, counselors, family friends, and clergy. In this scenario, the pedophilic perpetrator grooms the child over a period of time. He or she gains the friendship of children through enjoyable activities and gifts, introduces sexual activities that may seem innocent and even pleasurable, and progresses to more intrusive activities. The pedophile encourages secrecy.

A solo sex ring is a form of child sexual abuse that involves one adult perpetrator and multiple child victims, who may know about each other's sexual activities with the perpetrator. A sex ring may also involve multiple perpetrators and multiple victims.

Neurobiologic Consequences of Child Maltreatment

Severe physical abuse and repeated sexual abuse cause changes in the child's developing brain that persist into adulthood. Adult survivors of abuse are more likely to have abnormalities of their electroencephalograms (EEGs) that indicate limbic irritability. They are more likely to have abnormalities on magnetic resonance imaging (MRI) of the brain that indicate reduced size of the adult hippocampus. These abnormalities are more pronounced on the left side of the brain. Deficient integration exists between the left and right hemispheres, manifested by reduced size of the corpus callosum. These neurobiologic effects of child maltreatment probably mediate the behavioral and psychologic symptoms that follow abuse, such as increased aggressiveness, heightened autonomic arousal, depression, and memory problems.

EVALUATION PROCESS

The evaluation of a child or adolescent who may have been physically or sexually abused depends on its circumstances and context. Practitioners must consider whether they are conducting a forensic evaluation, which has legal implications and may ultimately be used in court, or a clinical evaluation, which is done for a therapeutic purpose. A forensic evaluation emphasizes collecting accurate and complete data to determine—as objectively as possible—what happened to the child. Was the injury an accident, was it self-inflicted, or was it a result of parental abuse? Was the child actually sexually abused, or was he or she indoctrinated to believe that he or she was abused? The data collected in a forensic evaluation must be preserved in a reliable manner through audiotape, videotape, or detailed notes. The results of the forensic evaluation are organized into a report that is read by attorneys, a judge, and others. On the other hand, the emphasis in a therapeutic evaluation is to assess psychologic strengths and weaknesses, make a clinical diagnosis, develop a treatment plan, and lay the foundation for continuing psychotherapy. The clinician may also be interested in determining what happened to the child, but it is not so essential to distinguish facts from fantasies. Compared with the forensic evaluation, the psychotherapist does not need to keep such detailed records and ordinarily does not prepare a report for court.

In addition to distinguishing a forensic examination from a therapy meeting, a number of factors can affect the evaluation of a child who was abused or may have been abused: whether one is a pediatrician in an emergency department or a child psychiatrist in an office, whether a parent or another person is suspected of the abuse, the severity of the abuse and the victim's relationship to the perpetrator, whether physical signs of abuse are obvious or absent, the age and gender of the child, and the degree of anxiety, defensiveness, anger, or mental disorganization that the child exhibits. Often, the examiner must be creative and persistent.

From the psychiatric perspective, the interview is usually the primary source of information and the physical examination is secondary. In practice, children who may have been neglected or sexually abused are interviewed first and are later given a physical examination and other tests. A child who has been physically abused is more likely to have a physical examination that may be followed by a psychiatric interview.

Parent Interviews

The evaluator obtains a history from the parents (separately, in most cases) and other pertinent informants, as well as from the child. The emphasis of the interview depends on the circumstances.

Suspected Physical Abuse. The examiner should consider the possibility that the parents are not telling the truth. The physician becomes a detective because the parents who bring the injured child to the emergency department may also be perpetrators of the abuse. To obtain treatment, the caregivers lie about how the injury occurred.

When the child is brought to the emergency room, a detailed and spontaneous account of the injury should be obtained promptly from parents or other caregivers before secondary details and rationalizations cloud the information provided. The interviewer should allow the caregiver to explain, to expound, to derail, or to detour the story line. An abuser or codependent parent may claim to have happened on the injured child in a coma or bleeding from some unknown trauma or to have noticed significant bruising, burns, or a crooked extremity while bathing the child. Comparing the parents' histories can provide valuable insight into how power is wielded in the family unit.

A 30-day-old girl was transferred from a rural hospital to a university medical center because of supposed near sudden infant death syndrome (SIDS). The child was unresponsive and required mechanical ventilation. A brain scan revealed bilateral subdural hematomas, subarachnoid hemorrhage, and hemorrhage in the parenchyma of the brain. An X-ray skeletal survey showed two posterior rib fractures. An ophthalmologist observed extensive retinal hemorrhages. After the child was admitted to the Pediatric Intensive Care Unit, the child abuse consultant interviewed the parents separately. The mother, 28 years of age, said that she had recently started a new job. The baby was perfectly fine when she left her in the care of her live-in boyfriend, the child's biological father. The father, 24 years of age, said that when he checked on the baby, he found her not breathing, blue, and unresponsive. He ran to report this to a neighbor and then called 911. The child abuse consultant told the father that the child must have been injured in some way and asked whether the father had any explanation for this injury. The father said, "I shook the baby after I found her not breathing." The consultant concluded that severe child abuse had occurred in the form of shaken-baby syndrome. The consultant notified child protective services and the local police department, so that they could initiate and coordinate their investigation. (Courtesy of William Bernet, M.D.)

Suspected Sexual Abuse. The examiner should consider the possibility that the parents are not telling the truth. This situation is more complex, however, than suspected physical abuse. For example, the mother may wish to avoid the discovery of father–daughter incest by blaming the child's genital injury on another child or a stranger. In another scenario, the mother may concoct an allegation of incest when the child had never been abused at all. The first version protects a father who is guilty; the second version implicates a father who is innocent.

The examiner should determine how the allegation originally arose and what subsequent statements were made. Determine the emotional tone of the first disclosure (e.g., whether the disclosure arose in the context of a high level of suspicion of abuse). Determine the sequence of previous examinations, the techniques used, and what was reported. Try to determine whether the previous interviews likely distorted the child's recollections. If possible, review transcripts, audiotapes, and videotapes of earlier interviews. Seek a history of overstimulation, prior abuse, or other traumas. Consider other stressors that could account for the child's symptoms. The examiner should also ask about exposure to other possible male and female perpetrators.

In Either Case. Whether physical or sexual abuse is involved, a pertinent psychosocial history should be collected and organized, including the following:

1. Symptoms and behavioral changes that sometimes occur in abused children
2. Confounding variables, such as psychiatric disorder or cognitive impairment, that may need to be considered
3. Family's attitude toward discipline, sex, and modesty
4. Developmental history from birth through periods of possible trauma to the present
5. Family history, such as earlier abuse of the parents, substance abuse by the parents, spouse abuse, and psychiatric disorder in the parents
6. Underlying motivation and possible psychopathology of adults involved

Collateral Information

The evaluator should consider requesting collateral information from the following, after obtaining authorizations: protective services, school personnel, other caregivers (e.g., babysitters), other family members (e.g., siblings), the pediatrician, and police reports.

Child Interview

Several structured and semistructured interview protocols have been introduced that were designed to maximize the amount of accurate information and to minimize mistaken or false information provided by children. These approaches include the Cognitive Interview, which encourages witnesses to search their memories in various ways, such as recalling events forward and then backward. The Step-Wise Interview is a funnel approach that starts with open-ended questions and, if necessary, moves to more specific questions. The interview protocol developed at the National Institute of Child Health and Human Development (NICHD) includes a series of phases and makes use of detailed interview scripts.

Although these protocols may be particularly important in a forensic context, experienced clinicians endorse flexibility and consistent good-hearted behavior by the interviewer. As when seeing any patient, the evaluator must size up the situation and use techniques that are likely to help the youngster become comfortable and communicative. One victim might need a favorite object (e.g., a teddy bear or a toy truck); another might need to have a particular person included in the interview. Some children are comfortable talking; others prefer to draw pictures. An unrelated joke, a shared cookie, or a picture on the evaluator's wall may lead to a disclosure of abuse. Important comments might be made while chatting during the break time instead of during the structured interviews.

CULTURAL CONSIDERATIONS IN CHILD MALTREATMENT

Parenting practices vary widely in U.S. society, and the cultural context of alleged abuse must be understood to facilitate helpful communication with families regarding discipline practices that contain characteristics of abuse. A recent study of the characteristics of child abuse among immigrant Korean families in Los Angeles who had active files with the Los Angeles County Department of Children and Family Services (LAC-DCFS) found that immigrant Korean families are more likely to be charged with physical abuse (49.4 percent) and less likely to be charged with neglect (20.6 percent) than any other group with active DCFS files in Los Angeles. That is, the circumstances under which physical abuse occurred most frequently was corporal punishment used by parents with an intention to discipline their children. The context of emotional abuse occurred most often among Korean families in which children witnessed domestic violence. A culturally sensitive approach was suggested to achieve effective child abuse prevention and interventions that will be accepted by Korean families.

GENOTYPE AND MALTREATMENT: RISKS FOR VIOLENT BEHAVIOR

Two recent studies of white males provided evidence that genotypes expressing high levels of monoamine oxidase A (MAOA) seem to protect against the malignant impact of childhood maltreatment on the development of conduct disorder and antisocial behavioral patterns. Subjects in a prospective cohort design involving court-substantiated cases of child abuse and neglect and matched comparison groups were followed into adulthood. A composite index of violent and antisocial behavior (VASB) was created based on arrest record, self-report, and diagnostic information. Genotypes associated with high levels of MAOA activity were correlated with less risk of violent and antisocial behavior in later life for whites, but this effect was not found for nonwhites. This result was not replicated in a group of adolescents with respect to the development of adolescent conduct disorder. Further studies are needed to understand the possible links between genotypes expressing high levels of MAOA and potential behavioral outcomes.

TREATMENT AND PREVENTION STRATEGIES

The immediate intent of strategic intervention is to ensure the child's safety, which may require the child's removal from an abusive or neglectful home environment. Physicians are among the groups of professionals who are mandated by law to report suspected child abuse or neglect to the local protective services agency.

Children who have been maltreated are at increased risk for further maltreatment, according to studies of child victims of abuse and maltreatment. Studies have shown that four factors were most consistently identified as predictors of future maltreatment: number of previous episodes of maltreatment; neglect as the form of maltreatment; parental conflict; and parental psychiatric illness. Maltreated children were found to be about six times more likely to experience recurrent maltreatment, and the risk of recurrence was highest within 30 days of the index experience. This underscores the importance of a careful examination of the protective factors in the home environment. Investigation has recently shown that even less striking forms of maltreatment, such as verbal aggression by parents, contribute to the malignant effects of child maltreatment.

Once a safe place is established for a maltreated child, a multimodal treatment strategy may begin, using components of psychoeducation, anxiety management, exposure related to the feared experiences, and cognitive-behavioral interventions. Given the multiple long-term effects of maltreatment, children may require monitoring and support for long periods of time after the abuse has ended.

▲ 20.4 Impact of Terrorism on Children

Over the last decade, children and adolescents in the United States have experienced large-scale domestic terrorist attacks, such as the September 11, 2001, attack on the World Trade Center in New York City, attacks against U.S. citizens in other parts of the world, and devastating violence toward peers in school shootings.

The U.S. Congress launched a series of initiatives in response to the threats and consequences of terrorism in the form the 2002 Public Health Security and Bioterrorism Preparedness and Response Act. Nonetheless, children and adolescents continue to view frequent media exposure to terrorist events throughout the world, which perpetuates a sense of danger.

The concept of terrorist acts is characterized by three distinct features: (1) They produce a societal atmosphere of extreme danger and fear, (2) they inflict significant personal harm and destruction, and (3) they undermine the perceived implicit social contract between citizens and the state that the state is able to protect them.

Child and adolescent reactions to exposure to terrorism is mediated by numerous factors, including personal appraisal of persisting danger, the likelihood of recurrent attack, and the perception of the relative safety of one's family and close friends. Children's responses to terrorist exposure are influenced by how their parents cope with the trauma and resulting turmoil and how well they understood the situation. Posttraumatic stress disorder (PTSD) has been studied in adolescents, with and without learning disabilities, who have been exposed to terror attacks. Findings from this study revealed that personal exposure to terror, past personal life-threatening events, and history of anxiety all contributed to the development of posttraumatic stress reactions. In addition, adolescents with learning disabilities who had difficulties in cognitively processing the traumatic events were at higher risk of developing PTSD when this was combined with the other high-risk factors, such as being personally exposed to the traumatic events.

Table 20.4–1 identifies the relationship between objective features of danger and subjective features related to exposure to terrorist acts.

The following summarizes data collected after the terrorist attack on the World Trade Center on September 11, 2001.

SEPTEMBER 11, 2001 ATTACKS

The U.S. Department of Education, through Project SERV, supported the New York City Board of Education in conducting a needs assessment of New York City schoolchildren. Christine W. Hoven and colleagues surveyed more than 8,000 randomly selected students 6 months after the September 11, 2001, attacks. Striking differences were seen in among students in the

Table 20.4–1
Experience of Danger Consequent to Terrorist Acts

Objective Features	Subjective Features
Actualized threat	Disruption of protective shield
Realistic threats	Appraisals of threat
False alarms	Fears of recurrence
Hoaxes	Living with uncertainty
	Ongoing worries about significant others
Official risk communication, media coverage, and personal exchanges of information	Modulation of information exposure
Heightened security	Safety and protective behaviors
Mobilization of prevention and response capabilities	Anxious and restrictive behaviors
	Aggressive and reckless behaviors
Attribution of responsibility	Categorization over discrimination of threat: risk of intolerance
Evacuation and rescue efforts	Themes of heroism and patriotism
Military mobilization	Political ideology
War	—
Additional dangers, terrorist acts, and personal tragedies	Changes in spiritual schema
	Parental demoralization

Courtesy of Robert S. Pynoos, M.D. M.P.H., Merritt D. Schreiber, Ph.D., Alan M. Steinberg, Ph.D., and Betty Pfefferbaum, M.D., J.D.

vicinity of Ground Zero as compared with students in the rest of the city with regard to exposure to smoke and dust, fleeing for safety, problems getting home, and smelling smoke in the days and weeks after September 11. Approximately 70 percent of all children, however, were exposed to at least one of these factors. Interpersonal exposure through direct victimization of a family member was greater among children attending schools outside the Ground Zero vicinity than those attending school in this area. Media exposure was extensive and prolonged. Signs of heightened security were visible throughout the city.

The study used several of the Diagnostic Interview Schedule for Children (DISC) predictive scales. In contrast to most disaster studies among children, which use continuous scale instruments, the abbreviated PTSD self-report diagnostic instrument uses a yes/no response format that overly emphasizes category C (avoidance) as the diagnostic discriminatory symptom. As a result, no age-, sex-, or exposure-related full symptom profiles were obtainable to more fully inform understanding of the nature, severity, and course of children's reactions to terrorism and public mental health response planning. In addition, higher estimated rates of PTSD (up to 20 percent among 4th- and 5th-graders) were found among school-age children, who are well documented to be the age group at most risk for avoidant behavior, than for high school students (6 percent), who, in pilot screenings in lower Manhattan, had low rates of avoidance and higher rates of irritability. No exposure-related differences were found in the rates of PTSD among high school students. Extremely high rates (52 percent) were found, however, among children who lost a parent or sibling, although no reported analysis was done of the contribution of symptoms of traumatic bereavement to this finding. Three sets of findings stand out from this study. First, similar to the findings by Armen K. Goenjian and colleagues after the catastrophic 1988 Spitak earthquake in Armenia, a significant degree of persistent separation anxiety was seen, especially among school-age children, but also among adolescents. Second, reflecting an age-related vulnerability to incident-specific new fears (e.g., subways and buses) and avoidant behavior of school-age children, a nearly 25 percent rate of agoraphobia was reported among 4th- and 5th-graders. Care must be taken, however, not to misrepresent *incident-specific new fears* as agoraphobia, because the course of recovery and intervention strategies may differ. Third, an enormous reservoir of prior traumatic experiences (more than one half of the total sample) was associated with severity of current PTSD symptoms, emphasizing the need to attend to prior trauma in conducting needs assessments, surveillance, and intervention strategies. Other risk factors, in addition to younger age, included female gender and Hispanic ethnicity. The finding of age-related increases in rates of conduct disorder also needs to be interpreted in light of adolescent response to an ecology of danger in which overly aggressive, reckless, and risk-taking behaviors are well documented and associated with posttraumatic stress reactions. A major strength of this study was the inclusion of self-reported impairment in addition to symptoms, setting an important standard for future studies.

J. Stuber and colleagues conducted a telephone survey of a random sample of adult residents of Manhattan 1 to 2 months after the September 11 attacks. The sample included more than 100 parents who were asked to describe the experiences and reactions of their children. Not surprisingly, given the time of the incident, most children were at school or day care when the events occurred. Many of the parents recalled concern about their children's safety at the time, and most were not reunited with their children for more than 4 hours. More than 20 percent of the parents studied reported that their children had received counseling related to the disaster. Receiving counseling was associated with male gender, parental posttraumatic stress, and having at least one sibling living in the household.

Also using parent report in a New York City telephone survey, Gerry Fairbrother and colleagues assessed predictors of posttraumatic stress reactions in children between the ages of 4 and 17 years, 4 to 5 months after the attacks. Almost 20 percent of children were reported by their parents to have experienced severe or very severe posttraumatic stress reactions, and approximately two thirds had moderate posttraumatic stress reactions. Parental reactions and viewing three or more graphic images of the disaster on television were associated with severe or very severe posttraumatic stress reactions in children.

More recently, Fairbrother and colleagues reported that 27 percent of children with severe or very severe posttraumatic stress reactions received some mental health care 4 to 5 months after September 11.

Exploring behavior problems in New York City children, Stuber and colleagues compared data from three cross-sectional telephone surveys of representative samples of adults. Two surveys were conducted after the September 11 attacks—the first between 4 and 5 months and the second between 6 and 9 months after the attacks. Behavior problems were related to the child's race or ethnicity, family income, living in a single-parent household, disaster event experiences, and parental reactions to the attacks. The results of these surveys were examined in light of findings from a representative survey conducted before September 11. The rate of behavior problems was lower in the first post–September 11 survey (4 to 6 months after the attacks) than in the pre–September 11 survey, but problems returned to pre–September 11 levels by the second post–September 11 study (6 to 9 months after the attacks). Consistent with findings in studies of the effects of Hurricane Andrew, these results suggest that behavior problems may actually decrease in the months after a disaster or that parents may be insensitive to them, but that they return to predisaster levels over time.

Media coverage of the September 11 attacks brought renewed debate about its impact, especially on children—even children with no direct exposure. Mark A. Schuster and colleagues reported extensive exposure to television coverage in children throughout the nation by using a representative survey of adults conducted in the first days after the attacks. Approximately one third of the parents surveyed attempted to limit or to prevent their children's viewing, but, among those whose parents made no attempt to restrict viewing, the number of hours of disaster coverage watched was related to the number of reported stress symptoms.

Using a Web-based, nationally representative sample of adults, William E. Schlenger and colleagues examined distress in children 1 to 2 months after the attacks by asking parents if their children were upset by the events. Of the children perceived as most upset, 20 percent had trouble sleeping, 30 percent were irritable or easily upset, and 27 percent feared separation from their parents. The mean age of children perceived as most upset was 11 years, with no statistically significant gender differences. The proportion of parents reporting at least one child upset did not differ by community in an analysis of data from the New York City metropolitan area, Washington, D.C., other major metropolitan areas, and the rest of the country.

A strength of these surveys was their examination of representative samples, but earlier work points to concern about assessing children by interviewing their parents. Furthermore, as with studies of the Oklahoma City bombings, the samples were composed mainly of indirectly exposed children, and the clinical significance of the findings is unclear.

Seven-year-old J survived the traumatic loss of two grandparents on the first plane into the World Trade Center. He was first seen in treatment 2 weeks after September 11, 2001. J's grandparents were on board American Airlines Flight No. 11 enroute to take care of J and his younger siblings. J and his siblings were preparing to leave for school when the family learned the news, and J observed the profound distress of his parents as they confirmed the presence of his grandparents aboard the aircraft. He observed the famous video segments of the second plane crashing into the second tower several times that morning before television access was limited. J was the first grandchild in his extended family, and he lived with his grandparents for the first 3 years of his life; thereafter, his grandparents spent approximately one half of the year with him and his family on the West Coast. They had enjoyed an exceptionally close relationship since his birth, and he participated in many activities (such as karate) solely with them until September 11th.

Almost immediately after the terrorist attacks, his parents became worried that J was taking the loss of his grandparents extremely hard, and they became increasingly concerned that he was preoccupied with the grisly nature of their deaths. He was becoming increasingly agitated as he talked about the gruesome aspects of their deaths. In treatment, he began to ask a continual series of questions about the nature of their deaths, including aspects of burning, fragmentation, pain, blood, and the exact moment of their deaths in comparison with what he had initially observed on television. This became the theme for the early phase of his care, which dealt with the questions about the nature of their deaths (i.e., whether they were intact or "blown up in a thousand pieces" and the sequence of fire, burning, pain, and death). J developed nightmares within days in which he awakened and called for his parents on the average of three times a night. J felt that he could not discuss the content of his dreams with his parents, given his observations of their own distress. He began to express fears that the "hijackers" would hurt his parents and other family members. He became focused on the concept that "half our freedom is gone," and he was concerned that one half of New York City was destroyed. His play centered on repetitively creating the World Trade Center with blocks and then crashing them down. Although he was able to resume sleeping through the night, he reported new troubling dreams with themes of ghosts "popping out" and "everyone is killed, and then I'm killed." This worsened after the onset of the war in Afghanistan, and he sought to reassure himself by repeatedly saying the "war is not here" (California) and by hoping that American forces would kill many.

He developed an intervention fantasy in which the therapist would have a time machine like "Jimmy Neutrino" and that he and the therapist could be transported back in time on board his grandparents' flight before it crashed. While his father (a former military pilot) flew the plane, he and the therapist overpowered the "hijackers" and threw them off the plane, and then his father landed the plane safely in Boston or at his home. After landing, his grandparents and their fellow passengers tell him "thank you," and they continue with their planned visit to see him. After expressing his wish verbally, he initiated play and used the same blocks to create the World Trade Center and then repeatedly had his "grandparents' plane" narrowly avoid the twin towers, as he and the therapist took control of the hijackers while his father deftly landed the plane safely. This appeared to be soothing and satisfying, and he began to recall many positive activities with his grandparents and a series of happy, highly detailed memories of himself and his grandparents, with profound sadness at the realization that these would be no more. While playing Candyland, he landed on a square that reminded him of his grandmother baking for him and the affectionate nicknames that they called him and that he called them, and he said "a piece of my heart is gone" and "I want them back."

He later expressed that they were more than grandparents, and he recalled living with them for a time in their home as both of his parents worked. At several phases, he alternately expressed rage and anger and confusion about the actions of "Osama Bin Laden." He acted out danger, aggression, and defense, repetitively using chess pieces to build a wall of protection between the opposing colors. This led to anxiety about his "plotting again" and concern for the safety of his parents. Around the Jewish holiday of Passover, J expressed to his family and friends that Passover was a celebration of "dead people" and "this night we have a cake, everyone eats a cake that represents people who died, it's sort of like a birthday party with special foods ... they take a picture with a candle, and they can scan the image of the person lost." (Courtesy of Robert S. Pynoos, M.D., M.P.H., Merritt D. Schreiber, Ph.D., Alan M. Steinberg, Ph.D., and Betty Pfefferbaum, M.D., J.D.)

Recently, Avraham Bleichman and colleagues, using a telephone survey of 512 Israeli citizens, found that 60 percent of the population reported that they believed that their lives were in danger. Approximately 38 percent of the sample of adults reported at least one symptom of traumatic stress, and more than one half reported feeling depressed, with 28 percent reporting being very depressed.

To respond to the mental health needs of children and adolescents who have been exposed to terrorism either through personal experience or through exposure to media depicting worldwide terrorism, the adverse psychologic reactions listed in Table 20.4–2 must be considered.

Table 20.4–2
Psychologic Disorders Associated with Terrorism

Acute stress disorder
Posttraumatic stress disorder
Depression
Anxiety
Separation anxiety disorder
Agoraphobia
Phobic disorders
Bereavement
Somatization
Irritability
Dissociative reactions
Sleep disturbances
Diminished self-esteem
Deterioration in school performance
Distress when exposed to traumatic reminders
Substance abuse

COMPONENTS OF MECHANISMS FOR RECOVERY FROM EXPOSURE TO TERRORISM

Perception of Safety

The notion of perceived safety is an important protective factor, as well as a component of recovery, for a child, adolescent, or adult who has been exposed to terrorism. A recent report of symptoms of PTSD, depression, and perceived safety in disaster workers 2 weeks after the September 11 terrorist attacks found that lower perceived safety was associated with increased symptoms of hyperarousal and intrusive fearful thoughts, but not avoidance. An expected diminished sense of safety was found in those individuals who had been in greater physical danger or who had worked with dead bodies compared with others who were physically less exposed. To regain a sense of security, reestablishment of a perception of safety is a necessary first step.

Reestablishment or Maintenance of Daily Routines

Although clearly it is not always possible to maintain usual daily routines amid war or exposure to terrorism, a study of Israeli adolescents found that those whose families were able to maintain their usual activities, such as attending school and family functions, were at lower risk for the development of posttraumatic reactions. On the other hand, adolescents' perception of family maintaining routine activities was a predictor of higher levels of avoidance and of posttraumatic reactions.

Proactive Interventions to Enhance Resilience

Perceived personal resilience has been shown in studies to be protective against symptoms of posttraumatic stress development. Proactive interventions aimed at enhancing a sense of personal resilience and an ability to cope with the stressful situation may serve to decrease the risk of psychiatric symptoms after exposure to terrorism. Interventions may include regaining a sense of perceived safety through reestablishing routines, altruistic tasks, family preparedness planning, and parental expression of security.

Index

Page numbers followed by t indicate tabular material.